NATURAL REMEDIES IN THE FIGHT AGAINST PARASITES

Edited by **Hanem Khater, M. Govindarajan**
and **Giovanni Benelli**

Natural Remedies in the Fight Against Parasites
http://dx.doi.org/10.5772/63275
Edited by Hanem Khater, M. Govindarajan and Giovanni Benelli

Contributors

Tebit Emmanuel Kwenti, Lilián Yépez-Mulia, Rosa María Ribas-Aparicio, Jonathan Isaí Andrade-Becerra, Ericka N. Pompa-Mera, Peng Liu, Jose Vega, Alison Wunderlich, Erica O.P. Zica, Vanessa F. S. Ayres, Anderson C. Guimarães, Renata Takeara, Nelissa Pacheco Vaz, Laurence Marchat, Esther Ramirez-Moreno, Jacqueline Soto-Sanchez, Gildardo Rivera, De La Garza, Cynthia Ordaz-Pichardo, Nidia Leon-Sicairos, Julio César Carrero, Hanem Fathy Khater

Published by InTech
Janeza Trdine 9, 51000 Rijeka, Croatia

Publishing Process Manager Edi Lipovic
Technical Editor SPi Global
Cover InTech Design team

First published July, 2017
Printed in Croatia
Legal deposit, Croatia: National and University Library in Zagreb

Additional hard copies can be obtained from orders@intechopen.com

Natural Remedies in the Fight Against Parasites, Edited by Hanem Khater, M. Govindarajan and Giovanni Benelli
p. cm.
Print ISBN 978-953-51-3289-9
Online ISBN 978-953-51-3290-5

For EU product safety concerns:
IN TECH d.o.o., Prolaz Marije Krucifikse Kozulić 3, 51000 Rijeka, Croatia,
info@intechopen.com or visit our website at intechopen.com.

Meet the editors

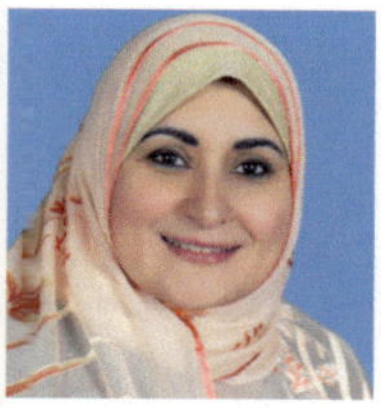

Prof. Dr. Hanem Khater is a professor of Parasitology working at Benha University, Egypt. She studied for her doctoral degree at the Department of Entomology, College of Agriculture, Food and Natural Resources, University of Missouri, Columbia, USA. She has completed her PhD degree in Parasitology at the Faculty of Veterinary Medicine, Zagazig University, Benha Branch, Egypt. She focused in her researches on novel control tools in the fight against arthropods of medical, veterinary, and agricultural importance such as mosquitoes, house flies, lice, green bottle fly, camel nasal botfly, soft and hard ticks, mites, and diamondback moth, as well as control of several parasites using safe and natural materials to avoid drug resistances and environmental contamination. She attended and presented research papers in many international conferences.

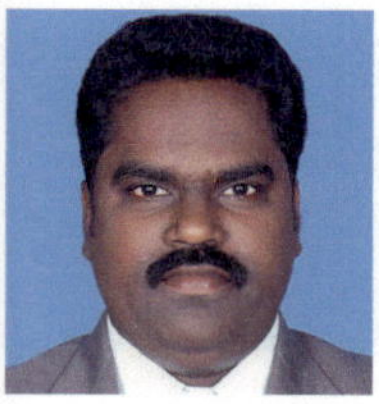

Dr. M. Govindarajan completed his BSc degree in Zoology at Government Arts College (Autonomous), Kumbakonam, and MSc, MPhil, and PhD degrees at Annamalai University, Annamalai Nagar, Tamil Nadu, India. He is serving as an assistant professor at the Department of Zoology, Annamalai University. His research interests include isolation, identification, and characterization of biologically active molecules from plants and microbes. He has identified more than 20 pure compounds with high mosquitocidal activity and also conducted high-quality research on photochemistry and nanosynthesis. He has published more than 150 studies in journals with impact factor and 2 books in Lambert Academic Publishing, Germany. He serves as an editorial board member in various national and international scientific journals.

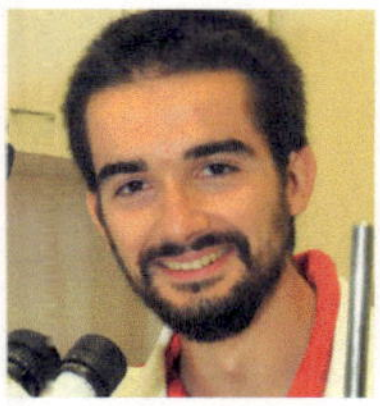

Dr. Giovanni Benelli is a research entomologist and an academic editor at the University of Pisa and an affiliate researcher at The BioRobotics Institute, Sant'Anna School of Advanced Studies (Pisa, Italy). Giovanni's research is focused on insect behavioral ecology as well as on the development of novel control tools in the fight against arthropod pests, including nanoformulated pesticides. Benelli is cooperating with more than 80 research projects worldwide and has published more than 250 studies on top-ranked international journals with impact factor.

Contents

Preface

Since millions of years, parasites had and still have to survive the struggle for life competed with individuals of their own species as well as with higher numbers of competitors. A noteworthy quote of the overall biodiversity found in any ecosystem can be attributed to parasitism since every species of animal is parasitized by at least another organism. The disease burden caused by parasites is significant and represents a challenging health problem, mainly in tropics and in developing countries. Chemical control is mostly effective, but there are some major limitations to face, including toxicity on nontarget organisms, the rapid development of drug and pesticide resistance, and high operational costs. Consequently, there is an urgent need for discovery of new, eco-friendly, and effective drugs. For centuries, medicinal and aromatic plants have been used to combat parasites in traditional medicine and, in many parts of the world, are still used for this purpose.

Besides the introductory chapter "Back to the Future: Solutions for Parasitic Problems as Old as Pyramids," this book discusses, in eight chapters, three major topics of natural parasitic control as biological, botanical, and miscellaneous control strategies.

Biological Control: A chapter reviews natural enemies or biological control agents including predators, parasites and parasitoids, and pathogens (covering viruses, bacteria, protozoa, fungi and nematodes); the effect of biocontrol agents on native biodiversity; case studies of the successful implementation of biocontrol methods; and challenges facing biological control strategies and their future perspectives.

Botanical Control: Three chapters highlight the advantages of the use of plant-derived compounds such as essential oils, plant extracts, and Mexican plants, as an alternative way to control and prevent parasites of humans, livestock, and wildlife.

Miscellaneous Biorationals: The last four chapters focus on other natural control methods including the benefits of involvement of gap junction proteins, permitting cellular communication in infectious diseases caused by parasites; lactoferricins (an iron-binding glycoprotein of the innate immune system) against intestinal parasitic diseases; plasmepsin for antimalarial drug development; and, finally , vaccination against *Trichinella spiralis*, highlighting its potential, limitations, and future perspective.

Natural product research shows a promising potential in finding new lead structures besides rational drug design. The editors of this book have a special research interest in natural control of parasites as well as arthropod pests. Therefore, we enthusiastically present this book with numerous updates on topics of vigorous timely research.

This textbook is designed for students and teachers at the same time. It emphasizes principles about natural control of the major parasites of humans, domestic animals, and crops. As always, we have strived for readability, enhancing chapters with figures and tables. Essential terms are defined and lists of abbreviations are provided. Numbered references at the end of each chapter make supporting data and further study easily accessible. Clear labeling makes all illustrations approachable and self-explanatory to the readers.

We thank the continuing efforts of the contributors to this book, exposing their thought about weaknesses in the biology of parasites and how nature contributes to solving parasitic problems. This knowledge, in turn, suggests safe materials for parasitic control. Then, we are grateful to the efforts of *all coworkers of each group* who kindly provided text and figures in their final format. Our sincere thanks are directed to *Mr. Edi Lipovic*, InTech Publishing Process Manager; *Prof. Dr. Azza A. Moustafa*, Research Institute of Medical Entomology, Egypt; *Galal Abouelella*, British University in Egypt; colleagues at Benha University, Egypt; *Prof. Dr. Adel Shaheen*, Department of Fish Diseases and Management, Faculty of Veterinary Medicine; *Dr. Ahmed Radwan*, Department of Parasitology, Faculty of Veterinary Medicine; and *Prof. Dr. Abdou Mahdi* and *Prof. Dr. Mohamed Hafez*, Plant Pathology Department, Faculty of Agriculture, for their valuable support and advice.

Prof. Dr. Hanem Khater
Department of Parasitology,
Faculty of Veterinary Medicine,
Benha University, Toukh,
Moshtohor, Egypt

Dr. M. Govindarajan M.Sc., M.Phil., Ph.D.,
Unit of Vector Biology, Phytochemistry and Nanotechnology,
Department of Zoology, Annamalai University,
Tamilnadu, India

Dr. Giovanni Benelli, Ph.D.,
Department of Agriculture, Food and Environment,
University of Pisa,
Pisa, Italy

Section 1

Introduction

Chapter 1

Introductory Chapter: Back to the Future - Solutions for Parasitic Problems as Old as the Pyramids

Hanem Fathy Khater

Additional information is available at the end of the chapter

http://dx.doi.org/10.5772/67554

1. Introduction

Parasitology is an interesting field of biology, and parasites have been the subjects of some of the most exciting discoveries among infectious diseases. A parasite is an organism that lives on or in a host organism and acquires its food from or at the expense of its host. There are three main classes of parasites: protozoa, helminths, and arthropods. All through history, the worldwide prevalence of selected parasitic diseases shows that there are more than enough existing infections for every living person to have one. Some serious parasites such as malaria, schistosomiasis, and African sleeping sickness have forward incalculable millions to their graves. In company with their bacteria, fleas destroyed a third of the European population in the seventeenth century [1].

Silently suffering, domesticated animals [2, 3] and birds [4, 5] are subject to a wide variety of parasites often in greater numbers than in humans for the reason that they are usually confined to the same pastures, pens, or farms, so that the infective stages of parasites turn out to be exceedingly dense in the soil, and the burden of parasites within each host grows to be overwhelming. Moreover, most wild animals can tolerate their parasite burdens fairly well, but crowdedness and malnutrition could subject infected herds to quick extinction unless a means of control of their parasites can be established in the near future [1].

Some other problems include food-borne illness and zoonosis, any disease or infection that is naturally transmissible from vertebrate animals to humans and vice versa, such as trichinosis, echinococcosis, and toxoplasmosis [6–9]. Furthermore, new zoonoses were recognized from time to time; Lyme disease, a bacterial infection transmitted by ticks, was long present in deer and white-footed mice, but recurrent transmission to humans was revealed in the 1970s [1]. Toxoplasmosis, a protozoan parasite transmitted by cats, increases rates of suicides and car accidents and leads to changes in personality profile exaggerated by schizophrenia; cultural changes could occur in populations where this parasite is very common, owing to mass personality modification regarding cultural aspects related to ego, work, rules, money, and material possessions [10].

2. Global burden of parasitic infection

Parasites bring about chronic debilitating, periodically disabling disease, are responsible for the overwhelming financial loss. In situations where it is prevalent, the number of hours of productive labor lost multiplied by the number of sufferer's yields a figure that can be charged as a loss in the manufacture of goods, in the production of crops, or in the earning of a gross national product [1]. Studies of 2010 and 2013 are enormous indicating that 832,900 yearly death estimates for parasitic infection including malaria, 584,000; cryptosporidiosis, 100,000; amebiasis, 55,000; leishmaniasis, 51,600; schistosomiasis, 11,700; Chagas disease, 10,300; cysticercosis, 1200; and food-borne trematodiases, 7000. The human population experienced a full amount of 2.5 billion Disability Adjusted Life Year (DALYs) in 2013, which is a large number of suffering but represents a significant reduction, ~25%, since 1990. DALYs are nearly the sum of Years of Life Lost (YLL) by the reason of premature mortality and Years Lost due to Disability (YLD) for people living with a health condition or its consequences [11].

3. Man-made problems

Without recognizing the ecological and environmental consequences, favorable conditions for parasites had been created, for instance, millions of people, especially children, die each year from preventable diseases through proper sanitation facilities. Urbanization is another problem as population shifts from rural to urban areas and high population densities commonly overload water and sewage capabilities of even major cities. Nightsoil (manure) is often used as fertilizer on food crops usually aggravates parasitic problems. Moreover, there are several examples of national and international efforts to enhance productivity and standard of living in less-developed countries that inadvertently increased parasitic diseases. Despite opposite advice from their own agricultural experts, The World Bank loaned the government of Brazil funds to pave highways into the Amazon region to inhabit poor urban workers for farming. As a consequence, the prevalence of malaria increased and spread to new foci when the migrants returned to the cities after their farms failed. Smaller dams for drainage and agriculture have promoted transmission of schistosomiasis, onchocerciasis, dracunculiasis, and malaria. In the same token, construction of the Aswan High Dam, an embankment dam built across the Nile, between 1960 and 1970, on the Nile River to control floods, provides water for irrigation and generates hydroelectricity, which is pivotal to Egypt's industrialization, resulted (unfortunately) in increased schistosomiasis in Egypt [1]. The unauthorized introduction of crayfish to the Nile Delta, Egypt, controlled snails biologically and broke the life cycle of *Schistosoma* spp.; however, it has helped in the decline of local fish populations (personal communication with Prof. Dr. Adel Shaheen, Department of Fish Diseases and Management, Benha University, Egypt).

http://dx.doi.org/10.5772/67554

4. Looking back for going full speed ahead

As the purpose of our book is to dig deeply and smoothly for the current alternative antiparasitics, it is wise to look back for ancient and traditional solutions to get the most of them and to go full speed ahead. In fact, many of the important parasites encountered today not only existed but were widespread in their distribution before written records began, and our early ancestors must have been aware of the presence of the largest and most common worms and of some of the diseases caused by parasites. Humans created high cultures in all continents, such as the peoples of the Egyptians, Sumerians, Babylonians, Mongolians, Chinese, Mayas, Aztecs, Incas, and so on. Medicinal plants had been time-honored everywhere and upgraded from generation to generation orally or through written documents (e.g., on dried/fired clay plates, papyrus), which was lost during wars and/or at the fall of high cultures after centuries of Excellency, so that only portions of all knowledge were retained until today.

Being the cradle of civilization, Ancient Egypt became synonymous with power, wealth, and technological advancement. I prefer taking about Ancient Egyptian Medicine, not only because I am very proud to be one of their ancestors and enthralled by eco-friendly alternatives in the interim but also because a great part of their stories are well documented and preserved, and they gave us the ever-standing pyramids, the mummies, the first solar calendar, hieroglyphics, and many more. Although abundant on historic ruins, the writings of Egyptians themselves were virtually indecipherable until the Rosetta stone was discovered in 1799 during Napoleon's conquest of Egypt. This basalt Stela bore a tribute to Ptolemy V (196 B.C.) carved in hieroglyphics and repeated in demotic, or simplified, characters, and also in Greek, providing Jean-Francois Champollion necessary keys to decipher the language [12]. It is said that when the young Frenchman realized the value of such stone, he fainted.

The credit should be given to Champollion for opening doors to a wider understanding of Ancient Egypt. So set back and be ready to travel back to ancient time, to hear the voices from the past, from the land of legend and mystery, known as "*The Mother of the World*," we have a story to tell. Set against the exotic backdrop of the Egyptian desert, the Step Pyramid of Djoser hearken our memories back to the days of pharaohs. The wind whispers to you some of the Egyptian secrets. The Step Pyramid was the first monumental stone building constructed in Egypt in the Third Dynasty by Imhotep (/ɪmˈhoʊtɛp/), means the one who comes in peace and he served as the Vizier of Djoser during the 27th century B.C. Ancient Egyptian medicine dates back to the days of Imhotep, the earliest known physicians, architects, and engineers [13].

5. Ancient Egyptian medicine

Ancient Egypt was not exclusively characterized by the construction of giant pyramids but as an epitome of medical knowledge that had a profound impact on Greek medicine and subsequently spread worldwide. If you were sick during the time of the pharaohs, no worries! There was a specialist doctor for your illness and the credit is given to Imhotep who diagnosed and treated well over 200 diseases that dealt with the abdomen, rectum, bladder, eyes, and more. He is known to have practiced surgery as well as dentistry. The Edwin Smith

Papyrus (carries the name of the man who purchased it from an Egyptian dealer in 1862) is the only medical papyrus of its time to reflect a scientific approach to medicine. Many Egyptologists credit the text to Imhotep, albeit he lived one millennium earlier, as the Papyrus is believed to be based on texts written earlier than 1600 B.C. [13].

To see the full vivid picture, the ancient Egyptians were very clean people who loved life and wanted to live their lives free of disease and pain. They bathed and purified their bodies often and shaved their body hair. Amusingly, they believed that human body consisted of passages that behaved like irrigation canals. When such canals became blocked, the person became sick. Therefore, they practice medicine in health and in sickness for preventative and curative health care. The first school dedicated to medicine dates all the way back to Egypt's first dynasty. Physicians studied at schools called "*The House of Life,*" and they were dedicated to one disease or one part of the body, and Egyptian doctors were everywhere. They were highly advanced in their awareness of the human body, suffering, and sickness; even the Greeks were green with envy of their expertise [13]. Proceeding their age, they designed the enema when they noticed the bird *Ibis* filling its beak with water and then injecting the water through its anus to wash its intestine. They also administered medications, with recommended doses, in the form of pills, cakes, suppositories, ointments, drops, gargles, fumigations, enemas, and baths. In addition, the liquid vehicles were water, milk, beer, and wine, each sweetened with honey, and the ingredients were expected to remedy a variety of problems and control flies and other insects as well [12].

Enchantingly, the green color used in eye makeup probably came from copper salts, which have an antiseptic effect, but whether they were effective inadvertently in preventing or treating the eye infections common in Egypt cannot be ascertained. Copper preparations, interestingly, are the main agents of the present century against trachoma [12], the world's leading cause of preventable blindness of infectious origin caused by the bacterium *Chlamydia trachomatis*, spread through direct personal contact, shared towels and cloths, and flies. This progressive culture was the perfect stage for innovative remedies as herbs (discussed briefly later on), minerals, metals, and oils. The Egyptian pharmacopeia included antimony, copper, salt, alum, carbon from charred wood, iron (possibly from meteorites), natron, malachite, desert oil, red ochre, and animal remedies, such as honey, white oil, ox fat, and goose fat [14].

6. Old and current: parasitic problems as old as pyramids

Illness is not a new thing, and sufferings and losses due to parasitic diseases are old as the Egyptian pyramids (**Figure 1**). Ancient Egyptians were aware of the impact of the environment on the everyday life, especially the River Nile (called *Ḥ'pī* or *Iteru*, meaning "river" and also called Ar or *Aur*, means "black," in reference to the black silt left behind after the yearly flooding), which is the longest river in the world approximately 4258 miles (6853 km) long and got its name from the Greek word "*Neilos*", means valley. Such a great river is a pleasant place to start in considering the health of the Egyptians, as the Nile is, the everlasting, the life- and health-giving source of water for drinking, cooking, washing, irrigation, and trading, till the degree that the negative confession said "*I have never stopped [the flow of] water*". By the way, there is a traditional Egyptian proverb says "*Once you drink from the Nile, you are destined to return*". In contrary, the other side of the story indicated that the Nile River, like other rivers, harbors parasites and other creatures that lead to illness [15], such as bilharziasis, filariasis, and

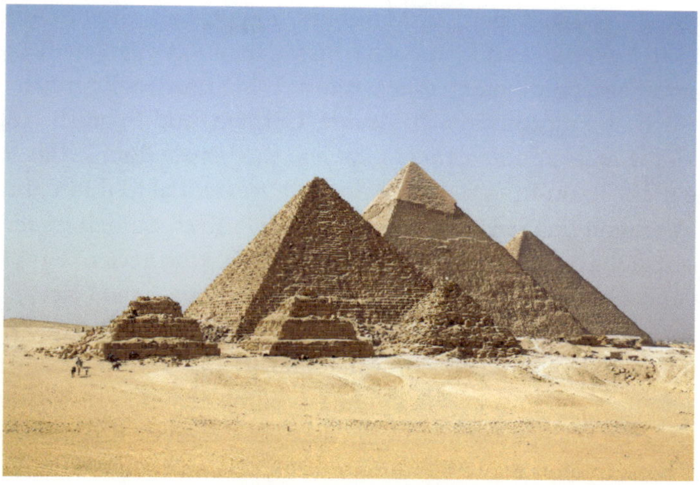

Figure 1. Solutions for parasitic problems as old as the Egyptian pyramids.

malaria. Before we proceed, it is worth to mention that many of the pharaoh's written orders that urged farmers to combat pests and protect the environment from pollution. Consequently, Egypt was one of the first countries that paid special attention to environmental problems and its impact on the individual who is considered the most important wealth. The Egyptians did not like pests which plagued them but accepted them as a legitimate part of creation;

Who creates that on which the mosquito lives,
worms and fleas likewise,
who looks after the mice in their holes
and keeps alive the beetles in every timber.

From the Hymn to Amen-Re, c.1600 BCE

After Jan Assmann
Ägypten - Theologie und Frömmigkeit einer frühen Hochkultur, p.73

6.1. Bilharziasis (aaa)

Schistosoma spp., the most famous trematode, has ancient roots in Egypt. Since the discovery of calcified *Schistosoma haematobium* eggs in a mummy by Ruffer [16] in 1910, *Paleoparasitology*, the study of parasites from the past and their interactions with hosts and vectors, has evolved. People waded through standing water, for the most part in the agricultural irrigation channels; parasites such as the *Schistosoma* infective stage could enter a human host, through feet or legs, and then lay eggs in the bloodstream. These worms caused a lot of damage as they traveled through various internal organs, bringing about sufferers weak and susceptible to other diseases [15]. Being experienced with bilharziasis, and called it "aaa," ancient Egyptians mentioned it 28 times in the Ebers, Berlin, Hearst, and London papyri. Ebers 62 says the disease is caused by *harrart* (*cercaria*). This is a parasitic worm with a complex life cycle alternating between two hosts, humans and that live on riverbanks [14]. This would explain the sentence by someone who, aware of the mode of infection, said, "*I have not waded in the water*" [17], as is reported in the negative confession in Chapter 125 of the Book of the Dead.

Paul Ghalioungui (1908–1987), born in Mansoura, Egypt, to a Greek Orthodox family, is famous for being an Egyptian endocrinologist, historian of Egyptian medicine, Egyptologist, and an authority on Pharaonic medicine; he wrote a vivid history of Egyptian medicine in several languages such as English, French, Arabic, German, and Spanish [18]. According to Ghalioungui [19], the male adult worm is 1 cm and the female double this length but much thinner than the male. In order to see the worms, it is essential to dilute the blood in water before clotting. A magnifying lens is considered crucial. Even though there is no proof that such lenses existed at that time, Elseesy [20] mentioned that the ancient Egyptians, who manufactured glass and fiberglass, also invented the magnifying lens. Elseesy opines that the penile sheaths are shown in some tomb murals, whether they were anticipated to prevent urination in water or to block the access of the parasite through the urethra, also have the same hygienic measures and effect. Schistosomiasis of the rectum is painful and may explain the high percentage of ancient Egyptian remedies for the anus. It is noteworthy here that the ancient Egyptians treated *aaa* with antimony chloride and such modern medicine up to about 40 years ago treated schistosomiasis using antimony tartrate [20]. **Table 1** presents more information about hepatoprotectives. Ancient Egyptians knew a lot of things about the Schistosoma's mode of infection, symptoms, and, surprisingly, treatments. They should be giving the credit for such discoveries, *aaa*, but the credit is given in Egypt again but to Theodor Bilharz, a German physician stationed in Egypt and became the first chief of the surgery at the Kasr-el-Aini Medical School and Kasr El Aini Hospital of Cairo. In 1851, he formally discovered, during an autopsy, the causative agent of hematuria and linked the parasite to urinary schistosomiasis, and then he identified it as *Distomum haematobium*. By the way, Bilharz discovered, in Egypt and in the same year, the dwarf tapeworm worm *Hymenolepis nana* living in the small intestine of an Egyptian male. At the age of 37, Bilharz died in 1862 from complications of typhoid fever after return to Cairo from an expedition to Massawa, a city on the Red Sea coast of Eritrea. He is buried in Cairo leaving a great legacy as *Bilharzia* is another term for schistosomiasis and The Theodor Bilharz Research Institute (TBRI) in Giza, Egypt, is named in his honor. The mission of TBRI is targeted toward control, diagnosis, and management of endemic diseases particularly urinary and hepatic schistosomiasis and their complications.

6.1.1. An unforeseen solution of schistosomiasis

Having an ancient root in Egypt, there was a long history of schistosomiasis control. Although the Aswan High Dam, the extension of perennial irrigation, and the increase of the Egyptian population afforded conditions favorable for its transmission, the national schistosomiasis control program that was gradually expanded after 1918, together with increased awareness, urbanization, diversification of the economy, and the changes in the rural villages, resulted in the accelerating decline of schistosomiasis [21]. Traditionally, Egyptians were consuming chicory in large amounts; it has been discovered that it purifies the liver and the blood and it helps in case of schistosomiasis.

Biologically, the unauthorized introduction of the crayfish, *Procambarus clarkii* known as freshwater lobsters, to the Nile Delta for aquaculture is a significant feature during the early 1980s leading to shocking consequences. The crayfish rapidly spread, became invasive, and colonized many areas. By 1996, it was estimated that 4.6 metric tons/year of *P. clarkii* could be harvested from the Nile; actually, crayfish could prey upon *Bulinus truncatus* and *Biomphalaria alexandrina* snails in the wild and was, therefore, likely a source of inadvertent biological control of schistosomiasis transmission [21]. Another biocontrol agent of nuisance snails in Egypt is the juvenile and adult black carp, *Mylopharyngodon piceus*, which is a species of cyprinid fish, feeding exclusively on snails. If you pass by a place having such fish, you will hear the sound of crushed snails; therefore, it is called "the snail carp" in Egypt." Black carp is formally introduced in Egypt by the General Authority for Fish Resources Development for controlling the intermediate hosts for human parasites as *Schistosoma* spp. as well as parasites relevant to cultures of freshwater fishes (personal communication with Prof. Dr. Adel Shaheen, Department of Fish Diseases and management, Benha University, Egypt and an expert in Aquaculture and Fish diseases in the African Union AU-IBAR).

Thus, crayfish and black carp played a biological role in reducing transmission of schistosomiasis and enabling praziquantel, the drug of choice to treat patients from the 1980s onwards distributed and funded By U.S. Agency for International Development (USAID), to make a dent in the prevalence rates by reducing transmission and re-infection in the meantime. In contrary to the situation in most other African countries where rates have increased, there is, fortunately, a great decline in schistosomiasis rates in Egypt in recent decades due to the intensive schistosomiasis control and water supply programs [21]. Hopefully, similar control measures cover all *Schistosoma* infested regions.

6.2. Mosquito-transmitted diseases

6.2.1. Filariasis

Filariasis is transmitted by mosquitoes and defined by swelling and thickening of the skin. Lymphatic filariasis was common along the Nile. While there are no written records, the swollen limbs of a statue of the Egyptian Pharaoh Mentuhotep II from about 2000 B.C. suggest that he was suffering from elephantiasis [22]. Some tomb pictures of servants illustrate enlarged male external genitalia and examination of the scrotal skin from the Leeds mummy, Natsef-Amun, evidenced the existence of filarial worms [14].

6.2.2. Malaria

The presence of malaria in Egypt from circa 800 BCE onwards has been confirmed using DNA-based methods [23] and antigens produced by *Plasmodium falciparum* (causing tertian fever) in mummies from all periods were detected, and all mummies were suffering from malaria at the time of their death (Nunn, 1997: 73). Elseesy [20] comments that the vast areas of land covered with River Nile water in the form of lakes and canals were indeed good media for the diseases. Herodotus wrote that the builders of the Egyptian pyramids (circa 2700–1700 BCE) were given large amounts of garlic [17] probably to protect them against malaria. The Pharaoh Sneferu, the founder of the Fourth dynasty of Egypt, who reigned from around 2613 to 2589 BCE, used bed-nets as protection against mosquitoes and Cleopatra VII, the last Pharaoh of Ancient Egypt, similarly slept under a mosquito net [18]. Whether the mosquito nets were used for the purpose of malaria prevention, or for avoiding the discomfort of mosquito bites, is unknown. The ancient Egyptians were using essential oils (having insect repellent effect) for medicinal benefits, beauty care, spiritual enhancement, and in literally all aspects of their daily life. More information about insect control is presented in Section 6.5 and **Table 1**.

Despite the African problems, Egypt, currently, almost eliminated malaria; there have been no cases of locally transmitted malaria in Egypt ever since June 14, 2014, because of the effort of The Egyptian Ministry of Health, local government, and health authorities who engaged in intensive malaria control activities in the affected areas as a village of Aswan Governorate, the latest appearance of malaria. They have recently completed active surveillance involving screening and treating, if needed, all villagers for malaria. Moreover, mosquito control activities have included entomologic surveillance, environmental management [23], and distribution of impregnated bed nets (personal communication with Prof. Dr. Azaa Abdel Fattah, Research Institute of Medical Entomology, Egypt, the authorized place doing the entomological part in malaria control).

6.3. Dracunculiasis

Confirmation of the presence of Guinea worm in ancient Egypt comes from the finding of a well-preserved female worm and a calcified worm in Egyptian mummies (205) [22]. The earliest descriptions of Guinea worms are from the Ebers papyrus from 1500 BC and include instructions for treating swelling in the limbs; they appear to refer to both the nature of the infection and techniques for removing the worm. Sometimes ancient Egyptians took in Guinea worms in their drinking water. The female worm would travel to the host's legs in order to lay her larvae, again causing ill health [15]. The solution is to wrap the exposed end of the worm on a stick and pulling it out. Amazingly, this remedy is still used nearly 4000 years later [13]. It worth mentioning that Dracunculiasis is not a problem in Egypt nowadays.

6.4. Enteric helminths

Enteric helminths were well known since ancient times. Evidence of eggs of the tapeworm, *Tenia* spp., was found in the mummy ROM (N AKHT) examined in Toronto, and roundworm infection was found in the mummy PUM II, unwrapped in the United States; the giant roundworm, *Ascaris lumbricoides*, is quite large and can be seen in stool. A piece of advice in Ebers Papyrus says that "*Do not eat unless you have an appetite for food.*" Because they are very clean, externally and internally, Herodotus mentioned that Egyptians were accustomed to cleanse their bodies by having purgatives on 3 days every month to clean their intestines. They applied castor oil as a purgative (applied traditionally in Egypt) and also prescribed it for cases of diarrhea as the goal of therapy was to hasten expulsion of the causative agents of diarrhea [24]. More herbal treatments such as pepper, cardamom, cumin, anise, almond, chamomile, fenugreek (*Helba* in Arabic), barley, cumin, pine oil, pomegranate roots, and so on were used by ancient Egyptians [14]. They also used coriander and onions to help against problems of the digestive system. Powdered cumin mixed with grease or lard was inserted as an anal suppository to disperse heat from the anus and stop itching; and leaves from many plants, such as willow, sycamore, and acacia, were also used [24].

For different gastrointestinal tract disorders, pomegranate and wormwood are well-known vermifuges in Egypt till now. It worth mentioning here that it is in Egypt where the first published studies have documented that traditionally used myrrh have molluscicidal effects on the intermediate hosts of trematodes as well as trematodicidal properties against *Fasciola, Dicrocoelium,* and *Heterophyes* spp. An Egyptian pharmaceutical company now produces a special myrrh preparation and markets it as gelatin capsules (Mirazid®) containing 300 mg of purified Commiphora (*Belsan* in Arabic) extract. The drug ameliorates all symptoms within a week and eliminates all worms within 4 weeks of treatment [25]. **Table 1** presents more information about anthelmintics, antidiarrheal, and laxatives.

6.5. Vermin

Ancient Egyptians suffered also from vermin (varmint or varmit), a plural noun means pests or nuisance animals, that spread diseases or destroy crops or livestock, till the degree of several plagues occurred during the time of Moses, such as plagues of locusts and lice infestations. The Ebers Papyrus mentions a few remedies against a number of pests. Generally speaking, tremendously clean people having rigorous notions of hygiene, the ancient Egyptians put remarkable effort and creativity into their battle against vermin.

6.5.1. Head lice

In response to the frustration and fear caused by lice, ancient Egyptians, men and women alike, typically kept their head shaved smooth. The beautifully lavish hairdos were usually wigs (an artificial covering of hair, and it was a fashion for the rich and the poor at that time), which control head lice in the mean time. Aromatic head louse formula includes one half-cup vinegar, one-half cup water, 12 drops essential oil of cinnamon, 12 drops essential oil of rosemary, and 12 drops essential oil of terebinth. Mix vinegar and water, add the essential oils and blend, and pour onto hair concentrating on areas near the scalp line, particularly near the ears and massage into the scalp. Comb thoroughly and very patiently with a fine tooth lice comb, rinsing or wiping the comb frequently. Even though head lice infestations are rare in the current decade, till the degree that the current youth know nothing about lice, Egyptians still prefer using what their ancestors did and use vinegar, essential oils, and fine-toothed comb for controlling head lice.

6.5.2. Fleas

In fact, a formula for driving vermin from homes has a modern ring as a solution of natron water was sprinkled to eliminate and repel fleas. It is worth mentioning that natron is a salt, and lavishly sprinkling carpets with salt and then vacuuming is a modern remedy against fleas [26].

Traditionally, Egyptians control insects through sprinkling fine salt over carpets or affected areas that dry out fleas as they walk over it and fleas will die over time. As fleas are attracted to light, a homemade light trap suspends a candle or a small light source over a shallow pan or bowl that is full of water and liquid soap. When fleas are attracted to light, they hop right into the bowl and drown. Having no idea about the synchronization phenomenon of flea occlusion, a pet (dog or cat) trap is also used to gather a huge number of fleas when introduced to a deserted house infested with fleas; then such pet was treated with essential oils or an insecticidal shampoo.

6.5.3. Cowling Insects

Some ancient Egyptian remedies for household pests include fumigation of the house with incense and myrrh and washing the house with a solution of natron or whitewashing the walls with *bebit* mixed with crushed charcoal. On the other hand, the traditional tricks of the Egyptians include adding bay leaves, as well as the tapering ends of cucumber to infested areas to repel roaches and ants. For killing any by-passing insects, (as fleas, bed bugs, cockroaches, ants, etc), vacuum the carpet and the floor, then mop them with water containing few drops of liquid soap (used for tiles, not dishes), a cup of vinegar, and a cup of kerosene. The odor of this mixture will disappear soon after aeration of the place; the result will surpass your expectations, the carpet, as well as the floor will shine again as new ones, and all crawling insects will die instantly. The other traditional solution is to fumigate the place with juniper for hidden creatures as bedbugs and rodents. To repel roaches and cloth-eating insects, dried levanter in small cloth buckets is added to wardrobe and naphthalene balls in semiopened small plastic bags, for nonstaining clothes, are added to the stored clothes.

6.5.4. Other vermin

Ancient Egyptians controlled the other vermin through fat of the oriole which is efficient in combating flies; fat of the woodpecker was used against fly stings; fresh palm wine would protect against gnats; loose ash spread around a grinding mill kills flour eating insects; natron, dried onion seeds or a dried Nile Tilapia were placed in front of the hiding hole of a snake to prevent it from leaving its lair; and fat of a cat spread on sacks and bundles keeps rats away, while grain is best protected from them by burning deer excrement. It worth to mention also that cats were being used by Ancient Egyptians to control rodents and protect grains; rodents were also hunted with ferrets and captured in traps [27]. Being praised for controlling vermin and its ability to kill snakes like cobras, the domesticated cat became an icon of grace and poise. More information was mentioned in **Table 1**. For repelling insects, rodents, and snakes, wormwood (*Sheeh* in Arabic) is the best traditional choice in Egypt by hanging small cloth pockets containing wormwood in the veranda, balcony, and plants to repel pests. Now, dear reader, I could expect that your feelings effortlessly came and went like clouds in a windy sky; therefore, could you please live in the moment, take a deep breath, and blow back after passing by your journey of the vivid story of the ancient and traditional Egyptian control strategies, as it is really time worthy to sharpen the saw and go full speed ahead for the best pest, vermin, control.

Target Effect	Used botanicals
Anthelmintics and vermifuge	Coriander; portulaca (*Regla* in Arabic); rue; lupinus (*Termes* in Arabic); sycamore fig (*Gemez* in Arabic); caper bush; carob (*Kharoob* in Arabic),; dodder (*pond weed* or *Hamool* in Arabic), lettuce seeds; date palm; camel's hay (*Halfa br* in Arabic); parley for round worm; and juniper (*Arar* in Arabic) for tape worm. Some recipes include: coriander, sandal wood and anise; portulaca, cow milk, and honey as herbal tea for 3 days; 1 spoon of carob seeds, 1 spoon of asafoetida (*Halteet* in Arabic),1 spoon of honey, 1 spoon of chuffa (groundnut or *Hab El Aziz* in Arabic), and one spoon of grape juice; small pieces of sycamore fig soaked in barley water; grape wine and frankincense for tape worm; 5 spoons of chuffa, 4 spoons of white oil and honey (used as a drink for one day); 5 spoons of artemisia (*Sheeh* in Arabic), 5 spoons of dodder, 20 spoons of barley water; and 12 gm of date palm seeds, 12 gm of carob and 25 table spoons of boiled barley. Moreover, the following recipe is used in case of worms and *Shistosoma spp*: equal amounts of *Ammi visnaga* (*Khela balady* in Arabic), Egyptian henbanes (*Hyoscyamus muticus* or *sakran* in Arabic), juniper, natron salt, pomegranate roots, and celery was used as herbal tea 3 times per day before meal.
Antidiarrheal (for dysentery)	Carob, pomegranate wine, tamarix (tamarisk, salt cedar), as well as herbal teas of the mixed ingredient as coriander, thyme and honey; and coriander, anise, and sandalwood.
Pesticides and repellents	Black peppercorns found in the nostrils of Ramses II for insect repellents; sulphurwort (*Al Qena* in Arabic) repel bed bugs; angelica fleas and ash were sprinkled as an insecticide and repellent; yellow sweet clover (yellow melilot) attract bees and repel cloth moth and garlic to repel snakes and scorpions. Some ingredients as myrh, spartium (scoparius or *alretm* in Arabic), rosemary, mastic, gum, *aloe vera*, Bahia rosewood, wild celery, and cardamom were ground and mixed with honey and uses as incense for air and cloth freshener and insect repellent.
Eye preparations	Portulaca; rue (*Sezab* or *Harmal* in Arabic); chuffa; carob; tamarix
Topical preparations	For skin problems and scabies: turmeric lotion; *aloe vera*, caper bush; portulaca, lupines, chuffa, pomegranate peel tea, and castor seed oil.
Laxatives	Linseed, cress (*Rashad* in Arabic, used also as poultices) and sycamore fig (used also as antiflatulent).
Hepatopr-otectives	Chicory (*Hendbaa, Sen El Assad* or *Serees* in Arabic), turmeric, and olive oil. Equal parts of juniper, lotus, *Ziziphus spina-christi* (*sedr* in Arabic), and *Citrullus colocynthis* (*hanzal* in Arabic)

N. B. The other antiparasitics used by Ancient Egyptians were discussed in the text.

Table 1. Some Antiparasitics used by Ancient Egyptians, Adapted from Abdel All [28].

7. No worries, Nature helps

Nowadays, farmers and growers are under huge pressure to decrease the use of chemical parasiticide without forfeiting yields or crop quality, in the mean time, parasitic control is becoming increasingly problematical due to the development of resistant populations and the decreasing availability of products. Substitutes for chemical control are needed urgently to be used as part of Integrated Parasite/Pest Management. Such *green movement* was the driving force to search for new environmentally compatible tools in the fight against parasites and vector insects because of the side effects of chemicals such as widespread of environmental contamination, toxicity to nontarget organisms, and negative effects on the health of humans and animals.

Biorational (biological and rational) parasiticides (**Figure 2**) are having limited or no adverse effects on the environment, nontarget organisms including humans. Such parasiticides, optimistically, are gaining popularity in the current climate of environmental awareness and public concern [29]. Biorationals include the following: biochemicals as botanicals [29–40], pheromones [29], photo insecticides [29, 41, 42], fatty acids [43], inorganics [44, 45], and insect growth regulators [29, 46]; biologicals, using competitors and natural enemies [29, 46] such as probiotics along with their prebiotics [47], parasitoids, predators, nematodes, and pathogens (virus, bacteria, fungi, or protozoa); and transgenic pesticides (genetically modified plants or organisms) [29, 46].

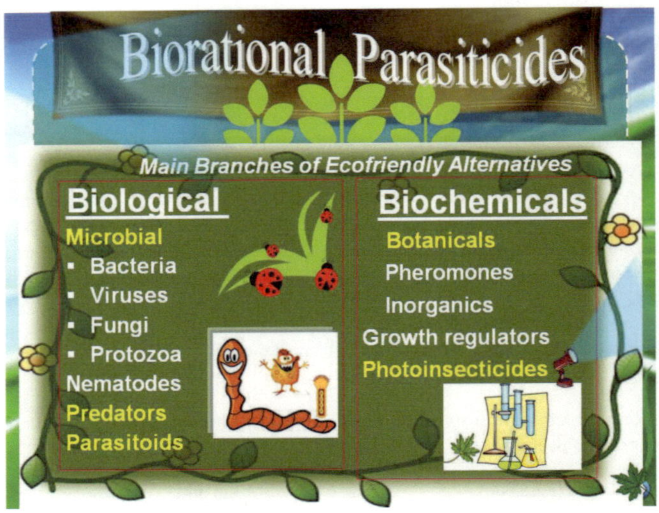

Figure 2. For fun and benefit, we should be ahead of parasites through using eco-friendly alternatives.

Nature is a smart skilled factory created to produce solutions to all our problems through an assortment of natural enemies and secondary metabolites produced by medicinal plants. Natural enemies take part in limiting potential parasite populations, and they are more likely to survive in the case of application of eco-friendly biopesticides [29]. Botanicals including plant extracts and essential oils are the most affordable tools [48, 49] for the poor and the rich since ancient times, as herbs constitute an alternative to conventional medicine in many developing countries. Ethnopharmacology can contribute to the exploration of phytotherapeutic resources for use in local contexts and countries of origin. Microencapsulation and nanotechnology include nanocapsules for vector and pest management and nanosensors for pest detection…etc [29] are used widely in agriculture and food plus their potential uses and benefits for parasite control are enormous as future trends [50–53]. Therefore, most biorationals will be straightforwardly thrashed out the whole time in this book.

8. For fun and Profit, we should be ahead of them

Parasites, from a biological perspective, are exciting, beautifully adapted, and complicated organisms. Recent decades witnessing emergence and re-emergence of disease agents, some of which are parasitic or transmitted by arthropods. *P. falciparum*, the most dangerous species of malaria organism, has become drug-resistant in many parts of the world, and there are numerous reports of drug resistance in *P. vivax*. Unfortunately, most parasites developed resistance to one drug after another, and many other examples are discussed later on throughout you expedition in this book. Money for research on tropical infections is very scant because pharmaceutical companies are reluctant to spend money to develop drugs for treating people who cannot pay for them, and the less-developed countries have many other urgent financial [1] and security problems.

An important role of parasitologists, together with that of other medical disciplines, is to break the deadly cycle by contributing to the global eradication of major parasitic diseases and pests while making possible more efficient use of the earth's resources especially botanicals; see Khater [29, 48, 54] for more information about their safety, commercialization, resource availability, barriers to commercialization, improving the efficacy, and future trends. Besides having medical, veterinary, and economic importance, controlling parasites naturally is enthralling (fun), which could be pursued for natural and safe products (profit). Despite being smaller than us and exquisitely adapted for life on or within the body of another (bigger) organism, parasites are smaller than us, they are smarter than us as they develop resistance faster than our ability to develop new drugs. Therefore, we should be ahead of them and try to win the never-ending battle via searching for safe and complex alternatives that parasites cannot defeat. All our efforts will be fruitful only when enveloped with hard work and great patience plus passion and ended with profits planned from the far beginning.

Author details

Hanem Fathy Khater

Address all correspondence to: hanemkhater@gmail.com; hanem.salem@fvtm.bu.edu.eg

Department of Parasitology, Faculty of Veterinary Medicine, Benha University, Moshtohor, Toukh, Egypt

References

[1] Schmidt GD, Roberts LS. Foundation of Parasitology. 8th ed. McGraw-Hill; 2009. 720p.

[2] Ramadan MY, Khater HF. Prevalence of *Eimeria* species infecting goats in Kalubyia governorate with trials of treatment by natural material (propolis) and toltrazuril. Egypt. Vet. Med. Soc. Parasitol. J. 2009; **5** (1): 1-10.

[3] Ramadan MY, Khater HF, Abd EL Hay AR, Abo Zekry AM. Studies on parasites that cause diarrhea in calves. Benha Vet. Med. J. 2015; **29**(1): 214-219.

[4] Khater HF. Some studies on enteric helminth parasites of poultry [Thesis]. Benha Branch: Zagazig University, Egypt; 1993.

[5] Ramadan MY, Khater HF, Seddiek SA, Abd El-Aty MA. Protozoal incidence in balady chicken flocks after viral vaccinations. Benha Vet. Med. J. 2015; **29**(1): 105-111.

[6] Khalifa NO, Khater HF, Fahmy HA, Radwan MEI, Afify JSA. Genotyping and phylogenetic analysis of cystic echinococcosis isolated from camels and humans in Egypt. Am. J. Epidemiol. Infec. Dis. 2014; **2**(**3**): 74-82.

[7] Khalifa NO, Khater HF, Nassief MZ. Genetic fingerprint of unilocular hydatidosis in Egyptian camels and humans using nested PCR. Pak. Vet. J. 2014; **34**(4): 522-526.

[8] Ramadan MY, Desoky AF, Khater HF. Seroprevalence and preliminary treatment of toxoplasmosis of pregnant goats in Kalubyia Governorate, Egypt. Acta Sci. Vet. 2007; **36** (3): 295-301.

[9] Khater HF, Khalifa NO, Barakat AMA. Serological and molecular studies of ovine and human toxoplasmosis with a trial of treatment of infected ewes. Sci. J. Vet. Adv. 2013; **2**(11): 157-168.

[10] Khater HF, Barakat AMA. Behavioral changes caused by toxoplasmosis (abstract). The Fifth International Conference of the Arab Society for Medical Research; 28-31 October 2016; Sharm El Sheikh, Egypt; 2016.

[11] Global Burden of Parasitic Disease. [Internet]. Available from: http://faculty.ucmerced.edu/kjensen5/index.php/research/global-burden-of-parasitic-disease/ [Accessed: 2016-12-18].

[12] Ancient Egypt [Internet]. Available from: http://www.healthguidance.org/entry/6310/1/Ancient-Egypt.html [Accessed: 2016-12-10].

[13] Ancient Egypt online [Internet]. Available from: http://www.ancient-egypt-online.com/ancient-egyptian-medicine.html [Accessed: 2016-12-10].

[14] Shafik A, Elseesy WR. Medicine in Ancient Egypt. In: Selin H, editor. Medicine Across Cultures: History and Practice of Medicine in Non-Western Cultures. Kluwer Academic Publisher; 2003. pp. 27-47.

[15] Filer JM. Ancient Egypt, BBC Report, Health Hazards and Cures in Ancient Egypt. 2011. [Internet]. Available from: http://www.bbc.co.uk/history/ancient/egyptians/health_01.shtml [Accessed: 2016-12-9].

[16] Ruffer MA. Note on the presence of "Bilharzia haematobia" in Egyptian Mummies of the Twentieth Dynasty. BMJ 1910; **1**: 16.

[17] Faulkner RO. The Ancient Egyptian Book of the Dead. London: British Museum Publications; 1972. 192p.

[18] Ghalioungui P. [Internet]. Available from: https://en.wikipedia.org/wiki/Paul_Ghalioungui [Accessed: 2016-12-9].

[19] Ghalioungui P. The Ebers Papyrus. Cairo: Academy of Scientific Research and Technology, 1987.

[20] Elseesy WR. Drugs in ancient Egypt. From a series of 100 articles on Egyptology. Rose-elYoussef Weekly Magazine 1999; 3706, June 19.

[21] Lopez M. A long history of schistosomiasis control. Stanford University [Internet]. 2015. Available from: http://schisto.stanford.edu/pdf/Egypt.pdf [Accessed: 2016-12-18].

[22] Cox FE. History of human parasitology. Clin. Microbiol. Rev. 2002; **15**(4): 595-612. Erratum in: Clin. Microbiol. Rev. 2003; **16**(1):174.

[23] History of Malaria [Internet]. Available from: https://en.wikipedia.org/wiki/History_of_malaria [Accessed: 2016-12-18].

[24] Ancient Egyptian Medicine in Sickness and in Health: Preventative and Curative Health Care [Internet]. Available from: http://www.reshafim.org.il/ad/egypt/timelines/topics/medicine.htm [Accessed: 2016-12-18].

[25] Abdul-Ghani RA, Loutfy N, Hassan A. Mini-review. Myrrh and trematodoses in Egypt: an overview of safety, efficacy and effectiveness profiles. Parasitol. Int. 2009;**58**: 210-214.

[26] A Modern Problem as Old as the pyramids [Internet]. Available from: http://www.touregypt.net/featurestories/lice.htm [Accessed: 2016-12-18].

[27] Vermin [Internet]. Available from: http://www.reshafim.org.il/ad/egypt/timelines/topics/pests.htm [Accessed: 2016-12-20].

[28] Abdel All A. Ancient Medicine. 3rd ed. Dar Agial for Publishing and Distribution: Egypt; 2007. 263 P.

[29] Khater HF. Ecosmart biorational insecticides: alternative insect control strategies. In Preveen F. editor. Insecticides—Advances in Integrated Pest Management. InTech: Croatia; 2011. pp. 17-60. DOI: 10.5772/27852.

[30] Khater HF, Shalaby AA. Potential of biologically active plant oils for control mosquito larvae *Culex pipiens* (Diptera: Culicidae) from an Egyptian locality. Rev. Inst. Med. Trop. S Paulo. 2008; **50**(2):107-112.

[31] Khater HF, Ramadan MY, El-Madawy RS. The lousicidal, ovicidal, and repellent efficacy of some essential oils against lice and flies infesting water buffaloes in Egypt. Vet. Parasitol. 2009; **164**: 257-266. doi:10.1016/j.vetpar.2009.06.011.

[32] Khater HF, Khater DF. The insecticidal activity of four medicinal plants against the blowfly *Lucilia sericata* (Diptera: Calliphoridae). Int. J. Dermatol. 2009; **48** (5): 492-497.

[33] Idris M, Abbas RZ, Masood S, Rehman T, Farooq U, Babar W, Hussain R, Raza A, Riaz U. The potential of antioxidant rich essential oils against avian coccidiosis. World's Poultry Sci J. 2016. doi:10.1017/S0043933916000787

[34] Khater HF, Hanafy A, Abdel-Mageed AD, Ramadan MY, El-Madawy RS. Control of the myiasis-producing fly, *Lucilia sericata*, with Egyptian essential oils. Int. J. Dermatol. 2011; **50**: 187-194. doi: 10.1111/j.1365-4632.2010.04656.x.

[35] Seddiek SA, Ali MM, Khater HF, El-Shorbagy MM. Anthelmintic activity of the white wormwood, *Artemisia herba-alba* against *Heterakis gallinarum* infecting turkey poults. J. Med. Plants Res. 2011; **5**(16): 3946-3957.

[36] Seddiek SA, Khater HF, El-Shorbagy MM, Ali MM. The acaricidal efficacy of aqueous neem extract and ivermectin against *Sarcoptes scabiei var. cuniculi* in experimentally infested rabbits. Parasitol. Res. 2013; **112**: 2319-2330.

[37] Khater HF, Ramadan MY, Abdel Mageid AD. In vitro control of the camel nasal botfly, *Cephalopina titillator*, with doramectin, lavender, camphor, and onion oils. Parasitol. Res. 2013; **112**:2503-2510. DOI 10.1007/s00436-013-3415-2

[38] Khater HF, El-Shorbagy MM, Seddiek SA. Lousicidal efficacy of camphor oil, d-phenothrin, and deltamethrin against the slender pigeon louse, *Columbicola columbae*. Int. J. Vet. Sci. Med. 2014: **2**(1): 7-13.

[39] Khater HF. Bioactivities of some essential oils against the camel nasal botfly, *Cephalopina titillator*. Parasitol. Res. 2014; **113**(2): 593-605

[40] Seddiek SA, El-Shorbagy MM, Khater HF, Ali AM. The antitrichomonal efficacy of garlic and metronidazole against *Trichomonas gallinae* infecting domestic pigeons. Parasitol. Res. 2014; **113**(4): 1319-1329.

[41] Khater HF, Hendawy N. Photoxicity of rose bengal against the camel tick *Hyalomma dromedarii*. Int. J.Vet. Sci. 2014; **3**(2): 78-86.

[42] Khater HF, Hendawy N, Govindarajan M, Murugan K, Benelli G. Photosensitizers in the fight against ticks: safranin as a novel photodynamic acaricide to control the camel tick *Hyalomma dromedarii* (Ixodidae). Parasitol. Res. 2016; **115**: 3747. DOI: 10.1007/s00436-016-5136-9

[43] Ali AM, Seddiek SA, Khater HF. Effect of butyrate, clopidol and their combination on the performance of broilers infected with *Eimeria maxima*. Brit. Poultry Sci. 2014; **55**(4): 474-482.

[44] Khater HF, Ramadan MY. The acaricidal effect of peracetic acid against *Boophilus annulatus* and *Argas persicus*. Acta Sci. Vet. 2007; **35** (1): 29-40.

[45] Khater HF, Seddiek SA, El-Shorbagy MM, Ali MM. The acaricidal efficacy of peracetic acid and deltamethrin against the fowl tick, *Argas persicus*, infesting laying hens. Parasitol. Res. 2013; **112**(1): 259-269. DOI: 10.1007/s00436-012-3133-1 https://www.ncbi.nlm.nih.gov/pubmed/23090722

[46] Khater HF. Biocontrol of Some Insects [Ph.D. Dissertation]. Benha Branch: Zagazig University, Egypt; 2003.

[47] Ali MA, Khater HF, Seddiek SA, Nada MO. Comparative efficacy of synbiotic and diclazuril on broilers experimentally infected with *Eimeria acervulina*. Assiut Vet. Med. J. 2015; **61**(146): 24-33.

[48] Khater HF. Prospects of botanical biopesticides in insect pest management. Pharmacologia. 2012; **3**(12): 641-656.

[49] Khater HF. Bioactivity of Essential oils as green biopesticides: recent global scenario. In: Govil JN, Bhattacharya S, editors. Recent Progress in Medicinal Plants. Vol. 37; Essentials Oils II. Studium Press LLC: USA; 2013. pp. 153-220.

[50] Roni M, Murugan K, Panneerselvam C, Subramaniam J, Nicoletti M, Madhiyazhagan P, Dinesh D, Suresh U, Khater HF, Wei H, Canale A, Alarfaj AA, Munusamy MA, Higuchi A, Benelli G. Characterization and biotoxicity of *Hypnea musciformis*-synthesized silver nanoparticles as potential eco-friendly control tool against *Aedes aegypti* and *Plutella xylostella*. Ecotox. Environ. Safe. 2015; **121**: 31-38. Green Technologies for Environmental Pollution Control and Prevention (Part 1).

[51] Murugan K, Priyanka V, Dinesh D, Madhiyazhagan P, Panneerselvam C, Subramaniam J, Suresh U, Chandramohan B, Roni M, Nicoletti M, Alarfaj AA, Higuchi A, Munusamy MA, Khater HF, Messing RH, Benelli G. Predation by Asian bullfrog tadpoles, *Hoplobatrachus tigerinus*, against the dengue vector, *Aedes aegypti*, in an aquatic environment treated with mosquitocidal nanoparticles. Parasitol. Res. 2015; **114**(10): 3601-3610. doi: 10.1007/s00436-015-4582-0.

[52] Govindarajan M, Khater HF, Panneerselvam C, Benelli G. One-pot fabrication of silver nanocrystals using *Nicandra physalodes*: a novel route for mosquito vector control with moderate toxicity on non-target water bugs. Res. Vet. Sci. 2016; **107**: 95-101.

[53] Govindarajan M, Rajeswary M, Muthukumaran U, Hoti SL, Khater HF, Benelli G. Single-step biosynthesis and characterization of silver nanoparticles using *Zornia diphylla* leaves: a potent eco-friendly tool against malaria and arbovirus vectors. J. Photochem. Photobiol., B: Biol. 2016; **161**: 482-489.

[54] Khater HF. Spice up Your Life and Garden: Precious treasures in your kitchen", Kindle Direct Publisher, 2017, P. 135.

Section 2

Biological Control

Chapter 2

Biological Control of Parasites

Tebit Emmanuel Kwenti

Additional information is available at the end of the chapter

http://dx.doi.org/10.5772/68012

Abstract

Parasites (ectoparasites or endoparasites) are a major cause of diseases in man, his livestock and crops, leading to poor yield and great economic loss. To overcome some of the major limitations of chemical control methods such as rising resistance, environmental and health risks, and the adverse effect on non-target organisms, biological control (biocontrol) is now at the forefront of parasite (pests) control. Biocontrol is now a core component of the integrated pest management. Biocontrol is defined as "the study and uses of parasites, predators and pathogens for the regulation of host (pest) densities". Considerable successes have been achieved in the implementation of biocontrol strategies in the past. This chapter presents a review of the history of biocontrol, its advantages and disadvantages; the different types of biological control agents (BCAs) including predators, parasites (parasitoids) and pathogens (fungi, bacteria, viruses and virus-like particles, protozoa and nematodes); the effect of biocontrol on native biodiversity; a few case studies of the successful implementation of biocontrol methods and the challenges encountered with the implementation of biocontrol and future perspectives.

Keywords: biological control, biological control agents, parasites, humans, plants, livestock, case study, challenges

1. Introduction

In nature, the population size of every species is regulated by natural environmental factors. These factors are responsible for the "checks and balances" of a population of living organisms. The event where living organisms live and die a natural death unaided by man is termed "natural control". Weather (abiotic or non-living factors) is an important factor in natural control; temperature and humidity are determinants of the survival of living organisms. Availability of competition (biotic factors) is also an important determinant for the survival of living organisms [1]. Many organisms are killed by pathogens (disease-causing agents) such as bacteria, viruses, fungi, parasites (parasitoids) and predators [1].

Living organisms, which are considered undesirable, are generally referred to as pests. Environmental factors (such as weather, geography and soil conditions) which affect pest populations generally vary from one location to another and changes through time. A combination of these factors may substantially reduce the pest population in one geographical area and make it more abundant in another. Pests sometimes outwit their natural enemies and grow to very high population density. To keep their population in check will necessitate the manipulation of the population of their natural enemies by man. This is termed biological control or simply biocontrol. Biocontrol is therefore defined as "any activity of one species that reduces the adverse effect of another" [1]. Biocontrol can also be defined as "the study and uses of parasites, predators and pathogens for the regulation of host (pest) densities" [2]. Biological control differs from natural control in that the latter does not involve human manipulation. The organism that suppresses the pest population is generally referred to as a biological control agent (BCA).

A parasite is an organism that lives and feeds in or on a host [3]. Parasites that invade and live within the host are referred to as endoparasites; meanwhile, those that live on the surface without invading the host are referred to as ectoparasites. Endoparasites include helminths and protozoa, and ectoparasites are fleas, ticks, mites, insects and so on. Parasites are a major cause of disease in man, his livestock and crops, leading to poor yield and economic loss. The biocontrol of parasites therefore entails the use of BCAs to suppress the population of the parasites.

This chapter focuses on the biological control of parasites, providing a brief history of biocontrol; their advantages and disadvantages; types of BCAs including predators, parasites (parasitoids) and pathogens (fungi, bacteria, viruses and virus-like particles, protozoa and nematodes); their effect on the native biodiversity; a few case studies of successful implementation of biocontrol; challenges encountered with the implementation of biocontrol strategies and finally their future perspectives.

2. History of biological control

The concept of biological control is not entirely new. The ancient Egyptians were probably the first to employ biocontrol dating some 4000 years ago, when they observed that cats fed on rodents, which damaged their crops. This most likely led to the domestication of the house cat [4]. However, the first record of biocontrol is from China. As early as the third century, a nest of the ants *Oecophylla smaragdina* were sold near Canton (today known as Guangzhou in China) for use in control of the citrus insect pests such as *Tesseratoma papillosa* (Lepidoptera). By 1200 A.D., the usefulness of the ladybird beetles as biological control agents of aphids and scales had been recognized. Between 1300 and 1799 A.D., the importance of biological control tools was recognized. Van Leeuwenhoek was probably the first to describe insect parasitism, which he illustrated in his publication in 1701. In 1726, de Reaumur recognized the first insect pathogen, a Cordyceps fungus that infects noctuid. The mynah bird, *Acridotheres tristis*, was successfully introduced from India to Mauritius by the British and the French for the

http://dx.doi.org/10.5772/68012

control of the red locust, *Nomadacris septemfasciata,* in 1762 (see **Figure 1**). In 1776, in Europe, the control of the bedbug, *Cimex lectularius,* was successfully accomplished by the release of the predatory pentatomid, *Picromerus bidens.* Koller was the first to put forth the concept of "natural control" in 1837 [5].

Between 1850 and 1887, the concept of biological control switched to the United States. In 1870, Charles V. Riley was the first person to conduct the successful movement of parasitoids for biological control when parasitoids were moved from Kirkwood, Missouri, to other parts of the United States for the control of the weevil (*Conotrachelus menuphar*). In 1883, the US Department of Agriculture (USDA) imported *Apanteles glomeratus* from England to control *Pieris rapea* (the imported cabbageworm) parasites that were distributed in DC, Iowa, Nebraska and Missouri. This marked the first intercontinental shipment of parasites. It was not until the 1800s that well-thought-out biological control projects were implemented across Europe. In 1888, the cottony cushion scale project was launched to control the cottony cushion scale, *Icerya purchase,* which was threatening to destroy the infant citrus industry. This was the first project to be launched. Since then, many projects have been launched including the gypsy moth project in New England (1905–1911) [5].

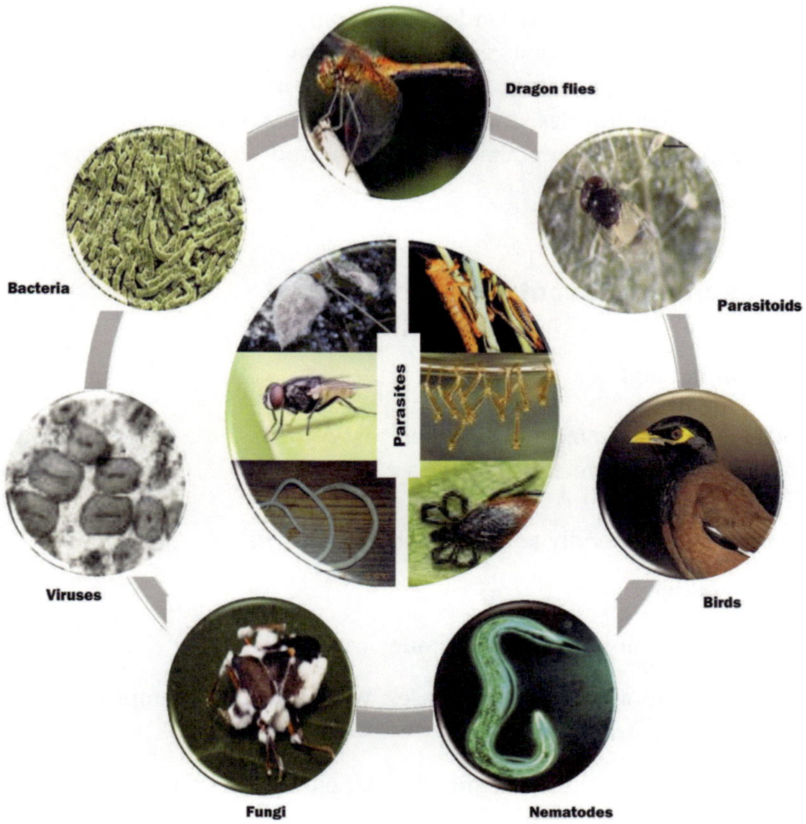

Figure 1. Images of some common parasites/pests (centre cycle) and biological control agents (external cycles) used in the biocontrol of parasites.

Between 1930 and 1940, there was a peak in biological control activity in the world with 57 different biological control agents established at various places. During World War II, there was a sharp drop in biological control activity and after the war, biological control did not regain popularity due to the production of relatively inexpensive synthetic pesticides. It was not until the late 1960s that the concept of integrated pest management (IPM) was implemented, and biological control was seen as a core component of IPM by some [5]. The other components of IPM are habitat manipulation, modification of cultural practices and the use of resistant varieties.

3. Importance of the biological control of parasites

Control of parasites nowadays is mainly by the use of chemicals (pesticides), but the commonly used chemicals are fast losing their effectiveness as a result of resistance arising from indiscriminate use. Moreover, pesticides present a danger to people, the environment, their residual build-up and their effect on non-target organisms such as beneficial insects, birds, domestic animals and sometimes the crop itself. A suitable alternative to the growing problem is biological (natural) control. Under ideal conditions, biocontrol has sustainability, which is lacking in the other methods of parasite control. There are several methods through which biological control of parasites could be achieved, including the use of predators (such as arthropods, mites, flies, beetles, amphibians, fish, birds, rodents, etc.), parasites (parasitoids) and pathogens (such as fungi, bacteria, viruses and virus-like particles, protozoa and nematodes).

4. Advantages and disadvantages of biocontrol

4.1. Advantages of biocontrol

Biocontrol offers some advantages over other pest-control strategies, particularly chemical pesticides. These advantages include as follows:

(1) It is environmentally friendly and safe to the applicator.

(2) There are no residues.

(3) Biocontrol could be very economical in some cases.

(4) Biocontrol is easy to apply; in many cases, we are merely manipulating something to favour naturally occurring controls.

(5) Biological control is sometimes lasting, thereby eliminating the needs for continuous re-application as is necessary with pesticides.

(6) Biocontrol is easily established

http://dx.doi.org/10.5772/68012

(7) BCAs are frequently very host specific.

(8) Unlike chemical methods, pests do not become resistant against BCAs.

4.2. Disadvantages of biocontrol

The disadvantages of biocontrol include as follows:

(1) Biocontrol is often slow. In biocontrol of pests, there is often a lag time between build-up of the pest population and build-up of the biocontrol agent. If a pest population is already at or above economically damaging levels, pesticides are the only alternative.

(2) BCAs do not completely eliminate their host [6]. If they do, they would also die. However, biological control may be integrated with other pest control strategies to achieve complete eradication.

(3) With biocontrol, there is the possibility that the BCA may tend to feed on the desired plants or insect, that is, crossovers [7–9]. Careful selection of the BCA will minimize this problem.

(4) BCAs are frequently ineffective in multiple weed complexes when used in biocontrol of weeds. This may be because the weed and the crop are so closely related that the control agent affects both the pest and the crop.

(5) The shipping, storage and application techniques of BCA can be relatively complex. Production of the BCA is also costly in some cases.

(6) Biocontrol sometimes may be costly compared to conventional methods. The high cost is usually attributed to the research that has to be done prior to implementation of the biocontrol strategy.

(7) Biocontrol if not well conceived may lead to dramatic changes in native biodiversity.

5. Types of biological control agents

Biocontrol of insects may include predators (e.g. spiders), parasites (parasitoids) or pathogens like viruses, bacteria, fungi, protozoa and nematodes (see **Figure 1**).

5.1. Predators

Predators can be vertebrates or invertebrates, some of which are arachnids, but deployment of insects is most common. The efficiency of predators in controlling populations of some ticks in different habitats varies and may reach up to 100% [10, 11]. For example, predation has been observed to be lower in tall grass areas than in short grass areas [12]. Likewise, predation has been observed to be two to eight times higher in open areas than in thick pasture areas and non-intensive pasture or agricultural areas [13]. The different types of predators can be classified as invertebrates and vertebrates.

5.1.1. Invertebrates

5.1.1.1. Spiders and insect herbivores

Spiders prey on many insects. Spiders have a defined habitat; a change in the habitat such as mulching may increase their population by as much as 60% [14, 15]. River prawns have been observed to prey on snails [16]. Insect herbivores including the cell-content feeder *Liothrips ludwigi* (Thysanoptera), the stem borers *Merocnemus binotatus* (Boheman) and *Tyloderma* spp. (Coleoptera) have shown promise in the control of weeds [17]. Both the adult and larval stages of the predatory thrips, *Scolothrips sexmaculatus,* are known to feed on spider mites and other thrips [18]. *S. sexmaculatus* prefers spider mite eggs but adult females will consume other mite stages as well [18].

5.1.1.2. Mites

Some mites are nematode predators. For example, some mites (*Phytoseiid* spp.) are capable of consuming *Ascaris* ova in the soil [19]. There are also a few mite species that are voracious predators of eggs and larvae of houseflies and other filth flies that develop in manure and faeces of livestock; for example, *Macrocheles muscaedomesticae* can eat up to 10 housefly eggs per day [20].

5.1.1.3. Flies

Use of the predatory fly, *Hydrotaea (Ophyra) aenescens,* which is commercially available in several northern European countries, presents a breakthrough in the indoor control of the housefly, *Musca domestica* [21]. Small flies such as *Mutilla glossinae* are important parasites of tsetse and are promising BCAs against the tsetse fly [22].

5.1.1.4. Ants

Around 27 species of ants from 16 genera mainly *Aphaenogaster, Iridomyrmex, Monomorium, Pheidol* and *Solenopsis* are known to prey on ticks, horn flies and different agricultural pests [23]. Application of the fire ant, *Solenopsis inucta,* in Louisiana in the USA markedly reduced the population of ticks (*Ixodes* spp.) transmitting anaplasmosis in cattle [23]. However, a wide applicability of fire ants may pose a challenge because of their painful sting.

5.1.1.5. Beetles

Dung beetles of the family Scarabaeidae (Scarabaeinae, Geotropinae and Aphodiinae) are useful in the control of pasture livestock flies since they breed primarily in cow pats. In addition, dung beetles such as *Onthophagus ganelle* and *Euniticellus intermedius,* introduced from Africa to Australia, are regarded as useful in the biocontrol of *Musca vetustissima* and the

http://dx.doi.org/10.5772/68012

buffalo fly *Haematobia exigua*. The African dung beetles are well adapted to cattle faeces and compete with fly larvae for food. Furthermore, the rapid burial of dung by the beetles reduces the breeding habitats for the flies [21]. The scarab beetle (*Scarabaeus sacer*), also referred to as sacred scarab among ancient Egyptians, was famous for its habit of rolling balls of dung along the ground depositing them in its burrows. The female would lay her eggs in the ball of dung. When they hatched, the larvae would use the ball for food. When the dung was consumed, the young beetles would emerge from the hole [24]. Dung beetles have been reported to reduce horn flies by as much as 95%, bush flies by 80–100% and result in nine times of fewer parasites produced [25, 26]. Dung beetles can also play a role in the biocontrol of bovine gastrointestinal nematodes (Trichostrongylidae). The spotted lady beetle (*Coleomegilla maculata*) is also able to feed on the eggs and larvae of the Colorado potato beetle *Leptinotarsa decemlineata* [27] and can be used in its control. The larvae of Coccinellids (ladybird or ladybug) are voracious predators of aphids and also consume mites, scale insects and small caterpillars.

5.1.1.6. Dragonflies and water bugs

Dragonflies (see **Figure 1**) may look like scary biters, but they are only dangerous to mosquitoes. Dragonfly larvae, "nymphs", feed on mosquito larvae, and adult dragonflies feed on adult mosquitoes [28]. On the other hand, water bugs, *Diplonychus indicus,* are also known to prey on mosquito larvae [29].

5.1.2. Vertebrates

5.1.2.1. Amphibians and fishes

The water tortoise *Pelomedusa subrufa* has been reported to be able to remove ticks from black rhinos in a streambed [30]. Also in some areas, the mosquito larvae may be controlled biologically by predatory fish such as *Gambusia affinis* and *Guppy poecilia* [31]. One study showed that introducing *Gambusia affinis* into water wells resulted in 98% reduction in the larval density of *Anopheles stephensi* [32]. Other predatory fishes such as the *Cyprinus carpio, Ctenopharyngodon idella, Aphanius dispar, Aplocheilus blocki, Tilapia* spp., *Catla catla, Labeo rohita* and *Cirrhinus mrigala* have also shown promise in the control of mosquitoes [33]. In China, for example, the presence of carp fish in certain rice fields reduced the number of malaria cases [34]. Another predatory fish, the black carp (*Mylopharyngodon piceus*), has shown promise in the biocontrol of the intermediate host snails of fish-borne zoonotic trematodes [35]. Snails (some of which are intermediate hosts of fascioliasis, paramphistomes and schistosomes) are eaten by some fishes as well.

5.1.2.2. Reptilians

Some lizards can eat arthropods. The lizard stomach may contain as many as 2.5–15 ticks/stomach. However, because there are few lizards near the bird nest, their effect on the tick population may be limited [21]. The Australian gecko *Gehydra dubia* and the exotic Asian house gecko *Hemidactylus frenatus* have been observed to prey on mosquitoes; in the laboratory, they have been observed to prey more on female mosquitoes and are therefore a promising tool for the biological control of malaria [28].

5.1.2.3. Birds

Birds are generally thought to be the main predators of insects. Some bird species are known to pick off ticks from the host during flight or collect them from the ground. Birds also eat the larvae of dung flies. One approach for biocontrol of trematodes is the control of the snail intermediate host. Domestic fowls and birds are predators of snails. Scrub jays have been observed to spend 89% of their time searching deer for ectoparasites [36]. In Africa, chickens are natural predators of ticks and actually pick ticks from the bodies of cattle as they lie down as well as from the vegetation [37].

5.1.2.4. Rodents and mammals

Some mammals are insectivorous. As an example, *Sorex araneus* preys on ticks and at times prefers them to alternative foods [12, 38]. Shrews seem to locate hidden ticks by their smell. Mice and rats are often cited as preying on ticks [39]. However, it is worth to mention here that it is not advisable to use rodents for controlling insects as they are more harmful and transmit more diseases than insects.

5.2. Parasites (parasitoids)

Parasites that attack other parasites are generally referred to as parasitoids. Parasitoids are very diverse in appearance, biology and the hosts they attack. Parasitoids lay their eggs on or in the body of an insect host, which is then used as food for the developing larvae. The host is ultimately killed. Most insect parasitoids are wasps or flies and may have a very narrow host range. The most important groups are the ichneumonid wasps, which prey mainly on caterpillars of butterflies and moths; braconid wasps, which attack caterpillars and a wide range of other insects including greenfly; chalcid wasps, which parasitize eggs and larvae of greenfly, whitefly [40], cabbage caterpillars and scale insects and tachinid flies, which parasitize a wide range of insects including caterpillars, adult and larval beetles and true bugs [37, 41–44].

5.3. Pathogens

5.3.1. Fungi

Pathogenic fungi can be classified into two: entomopathogenic fungi and nematopathogenic fungi.

5.3.1.1. Entomopathogenic fungi

Fungi that infect and kill arthropod (insects, ticks or mites) pests are referred to as "entomopathogenic fungi". Over 750 species of entomopathogenic fungi have been identified, a majority of them belong to the phylum Ascomycota and a few to the phylum Zygomycota and Ascomycotina [45]. Unlike the other BCAs, some fungi do not need to be ingested by the host [33]; entomopathogenic fungi produce spores as the insect comes in contact with these spores either on the body of dead insects or surfaces or in the air as airborne particles; the spores germinate in the presence of high humidity and produce germ tubes that allow them to penetrate the cuticle of the insect, usually at joints or creases where the insect's protective covering is thinner [46]. Death usually follows between 4 and 10 days, depending on the type of fungus and the number of infecting spores. Other fungi cause death by the production of toxins (mycotoxin). After death, the fungus produces thousands of new spores on the dead body, which disperse and continue their life cycle on new hosts. Some species go into a resting stage, which survive periods of adverse conditions before forming or releasing spores. The ascomycetes together with the mitosporic fungi are most widely used for biocontrol of pests.

The most commonly investigated entomopathogenic fungi belong to the genera *Metarhizium* and *Beauveria* and are increasingly being used in commercial formulation against arthropods. The Hyphomycetes, *Beauveria bassiana* and *Metarhizium anisopliae* (formerly known as *Enthomphthora anisopliae*) are the most common species known to cause natural outbreaks to a wide range of insect hosts, on their own under favourable conditions. These fungi provide a long-term strategy for larvae and puparia control since they may survive in the soil through recycling in insects or roots [47, 48]. *Metarhizium anisopliae* and *Beauveria bassiana* are also effective in the control of mosquitoes [49]. They infect mosquitoes early in life and kill them, depending on the exposure dose and fungus isolate after 3–14 days [50]. Fungal spores can be applied in outdoor attracting odour traps, on indoor house surfaces and on cotton pieces hanging from ceilings, bed nets and curtains [51, 52] to control adult mosquitoes. Commercially available products based on *B. bassiana* are Mycotrol O (Emerald BioAgriculture), Naturalis Home and Garden (H&G), Naturalis L (Troy BioSciences, Inc.) and Biosect® (Kafr El Zayat—KZ Chemicals, Egypt) [44]. For example, Khater [53] used Biosect® to control larvae of both *Musca domestica* and *Culex pepiens* in-vitro and observed that the total larval mortalities of mosquitoes were almost 100%.

Hyphomycetes of the genera *Fusarium* also contain some important pathogens. For example, Ghannam et al. [54] observed that certain species of *Fusarium* (*F. solani, F. oxysporum and F. arthrosporioides* strain E4a) were able to increase the dead spikes of the obligate holoparasitic weed, broomrape (*Orobanche* spp.), by 33.6–72.7%, thereby making it promising for broomrape control.

Other fungi species that are increasingly being used as BCAs include the Oomycetes, *Lagenidium giganteum* (formerly: *L. culicidum*), which are known to be pathogenic to the larvae of several mosquito genera [55]. Unfortunately, the fungus is not effective for mosquitoes in brackish or organically rich aquatic habitats. In contrast, *Lagenidium* spp. was isolated from Egypt for the first time from *Culex pipiens* larvae infesting a polluted creak in Miet El-Attar, Benha, Egypt, and it was observed to effectively control *Culex pipiens* [53]. As the fungi has the ability of self-propagation, it could be used for effective control of the vector of bancroftian filariasis and rift valley fever virus [46].

The entomophthorales are another group of fungi that are able to cause natural outbreaks in insect populations and are also promising as good BCAs [56]. Several different *Entomophthora muscae* sensu stricto genotypes have been documented, and each type has demonstrated a high degree of host specificity [56]. All available literature deal with *E. muscae* as a pathogenic fungi of adult *Musca domestica*, but Khater [53] isolated, for the first time in Egypt, from

Moshtohor, Toukh and Qlubia governorate a strain that has the unique ability to infect larvae of the house flies. Fungi such as *Leptolegnia* spp., *Coelomomyces* spp., *Hirsutella thomsonii, Nomuraea rileyi* and *Vericillum lecanii* are also being used in the control of insects [46].

The ascomycetes, *Trichoderma harzianum* and *T. viride,* have been shown to antagonize the fungi causing damping-off and wilt in bean plants [57].

5.3.1.2. *Nematopathogenic fungi*

Fungi that infect and kill nematodes (worms) are referred to as nematopathogenic fungi. Over 150 species of fungi are known to invade nematodes. Nematode-destroying fungi can be grouped into three: nematode-trapping fungi, the endoparasitic fungi and the fungal parasites of cyst and root-knot nematodes. Most nematopathogenic fungi fall in the group of nematode trapping; they use constricting (active) or non-constricting (inactive) rings, sticky hyphae, sticky knobs, sticky branches or sticky networks at intervals along the length of a widely distributed vegetative hyphal system to trap and kill nematodes by penetration and growth of hyphal elements within the host, for example, *Arthrobotrys candida, A. oligospora, Drechmeria coniospora* [58], *Harposporium anguillulae* [59] *and Monacrosporium* spp. [60]. The nematode-trapping fungi, *Duddingtonia flagrans,* which have demonstrated considerable superiority in the reduction of gastrointestinal nematodes parasitizing animals, produce thick-walled clamydospores that enable it to survive the passage through the gastrointestinal tract and is therefore effective in destroying the larval stages of parasitic nematodes in livestock [61, 62]. Feeding or field trials have clearly demonstrated that dosing with a few hundred thousand spores per kilogram of live birth weight (BW) of *D. flagrans* not only reduced the number of infective larvae but also increased the BW of the lambs compared with controls [63]. In another example, Araujo et al. [64] tested the nematode-trapping fungus *Arthrobotrys robusta* against *Cooperia punctate* larvae (L3) and observed a 53.81% reduction in the helminths eggs (EPG) in treated calves compared to non-treated calves as well as a 70.45% reduction in the number of recovered worms at necropsy in the treated calves compared to the control. Endoparasitic fungi infect nematodes by spores, which then develop and absorb the body contents, for example, *Harposporium anguillulae* [65]; meanwhile, the fungal parasites of cysts and root-knot nematodes exert their effect by invading eggs or females by ingrowth of vegetative hyphae, for example, *Verticillium chlamydosporum* [66–69]. Nematode-trapping fungi have increasingly been tested in the management of parasitic nematode infections of ruminants [70].

5.3.2. *Bacteria*

The most important entomopathogenic bacteria belong to the genera of *Bacillus* (see **Figure 1**). *B. thuringiensis* (Bt) is among the most widely used antagonist in the biological control of insects. After ingestion, target insects are killed by an enterotoxin released from a crystal protein in the bacterial spores. The mode of action of the toxin has been fully described [46]. Various subspecies of Bt has been used in biocontrol: *Bacillus thuringiensis* var *israelensis* (Bti), with activity against mosquito larvae, blackfly (Simuliid), sand fly, fungus gnats and related dipterans species; *B. thuringiensis* var *kurstaki* (Btk) and *B. thuringiensis* var *aizawai* (Bta) with activity against lepidopteran larval species; *B. thuringiensis* var *tenebrionis*

(Btt) with activity against coleopteran adults and larvae and *B. thuringiensis* var *japonensis* (Btj) strain buibui, with activity against soil-inhabiting beetles [46]. In some countries, commercial formulation of *B. thuringiensis var israelensis* is available for the control of mosquito larvae and the blackfly *Simulium damnosum* [71]. A study performed in Egypt comparing the activity of three *Bacillus thuringiensin* products in controlling ticks shows that Btk was more potent compared to Bti and *Bacillus thuringiensin* var *thuringiensin* in the control of ticks [72]. Several products of *Bacillus thuringiensin* are available in the market; a few examples of products include Dipel 2x (*B. thuringiensis* var. *kurstaki*), VectoBac (*B. thuringiensis* var. *israeliensis*) and HD 703 (*B. thuringiensis* var. *thuringiensis*) [72]. VectoBac, Bti (12 AS, Wady El Niel for agricultural development Co. Egypt) has been shown to be highly effective against *C. pipence* than *M. domestica* [53].

Mosquito larvae are also susceptible to *B. sphaericus*. *B. sphaericus* is effective in killing larvae of *Culex* spp. and *Anopheles* spp., especially those breeding in polluted water. Bti and *B. sphaericus* have been reported to successfully control certain species of sand fly (vector for the protozoa *Leshmania*) [73]. *B. penetrans* is also a well-known nematopathogenic bacterium of plant parasitic root-knot nematodes.

The bacterial pathogen, *Paenibacillus glabratella*, recently discovered by Duval et al. [74] has been observed to infect and cause high mortality in snails, therefore, making a promising BCA for the control of snails.

Another bacterium, *Streptomyces avermitilis*, produces toxins collectively called "avermectins" which are highly effective against several invertebrates from the classes Insecta, Arachnida and Nematodes [21]. *Streptomyces griseolus* has been shown in the laboratory to be able to control the trematode liver fluke, *Fasciola gigantica*, the causative agent of Fasciolosis [75]. Streptomyces are believed to kill parasites by the production of lytic enzymes such as α and β-glucanases, proteases, peptidases, cellulases, chitinases and lipases [75].

Bacteria belonging to the following genera have been tested for the control of plant parasitic nematodes including *Pasteuria* which are parasites of many plant-parasitic nematodes and water fleas [76]; *Brevibacillus laterosporus* strain G4 which is parasitic on *Heterodera glycines*, *Trichostrongylus columbriformis* and *Bursaphelenchus xylophilys* and the saprophytic nematode *Panagrellus redivius* [77, 78]; rhizobacteria (mainly *Bacillus* spp. and *Pseudomonas* spp.) are able to antagonize nematodes [79, 80] and the well-studied *Bacillus thuringiensis* (Bt) are also able to kill plant-parasitic nematodes [81]. More information about using bacteria as biocontrol agents has been extensively reviewed by Khater [46] and Tian et al. [82].

Nota bene: The Rickettsiae are a diverse group of bacteria, which cause diseases to humans and warm-blooded animals, and are transmitted by a number of arthropods such as ticks, fleas and so on. Some of these bacteria tend to parasitize these arthropods [83]. For example, ticks have become adapted as vectors, reservoirs and/or propagation sites of Rickettsiae [84] and often harbour generalized asymptomatic infections. Rickettsial infection may lead to alterations in tick behaviour, interfere with their development and cause pathological changes in salivary glands and ovarian tissues. In severe cases, infection may lead to death [85]. However, the use of Rickettsiae in biocontrol is not a reliable method.

5.3.3. *Viruses and virus-like particles*

Thousands of entomopathogenic viruses have been described but only a few, belonging to the families Entomopoxviridae (Entomopoxviruses, EPVs), Reoviridae (Cypoviruses, CPVs) and Baculoviridae (Baculoviruses, BVs), have been used successfully in controlling pest population [86]. The mode of pathogenesis and replication of entomopathogenic viruses varies according to the family, but infection nearly always occurs by ingestion [46]. The baculovirus (see **Figure 1**) is the most widely exploited virus group for biocontrol [87, 88]; they are very different from viruses that infect vertebrates and are considered very safe to use. The family Baculoviridae contains four genera: Alphabaculovirus (lepidopteran-specific NPVs), Betabaculovirus (lepidopteran-specific GVs), Gammabaculovirus (hymenopteran-specific NPVs) and Deltabaculovirus (dipteran-specific NPVs) [89]. At present, there are approximately 16 biopesticides based on baculoviruses available for use or are under development. The majority of these products are targeted against Lepidoptera. For example, codling moth granulovirus, CpGV (Cydia pomonella Granulovirus), is an effective biopesticide of codling moth caterpillar pests of apples, Gemstar LC (NPV of *Heliothis/Helicoverpa* spp. e.g. corn earworm, tobacco budworm and cotton bollworm); Spod-X LC (NPV of *Spodoptera* spp. e.g. beet armyworm); CYD-X and Virosoft CP4 (GV of *Cydia pomonella*, the codling moth) and CLV LC (NPV of *Anagrapha falcipera*, the celery looper) [46].

The leafhopper-infecting virus, Homalodisca coagulate virus-1 (HoCV-1, Dicistroviridae), has been shown to increase leafhopper mortality [90, 91]. The virus occurs in nature and spreads most readily at high population densities through contact among infected individuals, contact with virus-contaminated surfaces and/or as an aerosol in leafhopper excreta.

5.3.4. *Protozoa*

Very little attention has been given to entomopathogenic protozoans. Some protozoa such as *haemogregarina*, *Nosema*, *Babesia* and *Theileria* are pathogenic to some arthropods like ticks. Although there are no examples of effective direct biocontrol of protozoans, however, indirectly, some protozoans such as *Plasmodium* spp. and *Onchocerca volvulus* may indirectly be controlled by their intermediate hosts or vectors. The predatory soil amoeba *Theratromyxa weberi* is capable of ingesting nematodes. It flows over the nematode body and assimilates it within 24 h. This and other amoebae can be expected to have limited biocontrol capacities because they are slow-moving, as compared to nematodes. Other protozoa including *Nosema locustae* are pathogenic to grasshoppers and crickets; *Nosema pyrausta* (also known as *Perexia pyraustae*) is pathogenic to the European corn borer and *Vairimorpha necatrix* occurs naturally and infects corn earworm, European corn borer, armyworms, fall webworm and cabbage looper [92].

5.3.5. *Nematodes*

Numerous nematodes belonging to the genera *Steinernema* and *Heterorhabditis* are either obligate or facultative parasites of insects (including houseflies, fleas and other non-biting flies) and have been proven as effective BCAs [86] to control a wide range of insect pests including filth

http://dx.doi.org/10.5772/68012

flies, German cockroaches, cat fleas, armyworms, carpenter worms, crown borers, cutworms, flea beetles, leaf miners, mole crickets, plume moths, sciarid flies, root weevils, stem borers, webworms and so on [93]. They infect through penetration of the cuticle; invasion through the spiracles or anus or after ingestion by the host insect. The symbiotic bacteria contained within the nematode, when released into the body of the insect, cause septicaemia and death of the host. The bacteria then break down the insect body, which provides food for the nematodes. The nematode-bacterium relationship is highly specific; only *Xenorhabdus* spp. coexists with Steinermatids and only Photorhabdus bacteria coexist with heterorhabditids [46]. *Steinemema carpocapsae* (see **Figure 1**) has demonstrated effectiveness in the control of mosquitoes [49]. The host-specific entomoparasitic nematode, *Heterlylenchus autumnalis,* has been observed to parasitize *Musca autumnalis,* resulting in sterile female flies as nematode development occurs at the expense of egg production [94]. Entomopathogenic nematodes have been used commercially against insects during the last decades [95]. Seven species of nematodes have been commercialized worldwide and seven are currently available in the USA: *Steinernema carpocapsea, S. feltiae, S. glaseri, S. riobraus, Heterorhabditis bacteriophora, H. megidis* and *H. marelatus* [96]. There are two commercial nematode products available for termite control, Spear® and Saf T-Shield® [46].

The nematode *Paraiotonchium muscadomesticae* is also known to infect housefly larvae, but mortality is usually low except at high nematode concentrations. *P. muscadomesticae* infects housefly larvae and its descendants invade and damage the ovaries of adult female flies and are deposited in the larval habitat when the flies attempt to oviposit [46]. Furthermore, it has been observed that infected adults lived only about half as long as uninfected adults [97]. All these indirectly reduce housefly population.

Steinernema carpocapsae and *S. glaseri* have also been proven to be effective against *Teladorsagia* spp. and *Trichonstrongylus* spp. These nematodes are particularly useful on ground-inhabiting stages of fleas [98] and engorged females of numerous other ticks that fall to the ground [99–101]. Entomopathogenic nematodes are not harmful to humans, animals or plants and are generally regarded as remarkably safe to the environment [46].

Chaetogaster limnaei (Oligochaeta: Naididae) has long been observed to infect freshwater snails and protect the host from infection with various species of trematodes by eating both the miracidia and the cercaria. *C. limnaei* therefore has potentials in the biocontrol of parasitic diseases vectored by the freshwater snail (such as fascioliasis, schistosomiasis and related trematode infections) [102].

5.4. Earthworms

Earthworm population consume a large volume of soil and organic matter such as animal faeces. During feeding, they consume nematodes present in the soil and faeces. In different parts of the world, earthworms are responsible for natural biological control of trichostrongyle nematodes. For example, in northern Europe, earthworms play an important and often dominating role in removal of cattle dung from pastures and can be responsible for significant reduction of infective larvae of trichostrongyle nematodes on the pasture [103].

For more information about the life cycle, safety, production and genetically modified organisms (GMOs) of biological control agents, see Khater [46].

6. Effect of biological control on the native biodiversity

Biocontrol may have potential positive or negative effects on the diversity of native species. One of the major problems with biocontrol is the effect of the BCA on non-target species; the purpose of introduction of a BCA is to reduce the competitive advantage of exotic species that has previously invaded or been introduced there over the native species. However, the introduced BCA does not always target only the intended species; it can also target native species. Therefore, when introducing a BCA to a new area, a primary concern is its host specificity. BCA not targeting one species or a narrow range of species often makes for poor BCA and may become invasive species themselves. For this reason, potential BCA should be subject to extensive testing and quarantine before release to any environment. If an introduced species attacks the native species, this can lead to widespread changes in the biodiversity in that area. A classic example of biocontrol gone wrong is the cane toad that was introduced in Australia to control the introduced French's cane beetle and the Greyback cane beetle [104]. The toad instead was feeding on the native insect and soon took over native amphibian habitat and brought foreign disease to native toads and frogs, dramatically reducing their population.

Another notable example where biocontrol has gone wrong is in the introduction of the small Asian mongoose (*Herpestus javanicus*) found in the wild in South and Southeast Asia to Hawaii [105, 106]. *H. javanicus* was introduced to Hawaii over 100 years ago to control the rat population that were destroying the sugarcane plantations. Mongooses are entirely diurnal [107] meanwhile rats are nocturnal. The mongoose preyed on the endemic birds, especially their eggs, more often that it preyed on the rats. Both the mongoose and the rats now constitute a major threat to the bird's population in Hawaii. A few attempts have been made to eradicate these invasive mongooses but with limited success [108], and now the small Asian mongoose is regarded as one of the world's 100 worst invasive species [108, 109].

Furthermore, the sturdy and prolific eastern mosquitofish (*Gambusia holbrooki*), native to the eastern and southern United States, was introduced around the world in the 1930s and 1940s to feed on mosquito larvae and thus combat malaria. Unfortunately, it has thrived at the expense of local species, causing a decline of endemic fish and frogs through competition for food resources as well as through eating their eggs and larvae [110]. Many characteristics have been identified in Gambusia that contribute to their invasiveness: mosquitofish have short breeding periods and high fecundity [111], they exhibit higher feeding rates than their non-invasive relatives [112] and also show evidence of plastic responses to salinity-related stress; they produce more offsprings in higher salinities [113].

On the other hand, the replacement of the target species with another species which constitute more of a nuisance and for which the BCA does not normally attack is another challenge of biocontrol. This has happened in the past, for example in Douglas county, Oregon, USA, where Klamath weed populations were sharply reduced by biocontrol agents only to be replaced by tansy ragwort (*Senecio jacobaea*), which was in turn sharply reduced by BCAs only to be replaced by the Italian thistles (*Carduus pycnocepahalus*) [114].

7. Approaches to biocontrol

There are three broad approaches to biocontrol.

7.1. Importation

Importation involves the importation, screening and release of natural enemies to permanently establish effective natural enemies in a new area. Importation (also referred to as "classical biological control") usually targets introduced (non-native) pests in an area where their natural enemies normally do not exist. Native pests that are not adequately controlled by existing natural enemies may also be the target of classical biocontrol. The introduction of natural enemies to control the population of a pest is usually tightly regulated and is conducted solely by the federal or state agencies compared to the following two approaches that can be done by anyone [115]. This is necessary so that we do not import "solutions" that become more serious than the "problems" themselves.

7.2. Augmentation

Augmentative biological control typically involves the purchase and release of natural enemies that are already present in an area but not in quantity, enough to adequately keep in check the pest population in a particular location. The goal of this approach is simply to increase the number of natural enemies temporarily and therefore decrease the pest population in the area [115].

Release of natural enemies may take one of these forms: inundation or inoculation. With inundation, the target area is flooded with a large number of the natural enemies. Ideally, such a release will bring the pest(s) under control quickly, and it is hoped that the natural enemies will become permanently established in the area. Meanwhile, inoculation of an area usually involves much lower numbers. It is designed to allow establishment of a biological control agent in an area. Or such a release may be used merely to improve the natural enemy/pest ratio [116].

7.3. Conservation

This involves practices to conserve the population of natural enemies, thereby improving their effectiveness in the control of pests. Such practices include farming and gardening that provide the necessary resources for their survival and protect them from toxins and other adverse conditions. These conservative practices will benefit all natural enemies, whether native or imported or released through augmentation. This approach is frequently overlooked, yet it is just as important as the other two approaches [115].

8. Case studies of biocontrol

One of the most foretold stories of the success of biocontrol on a large scale is the eradication of the cottony cushion scale (origin: Australia) which was a serious threat to the citrus industry. The cottony cushion scale (*Icerya purchasi* Maskell) was introduced into North America and India and it rapidly spread, threatening the citrus crop. Chemical methods were either ineffective or too expensive to control the pest. The coccinellid beetle, *Rodolia cardinalis*, which is the natural enemy of the scale in its native Australia was introduced into the areas affected by the scale in North America and India, and it successfully controlled the cottony cushion scale [5]. Since then, other successes on a similar scale have been recorded, most in the biocontrol of parasites (pests) of plants. Biocontrol of parasites of medical and veterinary importance is still at its infancy, that is at the level of research, and as such no success story has been described. A few success stories in the biocontrol of parasites of agricultural importance are described below.

8.1. Case study 1: biocontrol of water hyacinth *(Eichhornia crassipes)*

Water hyacinth is a free-floating aquatic weed of South American origin and ranks among the top 10 weeds worldwide. It is one of the most noxious weeds known to man and has spread to at least 50 countries around the globe. The weed grows and occupies water surfaces of ponds, tanks, lakes, reservoirs, streams, rivers and irrigation channels. It was also a menace in flooded rice fields, considerably reducing yield. It interferes with the production of hydroelectricity, blocks water flow in irrigation channels, prevents the free movement of navigation vessels, interferes with fishing and fish culture and facilitates breeding of mosquitoes as well as fostering waterborne diseases [117]. Furthermore, water loss due to evapo-transpiration was a major concern especially in areas where freshwater shortage was common. Under ideal conditions, water hyacinth plants can propagate vegetatively and double their number in 10 days; the seeds can remain dormant for as long as 20 years before germinating [117]. The weed was indeed a major problem in India [117]. With this high growth rate, the weed defied most control methods.

Three exotic natural enemies were introduced in India, that is hydrophilic weevils—*Neochetina bruchi* (from Argentina) and *N. eichhorniae* (from Argentina)—and galumnid mite *Orthogalumna terebrantis* (from South America) in 1982 for the biological suppression of water hyacinth. Starting from October 1983, field releases of mass-bred weevils *N. eichhorniae* and *N. bruchi* in different water tanks in Karnataka, located at Byramangala (500 ha), Bellandur (344 ha), Varthuru (40 ha), Hebbal (20 ha), Nagavara (20 ha), Agram (20 ha) and others from October 1983 to December 1986; in an 8-ha tank at Nacharam in Hyderabad (Andhra Pradesh) in 1987; Ramgarh lake near Gorakhpur (Uttar Pradesh) in 1988; in 43-km-peripheral Surha lake, Balia, (Uttar Pradesh) in 1990 and Lakhaibill (Alengmore) and Assam in 2000, resulted in suppression of water hyacinth within 4 years. The weevils have cleared the Tocklai River and were proving very effective in most of the water bodies. Releases of the water hyacinth mites, like *O. terebrantis,* which are specific to water hyacinth were initiated in 1986 at Bangalore, Karnataka. About 25,000 adults were released in Agram, Kengeri and Byramangala tanks.

Establishment was obtained within 6 months in all the tanks. The mite was more efficient in water in which *N. eichhorniae* was also present [117]. Many other successes have been recorded in the biocontrol of weeds which can be found in the review by Cork et al. [118].

8.2. Case study 2: biocontrol of the glassy-winged sharpshooter *(Homalodisca virepennis* formerly known as *H. coagulata)*

The glassy-winged sharpshooter (*Homalodisca vitripennis*) is a large leafhopper insect from the family Cicadellidae. It is native to North America (northeastern Mexico) but has spread into the USA, where it has become an agricultural pest [119]. It is thought that the glassy-winged sharpshooter invaded and was established in the southern California sometimes around 1990 [120]. The glassy-winged sharpshooter usually lays a mass of eggs on the underside of leaves and covers them with the "brochosomes", a powdery white protective secretion kept in dry form. After hatching, the nymphs feed within the vascular system of small stems, molt several times and become adults which continue to feed on a wide variety of plants including grapes, citrus trees, almonds, stone fruit and oleanders resulting in enormous damage. Their feeding method along with their voracious appetite for so many different hosts makes them an effective vector for the bacterium *Xylella fastidiosa*, which causes plant disease. *X. fastidiosa* has been linked to many plant diseases including phoney peach disease in the southern USA; oleander leaf scorch and Pierce's disease in California and citrus X disease in Brazil. Plants not affected by the bacterium become a reservoir for other sharpshooters to pick up and carry to other plants [121].

The glassy-winged sharpshooter has a number of natural enemies, in particular egg parasitoids. Female parasitoids lay their eggs inside glassy-winged sharpshooter eggs and the developing parasitoid larvae kill glassy-winged sharpshooter eggs by feeding inside the egg. The parasitoid larvae pupate inside the glassy-winged sharpshooter egg and then chew a circular exit hole through which they emerge. The winged parasitoids can fly and after mating, they look out for more glassy-winged sharpshooter eggs to parasitize. In this manner, the egg parasitoids help keep the glassy-winged sharpshooter population in check [121]. In the southeastern USA and northeastern Mexico, glassy-winged sharpshooter eggs are parasitized by several species of mymarid and trichogrammatid parasitoids, including *Gonatocerus ashmeadi* Girault, *G. triguttatus* Girault, *G. morrilli* Howard and *G. fasciatus* Girault. Virtually, all species of parasitoid in the family Mymaridae (order: Hymenoptera) are the most common natural enemies associated with *H. vitripennis* eggs in the southeastern United States [122]. *Gonatocerus tuberculifemur* and *G. deleoni* are other species of parasitoids that attack the glassy-winged sharpshooter eggs and were introduced into California from Argentina [123, 124].

The glassy-winged sharpshooter has also successfully invaded French Polynesia (the Society Islands, Marquesas and Austral Island groups) where it became established in 1999 [125], Hawaii where it became established in 2004 [126], Easter Island and the Cook Islands. Glassy-winged sharpshooter became established in Tahiti French Polynesia in 1999 and was likely introduced accidentally on ornamental plants imported from California [121]. In contrast to California, no natural enemies for the glassy-winged sharpshooter existed there, and no obvious competitors existed in urban or natural settings. The glassy-winged sharpshooter populations underwent an exponential growth and were a complete nuisance to the population;

watery excreta known as sharpshooter rain literally rained from infested trees because there were so many glassy-winged sharpshooters feeding on trees, their noisy wings, their dead bodies littered in houses and their high populations retarded plant growth and reduced local fruit production [121]. Due to intense population movement, the glassy-winged sharpshooter spread to other areas in the region such as Raiatea (Leeward Islands) Moorea, Leeward Islands of Huahine, Bora Bora, Tahaa and Maupiti. At the end of 2004 and the beginning of 2005, the glassy-winged sharpshooter populations were discovered outside of the Society Islands in two other archipelagos of French Polynesia substantially distant from Tahiti: the Australs, where two islands were infested (Rurutu and Tubuai) and the Marquesas, where one island, Nuku Hiva, was found infested [121].

To combat the glassy-winged sharpshooter infestation in French Polynesia, the mymarid egg parasitoid *Gonatocerus ashmeadi* was imported from California, mass bred and released. Between May and October 2005, 13,786 parasitoids were released at 27 sites in Tahiti. The parasitoid established readily, and within 7 months of release, the glassy-winged sharpshooter had been completely controlled in Tahiti, and glassy-winged sharpshooter populations were reduced by over 95% [127]. The parasitoid also spread unassisted to every other island infested by the glassy-winged sharpshooter and parasitized their eggs [121], which led to a successful control of the glassy-winged sharpshooter in the area.

8.3. Case study 3: biocontrol of the velvet bean caterpillar (*Anticarsia gemmatalis*)

One of the most successful uses of baculoviruses in biological control has been in Brazil. The baculovirus AgMNPV has been successfully used in the control of the velvet bean caterpillar (*Anticarsia gemmatalis*), a pest of soybeans. Plots of soybeans that were naturally infested with *A. gemmatalis* were sprayed with the virus. The AgMNPV is highly virulent for *A. gemmatalis* and only needs to be applied once, which makes it a good BCA for the control of the velvet bean caterpillar. Furthermore, the virus can be spread by insect predators and survive passage through the digestive tract of beetles and hemipteran. In Brazil, virus preparations were applied at 1.5×10^{11} occlusion bodies per ha, that is, about 20 g or 50 larval equivalents. The programme, which was initiated in the early 1980s, by 2005, had seen the treatment of area of over 2 m ha [128].

In other examples, the granulovirus of the codling moth *Cydia pomonella* (CpGV) has been used in a number of countries in North America and Europe for the control of the insect on pear and apple crops [128]. In China, the baculovirus HearNPV has also been successfully used to control the cotton bollworm, *Helicoverpa armigera*, which was a major pest of cotton and had developed resistance to the chemical insecticides in many parts of the world [129].

9. Challenges in the biological control of parasites

Some challenges in the implementation of biocontrol strategies are listed below.

The introduction of exotic natural enemies raises concern regarding the effect it may have on non-target native species as mentioned above. Conservation biologists are typically concerned with the health and growth of a wide variety of organisms. If a BCA does in fact attack any native non-target species, its persistence and ability to spread to areas far from the site of release become a serious liability [130–132].

There are also concerns among conservation biologists about the release of BCA precisely because the agents themselves which are non-native may carry non-native parasites and commensal species [114].

BCAs are easily influenced by environmental factors such as temperature, humidity and oxygen extremes, which determine the success of the biological control strategy. BCA if applied when conditions are not favourable is bound to fail.

There are also challenges in the distribution of BCAs product, especially those containing living organisms. Most industries producing BCA products are often situated a considerable distance away from where the BCA is to be used. Before the BCA reaches its destination, most of the organisms are dead. There is therefore the need to develop a sizeable distribution network comprising a group of producers that will safeguard the quality of the products and provide advice for the users [133].

Another challenge, which may be faced with the implementation of a biocontrol strategy in pest control, is the lukewarm attitude among agriculturalists, who find it difficult to forego their fast-acting chemical pesticides over the sluggish BCA [134, 135].

10. Future perspective

10.1. Biotechnology

With the advances in biotechnology, there is the potential of identifying and manipulating "biocontrol genes" particularly in microbial agents to produce more effective BCAs. Furthermore, genes in BCAs responsible for their antagonistic effects will also be used to screen for more effective BCAs. Biotechnologists in many countries are experimenting with fungi, viruses, bacteria, nematodes and insects genetically modified to express toxins (scorpion toxin, mite toxin and trypsin inhibitor), hormones (eclosion hormone and diuretic hormone) or metabolic enzymes (juvenile hormone esterase) to increase the speed of killing, enhance virulent and extend host specificity of these organisms. The so-called third-generation genetically modified organisms (GMOs) have been engineered to control pests in agriculture, pathogens in human health and invasive species in the environment [136].

In one approach, to improve the efficacy of *Bacillus thuringiensis* var *israelensis* (Bti), genes encoding the potent insecticidal proteins from Bti, Btj and *B. sphaericus* have been spliced into new bacteria strains that are 10-fold more toxic than wild types species of Bti and *B. sphaericus* used in current commercial formulations. These new GMOs are safe to humans, animals and the environment and can be used as components in the integrated vector control programmes aimed at reducing malaria, filariasis and other diseases of medical importance [137]. These recombinant bacterial larvicides are much more efficient than the wild-type strains from which they are derived, their costs are similar to the new chemical insecticides and they are much more environmentally compatible than most chemical insecticides [46].

In another approach, biotechnologists are trying to develop new biopesticides based on fungi. Fungi tend to be host specific, can be mass produced on inexpensive media and are thought to be harmless to animals, humans and the environment. Unfortunately, naturally occurring fungi tend to kill insects slowly. Genetic technology holds the promise of producing biopesticides based on hypervirulent insect-specific fungi that kill quickly; for example, laboratory experiments have been performed where scorpion toxin gene has been spliced into the fungus that infect mosquitoes to enhance the killing efficiency of the fungus [138].

In yet another approach, biotechnologists are studying baculoviruses, a large variety of viruses that act specifically on hundreds of arthropods, including many agricultural pests, but appear to be safe to plants and vertebrates. But because baculoviruses typically kill much more slowly than chemical pesticides, their use is limited. Biotechnologists are experimenting to increase the killing efficiency of baculoviruses by splicing into them toxin-expressing genes isolated from mites, scorpions and spiders [139]. Baculovirus recombinants that produce occlusion bodies incorporating Bt toxin have also been constructed by making a fusion protein consisting of a polyhedron and Bt toxin [140]. Other constructs have been tested with varying success [141]. This new biopesticide is highly pathogenic than the wild-type baculovirus as it combines the advantages of the virus and the bacteria toxin.

However, the use of biotechnology raises some questions regarding the potential impact of those GMOs or plants to human, animal and the environment and other non-target species. This has presented a major hurdle to research and field testing and the introduction of these recombinant BCAs to users. Fortunately, the use of genetically engineered microbial pathogen products for control is increasingly being accepted by the society, and commercial production is gradually gaining grounds. In the near future, genetically engineered microbial BCAs will soon be the most common biocontrol products available in the market to circumvent the problem of growing resistance to chemical pesticides and the threats posed to public health and the environment by the chemical pesticides.

10.2. Nanotechnology

Nanotechnology is another field that holds wide applicability in biological control in the near future. Nanotechnology for control has been applied mostly in the control of agricultural pests. Its application in the control of agriculture pest offers some advantages over traditional methods by providing green and highly efficient alternatives for the management of insect pests without harming nature [142]. Nanoparticles are known to be effective against plant pathogens, insects and pests. Hence, nanoparticles can be used in the preparation of new formulations like pesticides, insecticides and insect repellents [143–146]. Nanomaterials come in many forms—porous hollow silica nanoparticles (PHSNs) loaded with validamycin (pesticide) [147], nano-silica prepared from silica, polyethylene glycol-coated nanoparticles loaded with garlic essential oil, silver nanoparticles synthesized from various plant extracts and so on.

One of the most studied nanomaterials for the control of agricultural pests is nano-silica. Nano-silica formulated as nano-pesticide can effectively be used in the control of insect pests. The mechanism of control of insect pests using nano-silica is based on the fact that insect pests use a variety of cuticular lipids to protect their water barrier and thereby prevent death from desiccation. But nano-silica gets absorbed into the cuticular lipids by physiosorption and thereby causes death of insects purely by physical means when applied on leaves and stem surfaces [142]. It has also been shown that in addition to agricultural insect pests, surface-charged modified hydrophobic nano-silica (~3–5 nm) could be successfully used to control animal ectoparasites of veterinary importance [148].

Silver nanoparticles (AgNPs) have been synthesized using various plant extracts as reducing and stabilizing agents. These AgNPs have been tested and shown to be of higher toxicity against the mosquito vectors of parasites of medical and veterinary importance. For example, an AgNP synthesized using extracts of *Artemisia vulgaris* leaves has been observed to be highly toxic to *Aedes aegypti* larval instars (I–IV) and pupae, with LC_{50} ranging from 4.4 (for the first instar) to 13.1 ppm (for the pupae) and was also observed to increase the predatory efficiency of the Asian bullfrog tadpole, *Hoplobatrachus tigerinus*, a natural predator on mosquito larvae [149]. AgNP synthesized using other plant extracts has also demonstrated similar or higher efficacy: AgNP synthesized using the aqueous leaf extract of the seaweed, *Hypnea musciformis*, has shown larvicidal and pupicidal toxicity against *Aedes aegypti* and the cabbage pest, *Plutella xylostella* [150]; AgNP synthesized using *Nicondra physalodes* has shown larvicidal toxicity against *Anopheles stephensi*, *Aedes aegypti* and *Culex quinquefasciatus*, with the maximum efficacy detected against *An. Stephensi* (LC_{50} = 12.39 μg/ml) [151] and AgNPs synthesized using *Zornia diphylla* have shown higher toxicity against *Anopheles subpictus*, *Aedes albopictus* and *Culex tritaniorhynchus* with LC_{50} values of 12.53, 13.42 and 14.61 μg/ml, respectively [152]. AgNPs are promising for the development of eco-friendly larvicides against mosquito vectors, with negligible effect against non-target species.

Yang et al. [153] have demonstrated that the efficacy of the insecticidal activity of polytherlene glycol-coated nanoparticles loaded with garlic essential oil against adult red flour beetle (*Tribolium castaneum*) insects found in store products was as high as 80%. In another example, Sabbour [154] tested two nanomaterials Aluminium oxide (Al_2O_3) and Titanium dioxide (TiO_2) against rice weevil *Sitophilus oryzae* and observed that under laboratory conditions, the mortality increased significantly to 50.6 ± 3.6 as compared to 3.0 ± 3.4 for the control and under store condition, the mortality increased significantly to 67.3 ± 1.4 after 45 days of storage as compared to 3.8 ± 3.8 in the control. Furthermore, accumulative mortality (%) of *S. oryzae* beetles increased gradually by increasing the period of exposure.

Nanotechnology has also been applied on BCAs. Nanoparticles as various formulations of essential oils, silica gels, powders and so on applied on BCAs have been shown to increase the effectiveness of BCAs in neutralizing some agricultural pests. For example, Sabbour [155] showed that in the laboratory, the nano-entomopathogenic fungi, nano-*Beauveria bassiana* and nano-*Metarhizium anisopliae*, formulated using dust carriers, were more effective in the killing of the insect pest of stored rice *Sitophilus oryzae* (L.) compared to control. The LC_{50} obtained were 45×10^4 and 57×10^4 conidia/ml for nano-*B. bassiana* and nano-*M. anisopliae*, respectively, lower than 66×10^4 and 77×10^4 conidia/ml for *B. bassiana* and *M. anisopliae*, respectively. There was a significant reduction of the number eggs laid/female as well as the number of emerged adults in stored bags that were treated with nano-entomopathogenic fungi nano-*B. bassiana* and nano-*M. anisopliae* compared to control. On the other hand, some BCAs are capable of producing nanoparticles. For example, there are a large volume of research reports that suggest that actinobacteria are capable of producing metal oxide nanoparticles. These can be exploited in the green synthesis of nanomaterials and utilized in biological systems [156]. Sabbour [157] tested the efficacy of nano-extracted destruxin from *Metarhizium anisopliae* against the Indian meal moth *Plodia interpunctella* (which is one of the most serious stored grain pest worldwide), and the LC_{50} obtained was 77 × 10^4 for nano-destruxin compared to 103 × 10^4 for destruxin. Under laboratory conditions, the number of eggs laid/female significantly decreased to 17.4 ± 3.8 and 10.6 ± 9.5 eggs/female after treatment with destruxin and nano-destruxin as compared to 99.9 ± 7.9 eggs/female for the control after 120 days. And under store conditions, the number of eggs laid/female decreased significantly to 13.1 ± 9.2 after nano-destruxin treatments after 120 days. Furthermore, the emerged adults decreased to 2% after nano-destruxin treatments after 120 days [157].

Nanotechnology also has promising applications in nanoparticle-mediated gene (DNA) transfer. It can be used to deliver DNA and other desired chemicals into plant tissue for protection of host plants against insect pests [158]. There is evidence that nanotechnology will revolutionize agriculture including pest management in the near future [159].

10.3. Microencapsulation

Microencapsulation is another new field that holds promise in biological control. Microencapsulation is a process in which active substances are coated by extremely small capsules [160]. Microencapsulation has numerous applications in areas such as the pharmaceutical, agricultural, medical and food industries, being widely used in the encapsulation of essential oils, colourings, flavourings, sweeteners and microorganisms, among others [161]. Microencapsulation in biological control can be used for the enhancement of the activity of BCAs in biocontrol, especially pathogens. The coating may impact stability, protection from UV radiation and/or other environmental conditions, enhance the attractiveness of the pesticide to the pest and/or serve to separate two different biologically incompatible pesticides within a mixture. For example, *Bacillus subtilis* has been widely used as a BCA in agriculture but their short shelf life limits their use. In a study in which *Bacillus subtilis* was microencapsulated using maltodextrin, it was observed that the mean survival rate of *B. subtilis* was more than 90%, when spray drying was performed at 145°C, with a feed flow rate of 550 mL h−1 and a spray pressure of 0.15 MPa. The shelf life was also significantly prolonged compared to wettable powders. Moreover, the biocontrol efficacy of the *B. subtilis* microcapsule reached 79.91% when a dosage of 300 g hm^{-2} was used; the microcapsule showed higher control efficacy than thiram wettable powder against the plant pathogenic fungus *Rhizoctonia solani* in tomato under field conditions [162]. This approach can be applied to other BCAs, especially pathogenic microorganisms, to enhance their effectiveness.

11. Conclusion

To date, many strategies have been used in the control of parasites including the use of chemicals. The chemical methods are limited in their application, partly as a result of the rising

http://dx.doi.org/10.5772/68012

resistance, environmental and health risks and the potential effect to non-target organisms. In addition to the previously mentioned biological control agents, parasites could also be controlled naturally through botanicals [163–167], photosensitizers [168, 169], symbiotic [170], organic [171] and short-chain fatty acids [172]. Biological control approaches hold promise as the most suitable alternative to the chemical pesticides and are now a core component of IPM. A good number of promising BCAs including predators, parasites (parasitoids) and pathogens (fungi, bacteria, viruses and virus-like particles, protozoa and nematodes) have been identified and proven to be efficacious against many parasites of medical, veterinary and agricultural importance, as highlighted in the chapter [25, 49, 85]. In the past, biological control has been applied successfully to control parasites especially in the agricultural sector [120]. However, there are still many challenges in the implementation of biological control strategies including their potential effects on native biodiversity [133–135], the unwillingness to ditch the chemical methods for BCAs by farmers [129] and challenges in the production and distribution of the BCAs [136]. With the recent advances in biotechnology and the application of most recent technologies such as nanotechnology [145] and microencapsulation [162], there are many opportunities for the continued use and expanded role of natural enemies in biological control; newer BCAs are being identified and older ones are being genetically engineered to make them more efficacious in their antagonism of parasites. There is, therefore, optimism that in the future, biological control will develop to overcome many of the challenges, and BCAs will become the mainstay for the control of parasites.

Abbreviations

IPM	Integrated pest management
BCA	Biological control agent
USDA	The US Department of Agriculture
Bt	*Bacillus thuringiensis*
BV	Baculovirus
GMO	Genetically modified organism
PHSNs	Porous hollow silica nanoparticles
DNA	Deoxyribonucleic acid
AgNPs	Silver nanoparticles
BW	Birth weight

Author details

Tebit Emmanuel Kwenti

Address all correspondence to: kwentitebit@yahoo.com

Faculty of Health Sciences, University of Buea, Buea, Cameroon

References

[1] Alston DG. General Concepts of Biological Control. Utah State University Extension and Utah Plant Pest Diagnostic Laboratory. Logan, Utah, US. IPM-015-11. 2011.

[2] DeBach P. Biological Control of Insect Pests and Weeds. London, UK: Chapman and Hall; 1964. p. 844

[3] Dreistadt SH. Biological control and natural enemies of invertebrates: Integrated pest management for home gardeners and landscape professionals. Statewide Integrated Pest Management Program. University of California, Davis, California, US; 2014; Pest Notes Publication 74140:1-6

[4] Du Roi IPM. Integrated Pest Management: The Concept [Internet]. Available from: http://www.duroibugs.co.za/about.htm [Accessed: 17 October 2016]

[5] van den Bosch R, Messenger PS, Gutierrez AP. The history and development of biological control. In: An Introduction to Biological Control. US: Springer; 1982. pp. 21-36. DOI: 10.1007/978-1-4757-9162-4_3

[6] Greathead DJ. Benefits and risks of classical biocontrol. In: Hokkanen HM, Lynch JM, editors. Biological Control: Benefits and Risks. Cambridge, UK: Cambridge University Press; 1995. pp. 53-63

[7] Lockwood JA. Environmental issues involved in biological control of rangeland grasshoppers (Orthoptera: Acrididae) with exotic agents. Environmental Entomology. 1993;**22**:503-518

[8] Lockwood JA. Nontarget effects of biological control: What are we trying to miss? In: Follett PA, Duan JJ, editors. Nontarget Effects of Biological Control. Boston, Massachusetts: Kluwer Academic Publishers; 2000. pp. 15-30

[9] McEvoy PB, Coombs EM. Why things bite back: Unintended consequences of biological weed control. In: Follett PA, Duan JJ, editors. Nontarget Effects of Biological Control. Boston, Massachusetts: Kluwer Academic Publishers; 2000. pp. 167-194

[10] Wilkinson PR. A preliminary note on predation on free-living engorged female rocky mountainwood ticks. Journal of Medical Entomology. 1970;**7**:493-496

[11] Wilkinson PR. Factors affecting the distribution and abundance of the cattle tick in Australia: Observations and hypotheses. Acarologia. 1970;**12**:492-507

[12] Mwangi EN, Dipeolu OO, Newson RM, Kaaya GP, Hassan SM. Predators, parasitoids and pathogens of ticks: A review. Biocontrol Science and Technology. 1991;**1**:147-156

[13] Krivolutsky DA. Eradication of larvae and nymphs of the tick Ixodes persulcatus by predators. In: Proceedings of the Conference on Ticks Encephalitis Hemorrhagic Fever viruses; December 10-13, 1963; Omsk, Izd. Minzdrav RSFSR. Omsk NII POI, Omsk: Otd. San. epidemiol. kontr.; 1963. p. 187-188

[14] Jackson RR, Pollard SD. Predatory behavior of jumping spiders. Annual Review of Entomology. 1996;**41**:287-308

[15] Riechert SE, Bishop L. Prey control by an assemblage of generalist predators: Spiders in garden test systems. Ecology. 1990;**71**:441-1450

[16] Sokolow SH, Lafferty KD, Kuris AM. Regulation of laboratory populations of snails (*Biomphalaria* and *Bulinus* spp.) by river prawns, *Macrobrachium* spp. (Decapoda, Palaemonidae): Implications for control of schistosomiasis. Acta Tropica. 2014;**132**:64-74

[17] Hernández MC, Walsh GC. Insect herbivores associated with Ludwigia species, Oligospermum section, in their Argentine distribution. Journal of Insect Science. 2014;**14**(1):201. DOI: 10.1093/jisesa/ieu063

[18] Mahr SER, Cloyd RA, Mahr DL, Sadof CS. Biological control of insects and other pests of greenhouse crops. University of Wisconsin Cooperative Extension. Lake street, Madison, Wisconsin, US. North Central Regional Publication **581**; 2001

[19] Lysek H. Effect of certain soil organisms on the eggs of parasitic roundworms. Nature. 1963;**199**:925

[20] Safaa, Abo-Taka M, Heikal HM, Abd El-Raheem AM. Macrochelid mite, *Macrocheles muscaedomesticae* (Acarina: Macrochelidae) as a biological control agent against house fly, *Musca domestica* (Diptera: Muscidae) in Egypt. International Journal of Zoological Research. 2014;**10**:30-36

[21] Pirali-Kheirabadi K. Biological control of parasites. In: Shah MM, editor. Parasitology. Rijeka, Croatia: Intech; 2012. p. 54-66.

[22] Oluwafemi R. Biological Control of Tsetse Fly Project (BICOT) in Lafia local government area of Nasarawa State, Nigeria, 1984-2000. The Internet Journal of Veterinary Medicine. 2008;**7**(1):1-5

[23] Jemal A, Hugh-Jones M. A review of the red imported fire ant (*Solenopsis invicta* Buren) and its impacts on plant, animal, and human health. Preventive Veterinary Medicine. 1993;**17**:19-32

[24] Egyptian Myths. Ancient Egypt: The Mythology [Internet]. 2014. Available from: http://www.egyptianmyths.net/scarab.htm [Accessed: 26 November 2016]

[25] Bornemissza GF. Insectary studies on the control of dung breeding flies by the activity of the dung beetle, *Onthophagus gazelle* F. (Coleoptera: Scarabaeidae). Australian Journal of Entomology. 1970;**9**(1):31-41

[26] Bornemissza GF. The Australian dung beetle project, 1965-1975. Australian Meat Research Committee Reviews. 1976;**30**:1-30

[27] Acorn J. Ladybugs of Alberta: Finding the Spots and Connecting the Dots. Edmonton, Alberta, Canada: University of Alberta; 2007. p. 15

[28] Canyon DV, Hii JL. The gecko: An environmentally friendly biological agent for mosquito control. Medical and Veterinary Entomology. 1997;**11**(4):319-323

[29] Sankaralingam A, Venkatesan P. Larvicidal properties of water bug *Diplonychus indicus* Venkatesan & Rao and its use in mosquito control.Indian Journal of Experimental Biology. 1989;**27**(2):174-176

[30] Mwangi EN, Newson RM, Kaaya GP. Predation of free-living engorged female *Rhipicephalus appendiculatus*. Experimental and Applied Acarology. 1991;**12**:153-162

[31] Walker K. A review of control methods for African malaria vectors: Activity Report 108 [thesis]. Washington DC, USA: Agency for International Development; 2002. p. 54. Available from: http://www.ehproject.org/PDF/Activity_Reports/AR108MalRevArch.pdf

[32] Menon PKB, Rajagopalan PK. Control of mosquito breeding in wells by using *Gambusia affinis* and *Aplocheilus blocki* in Pondicherry town. Indian Journal of Medical Research. 1978;**68**:927-933

[33] Kamareddine L. The biological control of the malaria vector. Toxins. 2012;**4**:748-767. DOI: 10.3390/toxins4090748

[34] World Health Organization. Manual on Environmental Management for Mosquito Control with Special Emphasis on Malaria Vectors. WHO Offset Publication No. 66. Geneva, Switzerland: World Health Organization; 1982. pp. 1-276

[35] Hung NM, Duc NV, Stauffer JR, Madsen H. Use of black carp (*Mylopharyngodon piceus*) in biological control of intermediate host snails of fish-borne zoonotic trematodes in nursery ponds in the Red River Delta, Vietnam. Parasites & Vectors. 2013;**6**:142. DOI: 10.1186/1756-3305-6-142

[36] Isenhart FR, DeSante DF. Observations of scrub jays cleaning ectoparasites from black-tailed deer. Condor. 1985;**87**:145-147

[37] Hassan SM, Dipeolu OO, Amoo AO, Odhiambo TR. Predation on livestock ticks by chickens. Veterinary Parasitology. 1991;**38**(2-3):199-204

[38] Short NJ, Norval RAI. Tick predation by shrews in Zimbabwe. Journal of Parasitology. 1982;**68**:1052

[39] Samish M. Pathogens and predators of ticks and their potential in biological control. Annual Review of Entomology. 1999;**44**:159-182

[40] Hoddle MS, Van Driesche RG, Sanderson JP. Biology and use of the whitefly parasitoid *Encarsia formosa*. Annual Review of Entomology. 1998;**43**:645-669

[41] Smith SM. Biological control with Trichogramma: Advances, successes, and potential of their use. Annual Review of Entomology. 1996;**41**:375-406. DOI: 10.1146/annurev.en.41.010196.002111

[42] Wajnberg E, Hassan SA. Biological Control with Egg Parasitoids. Wallingford, Oxfordshire, England: CABI Publishing; 1994

[43] Gullan PJ, Cranston PS. The Insects: An Outline of Entomology. 4th ed. Oxford, U.K.: Wiley-Blackwell; 2010

[44] Jian L, Dakshina RS. Parasitoids of Dipteran leafminers, Diglyphus spp. (Insecta: Hymenoptera: Eulophidae). EENY-484 (IN877). Entomology and Nematology Department, Florida Cooperative Extension Service, Institute of Food and Agricultural Sciences, University of Florida, Gainesville, Florida, US; 2010

[45] McCoy CW, Samson RA, Boucias DG. Entomogenous fungi. In: Ignoffo CM, editor. CRC Handbook of Natural Pesticides: Microbial Insecticides, Part A; Entomogenous Protozoa and Fungi. Florida, USA: CRCPress; 1988. pp. 151-236

[46] Khater HF. Ecosmart biorational insecticides: Alternative insect control strategies. In: Perveen F, editor. Insecticides—Advances in Integrated Pest Management. Rijeka, Croatia: InTech; 2012. pp. 18-61

[47] Leger RJS. Studies on adaptations of *Metarhizium anisopliae* to life in the soil. Journal of Invertebrate Pathology. 2008;**96**:271-276

[48] Quesada-Moraga E, Ruiz-Garcia A, Santiago-Alvarez C. Laboratory evaluation of entomopathogenic fungi *Beauveria bassiana* and *Metarhizium anisopliae* against puparia and adults of *Ceratitis capitata* (Diptera: Tephritidae). Journal of Economic Entomology. 2006;**99**:1955-1966

[49] Ebrahim AY. Biological control of vector born protozoan parasites of veterinary importance. Applied Scientific Reports. 2015;**10**(3):122-127. DOI: 10.15192/PSCP.ASR.2015.10.3.122127

[50] Knols BGJ, Bukhari T, Farenhorst M. Entomopathogenic fungi as the next-generation control agents against malaria mosquitoes. Future Microbiology. 2010;**5**(3):339-341

[51] Scholte EJ, Ng'habi K, Kihonda J, Takken W, Paaijmans K, Abdulla S, Killeen GF. An entomopathogenic fungus for control of adult African malaria mosquitoes. Science. 2005;**308**:1641-1642

[52] Okumu FO, Madumla EP, John AN, Lwetoijera DW, Sumaye RD. Attracting, trapping, and killing disease-transmitting mosquitoes using odor-baited stations—the Ifakara odor-baited stations. Parasites & Vectors. 2010;**3**:1-10

[53] Khater HF. Biocontrol of some insects [thesis]. Benha Branch, Egypt: Zagazig University; 2003

[54] Ghannam I, Barakat R, Al-Masri M. Biological control of Egyptian broomrape (*Orobanche aegyptiaca*) using *Fusarium* spp. Phytopathologia Mediterranea. 2007;**46**:177-184

[55] Sur B, Bihari V, Sharma A, Joshi AK. Studies on physiology, zoospore morphology and entomopathogenic potential of the aquatic oomycete: *Coelomomyces giganteum*. Mycopathologia. 2001;**154**:51-54

[56] Jensen AB, Thomsen L, Eilenberg J. Intraspecific variation and host specificity of *Entomophthora muscae* sensu stricto isolates revealed by random amplified polymorphic DNA, universal primed PCR, PCR-restriction fragment length polymorphism, and conidial morphology. Journal of Invertebrate Pathology. 2001;**78**(4):251-259

[57] Sallam NMA, Abo-Elyousr KAM, Hassan MAE. Evaluation of *Trichoderma Species* as biocontrol agents for damping-off and wilt diseases of *Phaseolus vulgaris* L. and efficacy of suggested formula. Egypt Journal of Phytopathology. 2008;**36**(1-2):81-93

[58] Santos CP, Charles TP. Effetio da aplicacao de conidios de *Drechmeria coniospora* em cultivos de fezes contendo ovos de *Haemonchus contortus* [Effect of an endo-parasitic fun-

gus, *Drechmeria coniospora,* in faecal cultures containing eggs of *Haemonchus contortus*]. Arquivo Brasileiro de Medicina Veterinária e Zootecnia. 1995;**47**:123-128

[59] Charles TP, Rouque MVC, Santos CD. Reduction of *Haemonchus contortus* infective larvae by *Harposporium anguillulae* in sheep faecal cultures. International Journal for Parasitology. 1996;**26**:509-510

[60] Gronvold J, Korsholm H, Wolstrup J, Nansen P, Henriksen SA. Laboratory experiments to evaluate the ability of *Arthobotrys oligospora* to destroy infective larvae of *Cooperia species* and to investigate the effect of physical factors on the growth of the fungus. Journal of Helminthology. 1985;**59**:119-126

[61] Mendoza de Gives P, Crespo JF, Rodriguez DH, Prats VV, Hernandez EL, Fernandez GEO. Biological control of *Haemonchus contortus* infective larvae in ovine faeces by administering an oral suspension of *Duddingtonia flagrans* chlamydospores to sheep. Journal of Helminthology. 1998;**72**:343-347

[62] Vilela VLR, Feitosa TF, Bragab FR, de Araújo JV, de Oliveira Souto DV, da Silva Santos HE, da Silva GLL, Athayde ACR. Biological control of goat gastrointestinal helminthiasis by *Duddingtonia flagrans* in a semi-arid region of the Northeastern Brazil. Veterinary Parasitology. 2012;**188**:127-133. DOI: 10.1016/j.vetpar.2012.02.018

[63] Larsen M. Biological control of nematode parasites in sheep. Journal of Animal Science. 2006;**84**:E133-E139

[64] Araujo JV, Gomes APS, Guimaraes MP. Biological control of bovine gastrointestinal nematode parasites in Southeastern Brazil by the nematode-trapping fungus *Arthrobotrys robusta*. Revista Brasileira de Parasitologia Veterinária. 1998;**7**(2):117-122

[65] De S, Sanyal PK. Biological control of helminth parasites by predatory fungi. VetScan. 2009;**4**(1): 387-395

[66] Tribe HT. Pathology of cystnematodes. Biological Reviews of the Cambridge Philosophical Society. 1977;**52**:447-508

[67] Lysek H, krajci D. Penetration of ovicidal fungus *Verticillium chlamydosporium* through the *Ascaris lumbricoides* egg-shells. Folia Parasitologica. 1987;**34**:57-60

[68] Lysek H, Sterba J. Colonization of *Ascaris lumbricoides* eggs by the fungus *Verticillium chlamydosporium* Goddard. Folia Parasitologica. 1991;**38**:255-259

[69] Kunert J. On the mechanism of penetration of ovicidal fungi through egg shells of parasitic nematodes, decomposition of chitinous and ascaroside layers. Folia Parasitologica. 1992;**39**:61-66

[70] Ranjbar-Bahadori SH, Razzaghi-Abyaneh M, Bayat M, Eslami A, Pirali-Kheirabadi KH, Shams-Ghahfarokhi M, Lotfollahzadeh S. Studies on the effect of temperature, incubation time and in vivo gut passage on survival and nematophagous activity *Arthrobotrys oligospora var. oligospora* and *A. cladodes var. macroides*. Global Veterinaria. 2010;**4**:112-117

[71] Ravensberg WJ. Biological control of pests: Current trends and future prospects. In: Brighton Crop Protection Conference-Pest and Diseases. Thornton Heath, UK: British Crop Protection Council; 1994. pp. 591-600

[72] Hassanain MA, el Garhy MF, Abdel-Ghaffar FA, el-Sharaby A, Abdel Megeed KN. Biological control studies of soft and hard ticks in Egypt. I. The effect of *Bacillus thuringiensis* varieties on soft and hard ticks (ixodidae). Parasitology Research. 1997;**83**(3):209-213

[73] Robert LL, Perich MJ, Schlein Y. Phlebotomine sand fly control using bait-fed adults to carry the larvicide *Bacillus sphaericus* to the larval habitat. Journal of the American Mosquito Control Association. 1997;**13**:140-144

[74] Duval D, Galinier R, Mouahid G, Toulza E, Allienne JF, Portela J, Calvayrac C, Rognon A, Arancibia N, Mitta G, Théron A, Gourbal B. A novel bacterial pathogen of *Biomphalaria glabrata*: A potential weapon for schistosomiasis control? PLoS Neglected Tropical Diseases. 2015;**9**(2):e0003489. DOI: 10.1371/journal.pntd.0003489

[75] El-Gammal EW, Shalaby HA, Ashry HM, El-Diwany AI. In vitro action of *Streptomyces griseolus* proteases as bio-control on *Fasciola gigantica* eggs. Journal of Bacteriology & Parasitology. 2014;**5**:1000192. DOI: 10.4172/2155-9597.1000192

[76] Bekal S, Borneman J, Springer MS, Giblin-Davis RM, Becker JO. Phenotypic and molecular analysis of a Pasteuria strain parasitic to the sting nematode. Journal of Nematology. 2001;**33**:110-115

[77] Oliveira EJ, Rabinovitch L, Monnerat RG, Passos LKJ, Zahner V. Molecular characterization of *Brevibacillus laterosporus* and its potential use in biological control. Applied and Environmental Microbiology. 2004;**70**:6657-6664

[78] Huang XW, Tian BY, Niu QH, Yang JK, Zhang LM, Zhang KQ. An extracellular protease from *Brevibacillus laterosporus* G4 without parasporal crystal can serve as a pathogenic factor in infection of nematodes. Research in Microbiology. 2005;**156**:719-727

[79] Rovira AD, Sands DC. Fluorescent pseudomonas—a residual component in the soil microflora. Journal of Applied Microbiology. 1977;**34**:253-259

[80] Krebs B, Hoeding B, Kuebart S, Workie MA, Junge H, Schmiedeknecht G, Grosch R, Bochow H, Hevesi M. Use of *Bacillus subtilis* as biocontrol agent. I. Activities and characterization of *Bacillus subtilis* strains. Zeitschrift für Pflanzenkrankheiten und Pflanzenschutz. 1998;**105**:181-197

[81] Feitelson JS, Payne J, Kim L. *Bacillus thuringiensis*: Insects and beyond. Bio/Technology. 1992;**10**:271-275. DOI: 10.1038/nbt0392-271

[82] Tian B, Yang J, Zhang K-Q. Bacteria used in the biological control of plant-parasitic nematodes: Populations, mechanisms of action, and future prospects. FEMS Microbiology Ecology. 2007;**61**:197-213

[83] Hsiao C, Hsiao TH. Rickettsia as the cause of cytoplasmic incompatibility in the alfalfa weevil, *Hypera postica*. Journal of Invertebrate Pathology. 1985;**45**:244-246

[84] Raoult D, Roux V. Rickettsioses as paradigms of newer emerging infectious diseases. Clinical Microbiology Reviews. 1997;**10**:694-719

[85] Sidorov VE. Some features of *Coxiella burnetii* interaction with argasid ticks (experimental morphological study). In: Grochovskaia IM, Melejaeva MA, editors. Razvitie Parazitologicheskoi Nauki v Turkmenistane. Ashchabad: Yilim; 1979. pp. 112-128

[86] Lacey LA, Kaya HK. Field Manual of Techniques in Invertebrate Pathology. 2nd ed. Dordrecht, The Netherlands: Springer; 2007

[87] Szewczyk B, Rabalski L, Krol E, Sihler W, Lobo de Souza M. Baculovirus biopesticides—a safe alternative to chemical protection of plants. Journal of Biopesticides. 2009;**2**(2): 209-216

[88] Szewczyk B, Lobo de Souza M, Batista de Castro ME, Moscardi ML, Moscardi F. Baculovirus biopesticides. In: Stoytcheva M, editor. Pesticides—Formulations, Effects, Fate. Rijeka, Croatia: InTech; 2011. pp. 25-36

[89] Jehle JA, Blissard GW, Bonning BC, Cory JS, Herniou EA, Rohrmann GF, Theilmann DA, Thiem SA, Vlak JM. On the classification and nomenclature of baculoviruses: A proposal for revision. Archives of Virology. 2006;**151**:1257-1266

[90] Hunter WB, Katsar CS, Chaparro J. Molecular analysis of capsid protein of *Homalodisca coagulata* virus-1, a new leafhopper-infecting virus from the glassy-winged sharpshooter, *Homalodisca coagulata*. Journal of Insect Science. 2006;**6**:28

[91] Hunnicutt LE, Hunter WB, Cave RD, Powell CA, Mozoruk JJ. Genome sequence and molecular characterization of *Homalodisca coagulata* virus-1, a novel virus discovered in the glassy-winged sharpshooter (Hemiptera: Cicadellidae). Virology. 2006;**350**(1):67-78

[92] Olson DM, Dinerstein E, Powell GVN, Wikramanayake ED. Conservation biology for the biodiversity crisis. Conservation Biology. 2002;**16**(1):1-3. DOI: 10.1046/j.1523-1739.2002.01612.x

[93] Smart GC Jr. Entomopathogenic nematodes for the biological control of insects. Journal of Nematology. 1995;**27**(4S):529-534

[94] Krafsur ES, Moon RD. Bionomics of the face fly, *Musca autumnalis*. Annual Review of Entomology. 1997;**42**:503-523

[95] Martin WRJ. Using entomopathogenic nematodes to control insects during stand establishment. Horticultural Science. 1997;**32**:196-200

[96] Kaya HK, Koppenhöfer AM. Biology and ecology of insecticidal nematodes. In: Polavarapu S, editor. Workshop Proceedings: Optimal Use of Insecticidal Nematodes in Pest Management. New Brunswick, NJ, United States: Rutgers University; 1991. pp. 1-8

[97] Geden CJ. Evaluation of *Paraiotonchium muscadomesticae* (Nematoda: Tylenchida: Iotonchiidae), a potential biological control agent of the housefly (Diptera: Muscidae). Biological Control. 1997;**10**:42-47

[98] Henderson G, Manweiler SA, Lawrence WJ, Templeman RJ, Foil LD. The effects of *Steinernema carpocapsae* (Weiser) application to different life stages on adult emergence of the cat flea *Ctenocephalides felis* (Bouche). Veterinary Dermatology. 1995;**6**:159-163

[99] Zhioua E, Lebrun RA, Ginsberg HS, Aeschlimann A. Pathogenicity of *Steinernema carpocapsae* and *S. glaseri* (Nematoda: Steinernematidae) to *Ixodes scapularis* (Acari: Ixodidae). Journal of Medical Entomology. 1995;**32**:900-905

[100] Samish M, Glazer I, Alekseev EA. The susceptibility of the development stages of ticks (Ixodidae) to entomopathogenic nematodes. In: Rodger M, Horn DJ, Needham GR, Welbourn WC, editors. Acarology IX. Columbus, Ohio: Ohio Biological Survey; 1996. pp. 121-123

[101] Kocan KM, Pidherney MS, Blouin EF, Claypool PL, Samish M, Glazer I. Interaction of entomopathogenic nematodes (Steinernematidae) with selected species of ixodid ticks (Acari: Ixodidae). Journal of Medical Entomology. 1998;**35**(4):514-520

[102] Ibrahim MM. Population dynamics of *Chaetogaster limnaei* (Oligochaeta: Naididae) in the field populations of freshwater snails and its implications as a potential regulator of trematode larvae community. Parasitology Research. 2007;**101**(1):25-33. DOI: 10.1007/s00436-006-0436-0

[103] Gronvold J. Field experiment on the ability of earthworms (Lumbricidae) to reduce the transmission of infective larvae of *Cooperra oncopnora* (Trichostrongylidae: Nematoda). Journal of Parasitology. 1987;**73**:1133-1137

[104] Clarke GM, Gross S, Matthews M, Catling PC, Baker B, Hewitt CL, Crowther D, Saddler SR. Environmental pest species in Australia. In: Australia: State of the Environment, Second Technical Paper Series (Biodiversity). Canberra: Department of the Environment and Heritage; 2000

[105] Hoagland DB, Horst GR, Kilpatrick CW. Biogeography and population biology of the mongoose in the West Indies. In: Woods CA, editor. Biogeography of the West Indies. Gainesville, Florida, USA: Sand Hill Crane Press; 1989. pp. 611-634

[106] Simberloff D, Dayan T, Jones C, Ogura G. Character displacement and release in the small Indian mongoose, *Herpestes javanicus*. Ecology. 2000;**81**(8):2086-2099

[107] Nellis DW, Everard COR. The biology of the mongoose in the Caribbean. Studies on the Fauna of Curaçao and Other Caribbean Islands. 1983;**1**:1-162

[108] Barun A, Hanson CC, Campbell KJ, Simberloff D. A review of small Indian mongoose management and eradications on islands. In: Veitch CR, Clout MN, Towns DR, editors. Island Invasives: Eradication and Management. Gland, Switzerland: IUCN; 2011. pp. 17-25

[109] IUCN. IUCN guidelines for the prevention of biodiversity loss caused by alien invasive species. In: Fifth Meeting of the Conference of the Parties to the Convention on Biological Diversity; Species Survival Commission of IUCN; Gland, Switzerland. 2000

[110] National Research Council (U.S.). Incorporating science, economics, and sociology in developing sanitary and phytosanitary standards in international trade. In: Proceedings of a Conference; June 2000. Washington DC, US: National Academies Press; 2000. p. 97

[111] Vila-Gispert A, Alcaraz C, Garcia-Berthou E. Life-history traits of invasive fish in small Mediterranean streams. Biological Invasions. 2005;**7**:107-116

[112] Rehage JS, Barnett BK, Sih A. Foraging behaviour and invasiveness: Do invasive Gambusia exhibit higher feeding rates and broader diets than their noninvasive relatives? Ecology of Freshwater Fish. 2005;**14**:352-360

[113] Alcaraz C, Garcia-Berthou E. Life history variation of an invasive fish (*Gambusia holbrooki*) along a salinity gradient. Biological Conservations. 2007;**139**:83-92

[114] Randall JM, Tu M. Biological control. In: Weed Control Methods Handbook. Virginia, US: The Nature Conservancy; 2001. pp. 1-24

[115] Mahr DL, Whitaker P, Ridgway NM. Biological Control of Insects and Mites: An Introduction to Beneficial Natural Enemies and Their Use in Pest Management. University of Wisconsin Cooperative Extension. Lake street, Madison, Wisconsin, US; 2008; No. A3842

[116] El-Ghany TMA, editor. Entomopathogenic Fungi and their Role in Biological Control. Foster City, CA, USA: OMICS Group eBooks; 2015. p. 46. DOI: 10.4172/978-1-63278-065-2-66

[117] Singh SP. Some Success Stories in Classical Biological Control of Agricultural Pest in India [Internet]. 2004. Available from: http://www.apaari.org/wp-content/uploads/2009/05/ss_2004_02.pdf [Accessed: 30 August 2016]

[118] Cock MJW, Day RK, Hinz HL, Pollard KM, Thomas SE, Williams FE, Witt ABR, Shaw RH. The impacts of some classical biological control successes. CAB Reviews. 2015;**10**(42):1-58

[119] Takiya DM, McKamey SH, Cavichioli RR. Validity of *Homalodisca* and of *H. vitripennis* as the name for glassywinged sharpshooter (Hemiptera: Cicadellidae: Cicadellinae). Annals of the Entomological Society of America. 2006;**99**(4):648-655

[120] Sorensen JT, Gill RJ. A range extension of *Homalodisca coagulata* (Say) (Hemiptera: Clypeorrhyncha: Cicadellidae) to Southern California. The Pan-Pacific Entomologist. 1996;**72**(3):160-161

[121] University of California, Riverside. Biological Control of the Glassy-winged Sharpshooter [Internet]. 2013. Available from: http://biocontrol.ucr.edu/irvin/gwssbiocontrol.html [Accessed: 19 October 2016]

[122] Triapitsyn SV, Phillips PA. First record of *Gonatocerus triguttatus* (Hymenoptera: Mymaridae) from eggs of *Homalodisca coagulata* (Homoptera: Cicadellidae) with notes on the distribution of the host. Florida Entomologist. 2000;**83**(2):200-203

[123] Triapitsyn SV, Logarzo GA, De León JH, Virla EG. A new Gonatocerus (Hymenoptera: Mymaridae) from Argentina, with taxonomic notes and molecular data on the *G. tuberculifemur* species complex. Zootaxa. 2008;**1949**:1-29

[124] Irvin NA, Hoddle MS. Comparative assessments of *Gonatocerus ashmeadi* and the "new association" parasitoid *Gonatocerus tuberculifemur* (Hymenoptera: Mymaridae) as biological control agents of *Homalodisca vitripennis* (Hemiptera: Cicadellidae). Biological Control. 2010;**55**(3):186-196

[125] Cheou D. Incursion of glassy-winged sharpshooter Homalodisca coagulata in French Polynesia. International Plant Protection Convention. Plant Protection Service Pest Alert No.24; 2002

[126] Hoover W. New Invader may Threaten Crops. Honolulu: The Honolulu Advertiser; 14 May 2004

[127] Hoddle MS, Grandgirard J, Petit J, Roderick GK, Davies N. Glassy-winged sharpshooter Ko'ed—first round—in French Polynesia. Biocontrol News and Information. 2006;**27**(3):47N-62N

[128] Szewczyk B, Hoyos-Carvajal L, Paluszek M, Skrzecz I, Lobo de Souza M. Baculoviruses—re-emerging biopesticides. Biotechnology Advances. 2006;**24**(2):143-160. DOI: 10.1016/j.biotechadv.2005.09.001

[129] Sun X, Peng H. Recent advances in biological control of pest insects by using viruses in China. Virologica Sinica. 2007;**22**:158-162

[130] Follett PA, Duan JJ. Nontarget Effects of Biological Control. Norwell, MA: Kluwer Academic Publishers; 2000. p. 316

[131] Bigler F, Babendreier D, Kuhlmann U, editors. Environmental Impact of Invertebrates for Biological Control of Arthropods: Methods and Risk Assessment. Wallingford: CABI Publishing; 2006

[132] van Lenteren JC, Bale JS, Bigler F, Hokkanen HMT, Loomans AJM. Assessing risks of releasing exotic biological control agents of arthropod pests. Annual Review of Entomology. 2006;**51**:609-634

[133] Nicot PC, Blum B, Köhl J, Ruocco M. Conclusions and perspectives for future research-and-development projects on biological control of plant pests and diseases. Classical and augmentative biological control against diseases and pests: critical status analysis and review of factors. 2011;**45**:68

[134] Heong KL, Escalada MM. Changing rice farmers' pest management practices through participation in a small-scale experiment. International Journal of Pest Management. 1998;**44**:191-197

[135] Thacker JRM. An Introduction to Arthropod Pest Control. Cambridge, England: Cambridge University Press; 2002

[136] Sagoff M. Third-generation biotechnology: A first look. Issues in Science and Technology. 2008;**25**(1): 70-74

[137] Federici BA. Recombinant bacterial larvicides for control of important mosquito vectors of disease. In: Atkinson PW, editor. Vector Biology, Ecology and Control. US: Springer; 2010. pp. 163-176

[138] Wang C, St. Leger RJ. A scorpion neurotoxin increases the potency of a fungal insecticide. Nature Biotech. 2007;**25**:1455-1456

[139] Bonning BC. Insect viruses: Biotechnological applications. In: Bonning BC, editor. Advances in Virus Research. New York: Academic Press; 2006. p. 68

[140] Chang JH, Choi JY, Jin BR, Roh JY, Olszewski JA, Seo SJ, O'Reilly DR, Je YH. An improved baculovirus insecticide producing occlusion bodies that contain *Bacillus thuringiensis* insect toxin. Journal of Invertebrate Pathology. 2003;**84**(1):30-37

[141] El-Menofy W, Osman G, Assaeedi A, Salama M. A novel recombinant baculovirus overexpressing a *Bacillus thuringiensis* Cry1Ab toxin enhances insecticidal activity. Biological Procedures Online. 2014;**16**:7. DOI: 10.1186/1480-9222-16-7

[142] Rai M, Ingle A. Role of nanotechnology in agriculture with special reference to management of insect pests. Applied Microbiology and Biotechnology. 2012;**94**:287

[143] Barik TK, Sahu B, Swain V. Nano-silica—from medicine to pest control. Parasitology Research. 2008;**103**:253-258

[144] Gajbhiye M, Kesharwani J, Ingle A, Gade A, Rai M. Fungus mediated synthesis of silver nanoparticles and its activity against pathogenic fungi in combination of fluconazole. Nanomedicine. 2009;**5**(4):282-286

[145] Goswami A, Roy I, Sengupta S, Debnath N. Novel applications of solid and liquid formulations of nanoparticles against insect pests and pathogens. Thin Solid Films. 2010;**519**:1252-1257

[146] Owolade OF, Ogunleti DO, Adenekan MO. Titanium dioxide affects disease development and yield of edible cowpea. The Electronic Journal of Environmental, Agricultural and Food Chemistry. 2008;**7**(50):2942-2947

[147] Liu F, Wen LX, Li ZZ, Yu W, Sun HY, Chen JF. Porous hollow silica nanoparticles as controlled delivery system for water-soluble pesticide. Materials Research Bulletin. 2006;**41**:2268-2275

[148] Ulrichs C, Mewis I, Goswami A. Crop diversification aiming nutritional security in West Bengal: Biotechnology of stinging capsules in nature's water-blooms. SATSA Annual Technical Issue. 2006;**10**:1-18

[149] Murugan K, Priyanka V, Dinesh D, Madhiyazhagan P, Panneerselvam C, Subramaniam J, Suresh U, Chandramohan B, Roni M, Nicoletti M, Alarfaj AA, Higuchi A, Munusamy MA, Khater HF, Messing RH, Benelli G. Predation by Asian bullfrog tadpoles, *Hoplobatrachus tigerinus*, against the dengue vector, *Aedes aegypti*, in an aquatic environment treated with mosquitocidal nanoparticles. Parasitology Research. 2015;**114**(10):3601-3610

[150] RoniaM, MuruganaK, PanneerselvamaC, SubramaniamaJ, NicolettibM, Madhiyazhagana P, Dinesha D, Suresha U, Khater HF, Weid H, Canalee A, Alarfaj AA, Munusamy MA, Higuchig A, Benellie G. Characterization and biotoxicity of *Hypnea musciformis*-synthesized silver nanoparticles as potential eco-friendly control tool against *Aedes aegypti* and *Plutella xylostella*. Ecotoxicology and Environmental Safety. 2015;**121**:31-38

[151] Govindarajan M, Khater HF, Panneerselvam C, Benelli G. One-pot fabrication of silver nanocrystals using *Nicandra physalodes*: A novel route for mosquito vector control with moderate toxicity on non-target water bugs. Research in Veterinary Science. 2016;**107**:95-101

[152] Govindarajana M, Rajeswary M, Muthukumaran U, Hoti SL, Khater HF, Benelli G. Single-step biosynthesis and characterization of silver nanoparticles using *Zornia diphylla* leaves: A potent eco-friendly tool against malaria and arbovirus vectors. Journal of Photochemistry and Photobiology B. 2016;**161**:482-489

[153] Yang FL, Li XG, Zhu F, Lei CL. Structural characterization of nanoparticles loaded with garlic essential oil and their insecticidal activity against *Tribolium castaneum* (Herbst) (Coleoptera: Tenebrionidae). Journal of Agricultural and Food Chemistry. 2009;**57**(21):10156-10162

[154] Sabbour MM. Entomotoxicity assay of two nanoparticle materials 1-(Al_2O_3 and TiO_2) against *Sitophilus oryzae* under laboratory and store conditions in Egypt. Journal of Applied Sciences. 2012;**1**(4):103-108

[155] Sabbour M. A novel pathogenicity of nano-*Beauveria bassiana* and *Metarihizium anisopliae* against *Sitophilus oryzae* (L.) (Coleoptera: Curculiondae) under laboratory and store conditions. International Journal of Scientific and Engineering Research. 2015;**6**(12):938-945

[156] Subramanian KS, Muniraj I, Uthandi S. Role of actinomycete-mediated nanosystem in agriculture. In: Subramaniam G, Arumugam S, Rajendran V, editors. Plant Growth Promoting Actinobacteria. Singapore: Springer; 2016. pp. 233-247. DOI: 10.1007/ 978-981-10-0707-1_15

[157] Sabbour MM. Laboratory and store efficacy of nano-extracted destruxin from *Metarhizium anisopliae* against Indian meal moth *Plodia interpunctella* (Lepidoptera-Pyralidae). Journal of Nanoscience and Nanoengineering. 2015;**1**(3):142-147

[158] Torney F. Nanoparticle mediated plant transformation. In: Emerging Technologies in Plant Science Research. Interdepartmental Plant Physiology Major. Fall Seminar Series (Phys 696). Iowa, US: Iowa State University; 2009

[159] Bhattacharyya A, Bhaumik A, Usha Rani P, Mandal S, Epidi TT. Nano-particles: A recent approach to insect pest control. African Journal of Biotechnology. 2010;**9**(24):3489-3493

[160] da Silva PT, Fries LLM, de Menezes CR, Holkem AT, Schwan CL, Wigmann EF, de Oliveira Bastos J, da Silva CB. Microencapsulation: Concepts, mechanisms, methods and some applications in food technology. Ciência Rural. 2014;**44**(7):1304-1311

[161] Azeredo HMC. Encapsulação: aplicação à tecnologia de alimentos. Alimentos e Nutrição. 2005;**16**(1):89-97

[162] Ma X, Wang X, Cheng J, Nie X, Yu X, Zhao Y, Wang W. Microencapsulation of *Bacillus subtilis* B99-2 and its biocontrol efficiency against *Rhizoctonia solani* in tomato. Biological Control. 2015;**90**:34-41

[163] Seddiek SA, Ali MM, Khater HF, El-Shorbagy MM. Anthelmintic activity of the white wormwood, *Artemisia herba-alba* against *Heterakis gallinarum* infecting turkey poults. Journal of Medicinal Plants Research. 2011;**5**(16):946-3957

[164] Seddiek SA, Khater HF, El-Shorbagy MM, Ali AM. The acaricidal efficacy of aqueous neem extract and ivermectin against *Sarcoptes scabiei var. cuniculi* in experimentally infested rabbits. Parasitology Research. 2013;**112**:2319-2330. DOI: 10.1007/s00436-013-3395-2

[165] Seddiek SA, El-Shorbagy MM, Khater HF, Ali AM. The antitrichomonal efficacy of garlic and metronidazole against *Trichomonas gallinae* infecting domestic pigeons. Parasitology Research. 2014;**113**:1319-1329. DOI: 10.1007/s00436-014-3771-6

[166] Khater HF. Bioactivities of some essential oils against the camel nasal botfly, *Cephalopina titillator*. Parasitology Research. 2014;**113**:593-605. DOI: 10.1007/s00436-013-3688-5

[167] Khatera HF, El-Shorbagy MM, Seddiek SA. Lousicidal efficacy of camphor oil, d-phenothrin, and deltamethrin against the slender pigeon louse, *Columbicola columbae*. International Journal of Veterinary Sciences and Medicine. 2014;**2**(1):7-13

[168] Khater HF, Hendawy NI. Photoxicity of Rose Bengal against the camel tick, *Hyalomma dromedarii*. International Journal of Veterinary Science. 2014;**3**(2):78-86

[169] Khater H, Hendawy N, Govindarajan M, Murugan K, Benelli G. Photosensitizers in the fight against ticks: Safranin as a novel photodynamic fluorescent acaricide to control the camel tick *Hyalomma dromedarii* (Ixodidae). Parasitology Research. 2016;**115**:3747-3758. DOI: 10.1007/s00436-016-5136-9

[170] Ali AM, Khater HF, Seddiek SA, Nada MO. Comparative efficacy of synbiotic and diclazuril on broilers experimentally infected with *Eimeria acervulina*. Assiut Veterinary Medical Journal. 2015;**61**(146):24-33

[171] Khater HF, Seddiek SA, El-Shorbagy MM, Ali AM. The acaricidal efficacy of peracetic acid and deltamethrin against the fowl tick, *Argas persicus*, infesting laying hens. Parasitology Research. 2013;**112**(1):259-269. DOI: 10.1007/s00436-012-3133-1

[172] Ali AM, Seddiek ShA, Khater HF. Effect of butyrate, clopidol and their combination on the performance of broilers infected with *Eimeria maxima*. British Poultry Science. 2014;**55**(4):474-482. DOI: http://dx.doi.org/10.1080/00071668.2014.920488

Section 3

Botanical Control

Chapter 3

Mexican Medicinal Plants as an Alternative for the Development of New Compounds Against Protozoan Parasites

Esther Ramirez-Moreno, Jacqueline Soto-Sanchez, Gildardo Rivera and Laurence A. Marchat

Additional information is available at the end of the chapter

http://dx.doi.org/10.5772/67259

Abstract

The protozoan parasites Plasmodium, Leishmania, Trypanosoma, Entamoeba histolytica, Giardia lamblia, and Trichomonas vaginalis, cause high morbidity and mortality in developed and developing countries. P. falciparum is responsible for malaria, one of the most severe infectious diseases in Africa. Hundreds of million people are affected by Trypanosoma and Leishmania that cause African and South American trypanosomiasis, and leishmaniasis. E. histolytica and G. lamblia contribute to the enormous burden of diarrheal diseases worldwide; trichomoniasis is the most common nonviral sexually transmitted disease in the world. Because of the important side effects of current treatments and the decrease in drug susceptibility, there is a renewed interest for the search of therapeutic alternatives against these pathogens. Natural products obtained from medicinal plants and their derivatives have been recognized for many years as a source of therapeutic agents. There are numerous reports about medicinal plants that are used by indigenous communities to treat gastrointestinal complaints. Importantly, phytochemical studies have allowed the identification of several secondary metabolites with anti-parasite activity. Our review revealed that Mexican medicinal plants have a great potential for the identification of new molecules with activity against protozoan parasites of medical importance worldwide and their potential use as new therapeutic compounds.

Keywords: *Plasmodium, Leishmania, Trypanosoma, Entamoeba, Giardia, Trichomonas,* Mexican medicinal plant

INTECH
open science | open minds

1. Introduction

Protozoan parasites represent a large public health problem worldwide, from tropical and developing regions to developed countries. Among them, *Plasmodium* spp. that produces malaria is considered as the first parasitic cause of death both in people living in endemic areas and travelers returning from these regions, affecting 240 million people in 2009 and producing more than 1 million deaths in children each year in Africa alone [1]. The hemoflagellates of the *Trypanosomatidae* family, *Leishmania* spp. and *Trypanosoma* spp. are responsible for three major human diseases, leishmaniasis (cutaneous, mucocutaneous, and visceral leishmaniasis), sleeping sickness (African trypanosomiasis), and Chagas disease (American trypanosomiasis), respectively [2]. Other highly prevalent infective parasites include the intestinal anaerobic protozoa, *Entamoeba histolytica* and *Giardia intestinalis* (commonly referred to as *G. lamblia* or *G. duodenalis*) that contribute to the enormous burden of diarrheal diseases worldwide, as well as *Trichomonas vaginalis*, which is the most common nonviral sexually transmitted disease in the world [3–5]. The control of these protozoan parasites is usually based on the improvement of sanitary conditions to avoid infection, and the treatment of infected individuals. Several drugs, such as metronidazole (MTZ), pentamidine, amphotericin B and derivatives, among others, are available for the treatment of these parasitic infections. However, significant side effects have been reported, and there is a decrease in drug susceptibility [6]. In the case of *Trypanosoma*, *Leishmania*, and *Plasmodium*, an alternative approach is the interruption of disease transmission by either preventing contacts between human beings and vectors, killing or altering the vector life cycle. However, the effectiveness of vector control is limited by the development of insecticide resistance [7–9]. Therefore, it is necessary to improve the current chemotherapy arsenal against these protozoan parasites and their vectors. Natural treatments based on probiotics [10, 11], propolis [12, 13], or lactoferrin [14] may represent potential therapeutic agents against protozoan parasites. The so-called "eco-friendly control tool of mosquito vectors" based on natural molecules derived from plants is another growing line of investigation [15–21]. The search for new, safe, and efficient agents usually involves the identification of a biochemical target in parasites and the development of specific inhibitors from *in silico* (computational), *in vitro*, and *in vivo* experiments. Another strategy relies on the screening of known and unknown molecules to identify active compounds. The identification of new drugs can result from chemical modifications of existing molecules, evaluation of drugs that are currently used to treat other diseases, screening of chemical libraries, and assessment of natural compounds derived from plants that are commonly employed in traditional medicine [22, 23].

Plants synthesize a large number of organic compounds also called primary metabolites that contribute to the production of carbohydrates, lipids, and proteins, among others, that are necessary for their growth. They also generate a small amount of a variety of secondary metabolites known as phytochemicals that are represented by alkaloids, carotenoids, flavonoids, saponins, hydroxycinnamic acids, and triterpenoids, among others. To date, more than 4000 of these compounds have been discovered; some of them are responsible for color and organoleptic properties of plants, such as the red color of grapes or the characteristic smell of lavender; others act as a natural protection system against pathogens or grazing animals [24]. Traditional medicines all around the world have identified the benefit of plants for human

http://dx.doi.org/10.5772/67259

health and have taken advantage of the biological properties of phytochemicals for the empiric treatment of common human diseases. More recently, a number of scientific experiments have been performed to determine how a specific phytochemical can act at the molecular and cellular levels to protect human cells against oxidative damage, to stimulate enzymes, to interfere with the DNA replication, or to affect infection processes. These works confirmed that natural molecules obtained from medicinal plants and their derivatives are a valuable source of new therapeutic agents for the treatment of common human diseases and the control of protozoan parasites and their vectors. Importantly, the key importance of natural product research was recently highlighted by the awarding of the 2015 Nobel prize to Youyou Tu for the discovery of the antimalarial drug artemisinin [25].

In this context, Mexico has more than 3000 species of medicinal plants that have been empirically used by indigenous communities for years [26]. Some of the herbal expertise of pre-Columbian Olmec, Toltec, Aztec, Maya, Zapotec, Mixteca and Perupecha civilizations has been used by European doctors and scientists from the time of the conquest, which contributed to increase the therapeutic arsenal and enrich the universal pharmacology through centuries. Although a number of Mexican plants are currently cultivated in most countries of Europa and other continents, there is still a large number of endemic species in Mexico that remain uncharacterized. As part of the efforts to explore their potential, several groups of investigation have initiated chemical, toxicological, pharmacological, or clinical investigations in order to provide rational elements for their therapeutic effects against diseases that affect the Mexican population, mainly central nervous system disorders, diabetes, metabolic syndrome, inflammatory processes, and gastrointestinal disorders [27]. Notably, extensive review of ethnobotanical data identified medicinal plants that are used by indigenous communities in Mexico to treat complaints that fit with symptoms of parasitic infections. In addition to terrestrial plants, marine algae represent a potential source of distinct secondary metabolites related to their specific metabolism. In most cases, a general *in vitro* evaluation of the selected plants was performed to confirm the traditional use. But in some cases, phytochemical studies have allowed the isolation and identification of secondary metabolites with antiparasitic activity (**Figure 1**). In this chapter, we describe the current knowledge about the effects of several

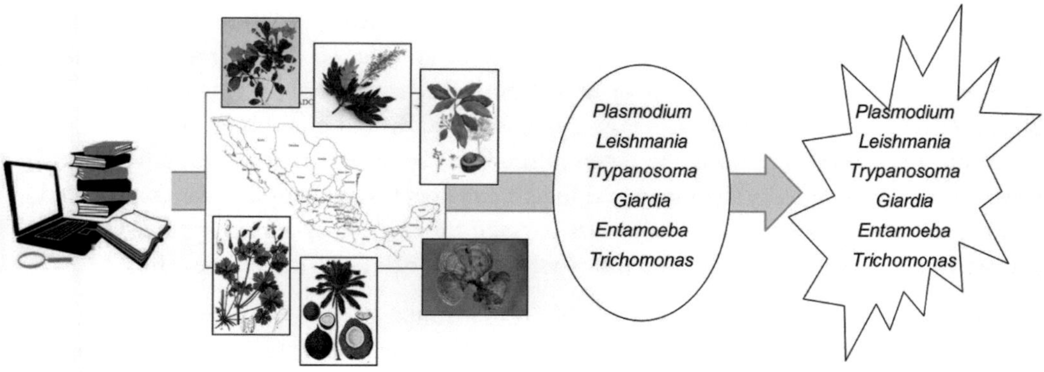

Figure 1. Strategy to search and review works about the evaluation of Mexican medicinal plants as an alternative for the development of new compounds against protozoan parasites.

Mexican plants against selected protozoan parasites of medical importance worldwide, including Mexico, namely *Plasmodium* spp., *Leishmania* spp., *Trypanosoma* spp., *G. lamblia, E histolytica,* and *T. vaginalis.* We also report the identification of some phytochemical compounds with antiparasitic activity.

2. Mexican medicinal plants against *Plasmodium falciparum*

2.1. *Plasmodium* and malaria

For decades, Malaria has been considered as the most important parasitic infectious disease worldwide, with high morbidity and mortality rates, as well as a huge socioeconomic impact in tropical and subtropical regions. In 2015, the World Malaria Report of the World Health Organization (WHO) estimated 214 million infected people and 438,000 deaths worldwide. Most cases and deaths occurred in Africa (88%), followed by the South-East Asia Region. However, for the first time, the incidence of malaria, which takes into account population growth, has been reduced by about 37% between 2000 and 2014, and the death rate has also been decreased by 60% worldwide. These encouraging numbers are the result of the efficient prophylactic and therapeutic management of malaria. Notably, the case number was reduced by 75% in several endemic countries from Asia region and South Africa and by 67.5% in Latin America. In this region, seven countries, namely Argentina, Belize, Costa Rica, Ecuador, El Salvador, Mexico, and Paraguay, are now in the elimination phase. In contrast, other countries including Panama, Nicaragua, Honduras, and Guatemala still maintain a significant transmission. Despite significant advances in the control of malaria worldwide, approximately 3.2 billion people in Asia, Latin America, and to a lesser extent, Middle East, i.e., nearly half of the world's population, were still at risk for malaria in 2015 [9, 28–30].

Malaria is caused by protozoan parasites of the genus *Plasmodium*. Among the five parasites known to infect human (*P. falciparum, P. malariae, P. ovale, P. vivax*, and *P. knowlesi*), *P. falciparum* is the most virulent, causing approximately 200 million clinical cases each year, while *P. vivax* is estimated to affect 13.8 million people [31]. *P. falciparum* is an intracellular parasite whose life cycle requires two hosts, *Anopheles* mosquito (sexual stages) and human (asexual stages). More than 70 different *Anopheles* species can transmit malaria, which contributes to the high spread of the disease [32]. Infection begins with the bite of an infected female mosquito; infective sporozoites rapidly move to the liver and proliferate (schizogony) in hepatocytes to form 30,000–40,000 merozoites that further escape into blood. In red blood cells, merozoites transform into trophozoites that invade new erythrocytes; some trophozoites differentiate themselves into microgametocytes (male) and macrogametocytes (female) that can be ingested by another *Anopheles* mosquito. These sexual parasite forms develop into a zygote, which progresses into an ookinete and an oocyst that releases sporozoites to infect a new host [33, 34].

The first symptoms of malaria also called the "primary attack" correspond to the hepatic phase and may resemble any febrile illness. In the erythrocytic phase, fever is accompanied by shivering, vomiting, joint pain, anemia, and retinal damage. Then, the typical symptoms of malaria, consisting in fever with sudden coldness and sweating, occur in periodic intervals of 2–3 days known as "short-term relapses." In some patients, "long-term relapses" of 20–60 days may occur due to reactivation of infection in the liver (*P. ovale* and *P. vivax*) or persistent infection in blood (*P. falciparum* and *P. malariae*) [35]. *P. falciparum* covers the surface of the infected blood cells with PfEMP1 proteins (*P. falciparum* erythrocyte membrane protein 1) to be sticked to blood vessels and escape destruction in the spleen. With time, this creates hemorrhagic events and obstruction of circulatory vessels, which leads to cerebral malaria [33].

WHO recommends artemisinin-based combination therapy (ACT) as the first-line treatment for *P. falciparum* malaria in all endemic regions. ACT combines a fast acting but rapidly cleared artemisinin derivative with a longer-lasting partner drug. The main combinations are lumefantrine (LMF) with artemether (ATM), which constitutes the most widely used ACT, mefloquine (MFQ) with artesunate (AS), amodiaquine (ADQ) paired with AS, and piperaquine (PPQ) combined with dihydroartemisinin (DHA). However, the increasing prevalence of artemisinin resistant *P. falciparum* across Southeast Asia and Africa threatens to destabilize malaria control worldwide. Artemisinin resistance is caused by over 20 different mutations in the *kelch13* gene [36]. The multridug resistance 1 gene (*Pfmdr1*) and chloroquine resistance transporter gene (*Pfcrt*) may also confer resistance to a great number of antimalarial drugs, including ATC [37, 38]. The recently developed vaccine, RTS,S/AS01 (RTS,S) (MosquirixTM) should help to protect young children against *P. falciparum* [39, 40]. However, malaria management in adult populations is still an extreme challenge and new antimalarials with distinct mechanisms of action are needed to circumvent existing or emerging drug resistance [41].

2.2. Relevant studies about Mexican plant with activity against *Plasmodium*

Plants are recognized as important sources of antimalarial compounds, such as artemisinin obtained from *Artemisia annua*, quinine present in western Amazonian *Cinchona* spp., as well as quassinoids and limonoids in plants of the *Simaroubaceae* and *Meliaceae* families, respectively [42, 43]. In Mexico, about 113 species are traditionally used to treat malaria symptoms, from which only several have been pharmacologically characterized (**Table 1**).

In 1990, Noster and Kraus performed the first investigations about the relevance of Mexican medicinal plants for the development of new antimalarial compounds. These authors examined two plants of the *Rubiaceae* family, *Coutarea latiflora* Sesse & Moc. ex. DC. (*Hintonia latiflora* Bullock) and *Exostema caribaeum* (Jacq.) Roem. et Schult. that were collected in Puebla, Mexico. Notably, *C. latiflora* also known as *Copalchi* is recommended to treat diabetes, stomachaches, gastric ulcers, diarrhea, skin problems, kidney problems, fever, typhus, and malaria. *E. caribaeum* is used for the treatment of gastritis, ulcers, diarrhea, stomachaches, to increase appetite and blood pressure, and to eliminate tapeworms; bark extracts are also efficient against fever, especially fever related to malaria. The hydrolyzed ethyl acetate extracts of the stem bark were shown to have the most potent antimalarial activity *in vitro*. Notably, one phenylcoumarin derivative isolated from the ether extract of *E. caribaeum* showed a moderate activity against chloroquine and pyrimethamine-sensitive FCH-5/*Tanzania* strain of *P. falciparum* [44]. Later, fractionation of lipophilic and hydrophilic extracts from the stem bark and branches of a related species, *E. mexicanum*, revealed the presence of two new 4-phenylcoumarins: 4',8-dihydroxy-5,7-dimethoxy-4-phenylcoumarin (exomexin A) and 3',4'-dihydroxy-5,7,8-trimethoxy-4-phenylcoumarin (exomexin B). Exomexin

Scientific names	Common names in Mexico	Portions	Extracts	Properties	Metabolites	References
Mexican medicinal plants against *Plasmodium*						
Exostema caribaeum	*Quina, melena de león*	Stem bark	Ethyl acetate	IC50 = 3.2 μg/ml	Phenylcoumarin derivative	[32]
Hintonia latiflora (= Cuntarea latiflora)	*Copalchi, palo amargo*	Stem bark	Ethyl acetate	IC50 = 7.3 μg/ml *In vivo* activity against schizonts at 40 mg/kg. IC50 = 24.7 and 25.9 μM IC50 = 25.9 μM	Phenylcoumarin derivative 5-O-β-D-glucopyranosyl-7,4′-dimethoxy-3′-hydroxy-4-phenylcoumarin 5-O-β-D-glucopyranosyl-7-methoxy-3′,4′-dihydroxy-4-phenylcoumarin	[32] [34]
Mexican medicinal plants against *T. cruzi*						
Aristolochia taliscana	*Guaco*	Roots	Methanol	*In vitro* activity on epimastigotes at 0.5 mg/ml	Neolignans (aupomatenoid-7 licarin A, aupomatenoid-1 and licarin B) and lignans (austrobailignan-7, and fragransin E1).	[42]
Persea americana	*Aguacate*	Seeds	Methanol	IC50 (epimastigotes) = 82 μM IC50 (trypomatigotes) = 49 μM	1,2,4-Tri-hydroxyheptadec-16-ene, 1,2,4-tri-hydroxyheptadec-16-yne and 1,2,4-trihydroxinonadecane derivatives	[43]
Senna villosa	*Booxsaal che, saal che, black bean*	Leaves	Chloroform	*In vitro* activity on epimastigotes at 1.6 mg/ml	8-Hydroxymethylen)-triecosanyl	[44]
Haematoxylum brasiletto	*Palo de brasil*	Leaves and aerial parts	Methanol	*In vitro* activity on epimastigotes at 7.92 mg/ml	Hematoxylin, Brazilin, Caffeic acid, Gallic acid, Methyl gallate, phloroglucinol, 4-hydroxycinnamic acid and 5-methoxypsoralen	[46]
Mexican medicinal plants against *Leishmania*						
Pentalinon andrieuxii	*Bejuco guaco, cantibtec, contrayerba*	Leaves and roots	Water	*In vitro* activity on promastigotes at 10 μg/ml	6,7-Dihydroneridienone, Cholest-4-en-3-one	[53]
Laennecia confusa	ND	Aerial parts	Water Chloroform	IC50 ~20 μg/ml	Flavonoids, Cyanogenic Glycosides and Cardiotonic Saponins, Sesquiterpene Lactones and Triterpenes	[55]

Scientific names	Common names in Mexico	Portions	Extracts	Properties	Metabolites	References
Mexican medicinal plants against *G. lamblia* and *E. histolytica*						
Zanthoxylum liebmannianum	*Colopahtle*	Leaves	Ethanol	IC50 (Eh) = 503.48 μg/ml IC50 (Gl) = 58 μg/ml	Asarinin	[64]
Teloxys graveolens	*Epazote de zorrillo*	Aerial parts	Methanol	IC50 (Eh) = 12.5 μg/ml IC50 (Gl) = 16.8 μg/ml IC50 (Eh) = 17.2 μg/ml	Melilotoside Narcissin	[65]
Rubus coriifolius	*Zarzamora*	Aerial parts	Methanol:dichloro methane	IC50 (Eh) = 11.6 μg/ml IC50 (Gl) = 55.6 μg/ml	(-)-Epicatechin	[66]
Geranium mexicanum	*Pata de León*	Roots	Dichloromethane–MeOH	IC50 (Eh) = 1.9 μg/ml IC50 (Gl) = 1.6 μg/ml	(-)-Epicatechin	[68]
Decachaeta incompta	*ND*	Leaves	Dichloromethane	IC50 (Eh) = 2.6 μg/ml IC50 (Gl) = 18.1 μg/ml	Incomptine A	[71]
Salvia polystachya	*Chia*	Aerial parts	Acetone	IC50 (Eh) = 22.9 μM IC50 (Gl) = 28.2 μM IC50(Eh) from 117.0 to 160.6 μM IC50 (Gl) from 107.5 to 134.7 μM	Linearolactone Polystachynes A, B and D	[73]
Lepidium virginicum	*pich' tuluk'*	Roots	Methanol	IC50 (Eh) = 100.1 μg/ml	Benzyl glucosinolate	[76]
Lippia graveolens *Ruta chalepensis*		Aerial parts	Methanol	IC50 (Eh) = 44.3 μg/ml IC50 (Eh) = 45.95 μg/ml	Carvacrol Chalepensin	[77]
Adenophyllum aurantium	*Arnica silvestre*	Roots	Ethyl acetate	IC50 (Eh) = 230 μg/ml	Thiophenes	[78]
Hippocratea excelsa	*Cancerina*	Roots	Hexane/ethanol	IC50 (Gl) = 0.11 μM IC50 (Gl) = 0.74 μM	Pristimerine tingenone	[83]
Geranium mexicanum *Rubus coriifolius* *Cuphea pinetorum* *Helianthemum glomeratum*	*Pata de léon* *Zarzamora* *Cenicilla o hierba de la gallina*	Roots Aerial parts Aerial parts Leaves	Dichloromethane/ methanol	ED50 (Gl) = 0.072 μmol/kg ED50 (Gl) = 2.057 μmol/kg ED50 (Gl) = 1.429 μmol/kg	(−)-Epicatechin Kaempferol Tiliroside	[84]

Scientific names	Common names in Mexico	Portions	Extracts	Properties	Metabolites	References
Mexican medicinal plants against *T. vaginalis*						
Carica papaya	*Papaya*	Seeds	*Methanol*	IC50 = 5.6 μg/ml	Sanguinarine alkaloid	[99]
Cocos nucifera	*Cocotero, coyolli*	husk fiber		IC50 = 5.8 μg/ml		
Bocconia frutescens	*ts'ixte'*	Aerial parts		IC50 from 30.9 to 60.9 μg/ml		
Geranium mexicanum	*Geranio de olor, Pata de león*	Roots				
Lygodium venustum	*Bejuco chino, crispillo*	Aerial parts				
Lobophora variegata	ND	Whole	Dichloromethane/ methanol	IC50 = 1.3 ± 0.7 μg/ml	Sulfoquinovosyl-diacylglycerols 1-3	[100, 101, 103]
Udotea conglutinata	ND			IC50 = 1.6 ± 0.1 μg/ml		

ND = not determined.
ED50, effective dose 50; IC50, half-maximal inhibitory concentration; MC100, concentration inducing 100% of the maximum response.
Gl, *G. lamblia*; Eh, *E. histolytica*.

Table 1. Names and metabolites of the most relevant Mexican medicinal plants with activity against selected protozoan parasites.

A, the most lipophilic molecule, had the strongest *in vitro* activity against the chloroquine-sensitive strain (poW) and the chloroquine-resistant strain (Dd2) of *P. falciparum,* with half-maximal inhibitory concentration (IC50) values of 3.6 and 1.6 μg/ml, respectively [45]. In another study, Argotte-Ramos et al. [46] confirmed that ethyl acetate extract of the stem bark of *H. latiflora* was also able to suppress parasitemia in mice infected with *P. berghei.* Bioassay-directed fractionation of the extract showed that this activity was due to two 4-phenylcoumarins, the new 5-O-β-D-glucopyranosyl-7,4′-dimethoxy-3′-hydroxy-4-phenylcoumarin and the previously reported 5-O-β-D-glucopyranosyl-7-methoxy-3′,4′-dihydroxy-4-phenylcoumarin.This latter molecule suppressed the development of schizonts by 70.8% at the dose of 40 mg/kg in the *in vivo* model. Both compounds were also effective against *P. berghei* schizonts in *in vitro* experiments with IC50 values of 24.7 and 25.9 μM, respectively. More recently, Rivera et al. [47] reported that methanolic extract of *H. latiflora* stem bark (HlMeOHe) also has an antimalarial efficacy. Toxicity assays showed that median lethal dose (LD50) was 2783.71 mg/kg. *P. yoelii yoelii*-infected mice treated with 600 and 300 mg/kg died after 6 and 7 days, respectively, with parasitemia around 45% versus 70% in untreated mice. Interestingly, treatment with 1200 mg/kg led to a 23 days survival time with a residual parasitemia of 23.6%. However, HlMeOHe seemed to be mutagenic since the average number of micronuclei significantly increased from 0.9 in untreated to 4.8 in treated mice. The authors concluded that the identification of the chemical composition of HlMeOHe should help to reduce its genotoxic potential.

Artemisia ludoviciana ssp. mexicana of the *Compositae* family has been empirically used for the treatment of intermittent fever and other symptoms. Malagon et al. [48] prepared ethanolic extracts from steams, leafs, and flowers to evaluate their activity in mice infected with *P. yoelii yoelii.* Results showed that parasite reproduction was inhibited up to 98.6% at the 5th day; the effective dose 50 (ED50) was of 29.2 mg/kg with a security margin 50 (SM50) of 28.7. Surprisingly, this extract did not seem to contain the artemisinin molecule discovered in the leaves of *A. annua* and that is the basis of ACT, which suggests the anti-*Plasmodium* effect may be due to another active molecule.

As part of an ethnobotanical study in Yucatan, Mexico (February 1994–June 1995; September 1996–October 1996), medicinal plants used by Mayan communities were collected from Chikindzonot, Ekpedz, and Xcocmil villages and surroundings to confirm their pharmacological relevance [49]. Notably, several species that are commonly recommended against fever or pain were screened *in vitro* for antimalarial activity, such as *Cestrum nocturnum,* also known as night-blooming jasmine, an evergreen woody shrub of the *Solanaceae* family, *Casearia corymbosa,* a 15-m high tree belonging to the *Salicaceae* family, and *Caesalpinia gaumeri,* a tree with deeply fluted and perforated trunk that belongs to the *Fabaceae* family. They also evaluated *Ehretia tinifolia,* a 25-m tree of the *Boraginaceae* family, whose pinguicas are traditionally used for nervous disorders and kidney problems, while the bark is used for wound healing, as well as *Manilkara zapota,* commonly known as the *sapodilla,* a long-lived, evergreen tree native from southern Mexico, Central America, and the Caribbean, which has curative properties against dysentery and diarrhea, fever, diuretics, high blood pressure, and pain caused by picket scorpion. Interestingly, nonpolar extracts of leaves from *C. nocturnum, C. corymbosa, C. gaumeri* and *E. tinifolia* showed different levels of antimalarial activity against both chloroquine-sensitive HB3 and chloroquine-resistant K1 strains of *P. falciparum,* with IC50 ranging from

172.49 to >500 μg/ml. In the case of *M. zapota,* nonpolar extract of stem bark was the most effective with an IC50 value higher that 500 μg/ml.

3. Mexican medicinal plants against *Trypanosoma cruzi*

3.1. *Trypanosoma cruzi* and American trypanosomiasis

T. cruzi is the causative agent of American trypanosomiasis or Chagas disease, which is the third cause of death in Latin America after malaria and schistosomiasis. Between 16 and 18 million people are affected by this disease that kills annually about 50 thousand people; importantly, 100 million people (25% of the population of Latin America) are at risk of contracting this infection [50].

T. cruzi is mainly transmitted by a triatomine bug (*Triatoma infestans*). In the vector, trypomastigote goes into the epimastigote stage that reproduces through binary fission in midgut to form metacyclic trypomastigotes. This infectious stage enters the human host through the bite wound or by crossing mucous membranes, and transforms into amastigotes in infected cells. Intracellular amastigotes can evolve into trypomastigotes that burst out of the cell and enter the blood stream to be transmitted to another triatomine bug. Nonvector transmission has also been described, mainly through oral infection, blood transfusions, congenital transmission, organ transplantation, and laboratory accidents [51].

Chagas disease has an acute and a chronic phase. The acute phase lasts for the first few weeks or months of infection; it can be asymptomatic or include fever, fatigue, and local swelling (called chagoma). In the chronic phase, patients usually have cardiac abnormalities, as well as digestive, neurological, or mixed alterations; recently, it has been shown that they also have behavioral changes, such as psychomotor alterations, attention and memory deficits, as well as depression [52]. Chemotherapy involves the use of two drugs: nifurtimox and benznidazole. However, both agents have variable efficacy in the acute phase and are ineffective in the chronic stage; moreover, they produce severe adverse effects [53].

3.2. Relevant studies about Mexican plant with activity against *Trypanosoma cruzi*

Because of the epidemiologic relevance of Chagas disease in Mexico, the traditional medicine has identified several Mexican plants that can help to control this infection (**Table 1**). Based on this knowledge, Abe et al. [54] performed a screening of crude methanolic extracts of several medicinal plants (20 families and 37 species) against epimastigotes of *T. cruzi.* Results showed that 18 extracts had a trypanocidal effect at a concentration of 2 mg/ml, and 13 extracts showed a trypanocidal activity at 1 mg/ml. The methanolic extract of root from *Aristolochia taliscana,* a medicinal species known as *guaco* that is used to treat bites of snakes, cough, diarrhea, and dermatological conditions, had the highest biological activity immobilizing all epimastigotes at a concentration of 0.5 mg/ml. Phytochemical study allowed the identification of six secondary metabolites: four neolignans (aupomatenoid-7 licarin A, aupomatenoid-1, and licarin B) and two lignans (austrobailignan-7 and fragransin E1). The best trypanocidal activity was found for aupomatenoid-7 and fragrasin E1, with a minimum concentration (MC100) value of 25 and 50 μg/ml, respectively. The structure-activity relationship (SAR) analysis determined that loss of the hydroxyl group reduces the trypanocidal activity. In addition, the authors suggested that steric effects might be affecting the biological behavior.

Following with the search of new options for the treatment of Chagas disease, Abe et al. [55] studied another set of Mexican medicinal plants belonging to 41 families and 65 species. Only one extract had a strong trypanocidal activity against epimastigotes of *T. cruzi*, while 10 extracts presented a weak activity. However, 39 extracts showed a good activity against trypomastigotes since concentrations inducing 100% of the maximum response (MC100) were between 125 and 500 μg/ml. The methanolic extract of seed from *Persea americana* (*Lauracea* family), a tree native from Central Mexico that produces avocado, showed the best activity on epimastigotes. The phytochemical analysis of the extract identified three 1,2,4-tri-hydroxyheptadec-16-ene derivatives, three 1,2,4-tri-hydroxyheptadec-16-yne derivatives, and two 1,2,4-trihydroxinonadecane derivatives. The most active compound was a 1,2,4-tri-hydroxyheptadec-16-ene (IC50 = 82 and 49 μM against epimastigotes and trypomatigotes, respectively). The SAR analysis determined that the transformation of the group 16-ene terminal by a group 16-yne reduces the activity.

Senna villosa is a leguminous plant of southeastern Mexico, with antifungal and antimicrobial activities, usually used to treat stomach disorders (laxative), dysmenorrhea, or fungal infection. Phytochemicals analysis has identified alkaloids, sterols, flavonoids, and anthraquinones as secondary metabolites. Particularly, Jimenez-Coello et al. [56] showed that crude chloroformic extracts had trypanocidal activity *in vitro* against epimastigotes of *T. cruzi* at a concentration of 1.6 mg/ml. The main metabolite responsible for the activity in *in vitro* experiments and *in vivo* models (33.6 mg/g) was (8-hydroxymethylen)-trieicosanyl acetate. Therefore, the same group of investigations tested chloroformic extracts of *S. villosa* leaves against amastigotes of *T. cruzi* during the acute phase of infection. Results showed a reduction in the number of amastigotes in cardiac tissue at a dose of 3.3 mg/g compared with untreated mice [57].

Molina-Garza et al. [58] evaluated the trypanocidal activity of 10 plants used in traditional Mexican medicine for the treatment of parasitic infections: *Artemisia Mexicana, Castela texana, Cymbopogon citratus, Eryngium heterophyllum, Haematoxylum brasiletto, Lippia graveolens, Marrubium vulgare, Persea americana, Ruta chalepensis*, and *Schinus molle*. Methanolic extracts (150 mg/ml) of *E. heterophyllum, H. brasiletto, M. vulgare*, and *S. molle* produced growth inhibition (88–100%) of *T. cruzi* epimastigotes. *C. citratus* and *A. mexicana* led to 83% inhibition, *P. americana* and *R. chalepensis* to 70%, and *C. texana* and *L. graveolens* to 33% inhibition. The highest values of trypanocidal activity (7.92 and 11.24 mg/ml) were for *H. brasiletto* and *E. heterophyllum*, respectively. The phytochemical characterization of *H. brasiletto* indicated the presence of hematoxylin, brazilin, caffeic acid, gallic acid, methyl gallate, phloroglucinol, 4-hydroxycinnamic acid, and 5-methoxypsoralen. Constituents of *E. heterophyllum* extracts have not been described yet, although the presence of (*E*)-2-dodecanal, a metabolite with trypanocidal activity, has been found in the related specie *E. foetidum*. *H. brasiletto* extracts also have unsaturated compounds, including carbonyl groups, carboxyl groups, triterpenes, sesquiterpene lactone, quinones, flavonoids, and tannins [59].

Carica papaya, a giant herbaceous plant in the *Caricaceae* family, is originated in Central America and widely distributed in southern Mexico. It is traditionally used for diabetes treatment and birth control, as antiseptic, antimicrobial, or diuretic, to control parasites, lower blood pressure and cholesterol, and reduce inflammation, among others. Some data also indicated that it has antiprotozoal activity. Therefore, Jimenez-Coello et al. [60] evaluated the effects of extracts and a mixture of the main components of *C. papaya* against *T. cruzi* amastigotes during subacute phase and chronic disease. Results showed that chloroformic extract was able to reduce the number of amastigotes (55.5 and 69.7%) in cardiac tissue of infected mice during the subacute phase at a concentration of 50 and 75 mg/kg, respectively. The fatty acids mixture also exhibited a similar trypanocidal activity (56.45%); however, the total elimination of the parasite was not achieved. In the chronic phase of infection, the number of amastigotes was only reduced to 46.8 and 5.13% using the same concentrations. Therefore, the authors suggested the use of this extract in combination with other reference drug for a more efficient pharmacological treatment of Chagas disease.

T. brucei is the other pathogen genus that is responsible for the African trypanosomiasis also known as sleeping sickness. Due the medical relevance of this parasitic infection and problems with conventional treatments, medicinal plants have been investigated to develop alternative drugs. Unfortunately, the potential of Mexican medicinal plants against this parasite does not seem to have been investigated yet; therefore, we did not include this topic in the present review.

4. Mexican medicinal plants against *Leishmania*

4.1. *Leishmania* and leishmaniasis

Cutaneous, mucocutaneous, and visceral (kala-azar) leishmaniasis are caused by more than 20 species of *Leishmania*, mainly *L. donovani*, *L. infantum*, or *L. chagasi*, in the case of visceral disease, while cutaneous forms can be due to more than 15 different species. All species are morphologically identical, but specific biochemical and molecular characteristics allow their identification through isoenzyme analysis, molecular methods, or monoclonal antibodies. This set of parasitic infections affects 88 countries worldwide, 67 in the old world, and 21 in America. The large majority (90%) of visceral leishmaniasis cases is reported in only five countries: Bangladesh, India, Nepal, Sudan, and Brazil, while cutaneous leishmaniasis mainly affects seven countries: Afghanistan, Algeria, Brazil, Iran, Peru, Saudi Arabia, and Syria. The annual incidence is estimated at 1.5 million cases of cutaneous, mucocutaneous, and diffuse cutaneous leishmaniasis and, 500,000 cases of visceral leishmaniasis. There are 350 million people at risk of contracting the disease, which is associated with about 2.4 million people with disabilities and about 70,000 deaths per year [61, 62].

Leishmania infection begins with the inoculation of promastigotes by a sand fly from *Phlebotomus* or *Lutzomyia* genus during blood meals. After being phagocytized by macrophages or other mononuclear phagocytic cells, parasite evolves to amastigotes that multiply and infect other mononuclear cells. The life cycle is continued when a sand fly feeds on an infected person and ingests amastigotes within macrophages. In the insect gut, amastigotes transform into promastigotes that migrate to the proboscis to be transmitted to another human host [63].

Cutaneous leishmaniasis is characterized by skin ulcers that are be cured by themselves, while mucocutaneous leishmaniasis is associated with progressive infection with invasion and destruction of the nasopharyngeal mucosa. Symptoms of visceral leishmaniasis mainly include fever, weight loss, enlargement of spleen and liver, as well as low blood counts. Treatment depends on the *Leishmania* species, the clinical signs, the geographic region, and the immunologic status of the patient. Visceral leishmaniasis is usually treated with liposomal amphotericin B, and recently by miltefosine (Miltex), although the pentavalent antimony (SbV) and paromomycin (Humatin) are also used in developing countries. The same treatments can also be used for severe cases of cutaneous or mucocutaneous disease. Most of these drugs cause serious problems, including renal insufficiency. In addition, their high cost makes treatment unaffordable for most infected people. Therefore, a large number of patients discontinue the treatment, which promotes the emergence of resistant strains [64].

4.2. Relevant studies about Mexican plant with activity against *Leishmania*

Besides the relevance of Leishmaniasis in Mexico, the study of Mexican plants as an option for the treatment of this infectious disease has been limited (**Table 1**). *Pentalinon andrieuxii*, a flowering plant in the *Apocynaceae* family, is a native plant of the state of Yucatan, Mexico that has been commonly used for the treatment of cutaneous leishmaniasis in southeastern Mexico. Lezama-Davila et al. [65] reported that aqueous and organic extracts of *P. andrieuxii* root (10 μg/ml) have activity on promastigotes of *L. mexicana in vitro*. The extracts of leaves and roots contain various secondary metabolites, mainly cardenolides, flavonoids, pregnane sterols, trinorsesquiterpenoids, and triterpenoids. Phytochemical analyses of root hexane extract revealed 16 sterol derivatives, three coumarins, and one triterpenoid. The evaluation of their effect on promastigotes and amastigotes of *L. mexicana* showed that five sterols have a greater inhibitory effect than the reference drug, pentostam, after 48 h exposure on promastigotes; notably, 6,7-dihydroneridienone was the most active metabolite with an IC50 value of 9.2 μM. These compounds were as effective as pentostam against amastigotes, with IC50 values from 1.4 to 3.5 μM versus 2.7 μM, respectively. Cholest-4-en-3-one was the most active metabolite with an IC50 value of 0.03 μM against the amastigote form. The SAR analysis showed the importance of fragment 4-ene-3-oxo in the steroidal system for the leishmanicidal effect, while the 3-ol-5-ene system reduced the antiparasitic activity. Variations in chain size on D ring of five members also influenced the activity. Interestingly, none of these compounds showed cytotoxic effects (IC50 >100 μg/ml) on noninfected bone marrow-derived macrophages from C57BL16 mouse. Authors suggested that these compounds may act as antagonists of endogenous sterols, interfering or inhibiting sterol biosynthesis, causing alterations in membrane of *L. mexicana*, and leading to morphological abnormalities and destruction of amastigotes [66].

Infusion of *Laennecia confusa* (*Asteraceae* family), native of the states of Chihuahua and Chiapas, Mexico, is used as sedative and treatment for alcohol addiction. The genus *Laennecia* contains several secondary metabolites, such as terpenoids, terpenes, saponoides, flavonoids, sterols, lactones, and tannins, among others. When Martínez-Ruiz et al. [67] evaluated the trypanocidal potential of *L. confusa*, they confirmed the presence of flavonoids, cyanogenic glycosides and cardiotonic, saponins, sesquiterpene lactones, and triterpenes, in 71 fractions obtained from aqueous, hexanic, methanolic, and chloroformic extracts. Aqueous and chloroformic extracts caused a significant growth reduction of *L. donovani* with IC50 values around 20 μg/ml; interestingly, the IC50 value decreased to 200 μg/ml for a specific fraction of the chloroformic extract. Unfortunately, all compounds exhibited toxicity on macrophages.

Lopezia racemosa (also known as *L. mexicana, L. hirsute* Jacq.), widely distributed in Mexico, is traditionally used for skin infections, stomach cancer, and urinary retention, among others. It has been reported that plants of the *Onagraceae* family contain tannins, flavonoids, and sterols as metabolic constituents; however, *L. racemosa* has not been submitted to phytochemical studies yet. Cruz-Paredes et al. [68] evaluated the effect of hexane, chloroform, and methanol extracts (HE, CE, and ME) of *L. racemosa* and their fractions on *L. donovani* promastigotes. Interestingly, HE 11-14b and ME 28-36 fractions and CE produced a high reduction (88%) in parasites number when compared with untreated controls. However, most extracts and fractions had a toxic effect on human-derived macrophages (THP-1); only fraction 28–36 ME showed no significant cytotoxicity (below 25%) (IC50 = 770 μg/ml). The authors hypothesized that the high amount of polyphenols (tannins and flavonoids) present in this plant may be responsible for the biological activity.

5. Mexican medicinal plants against gastrointestinal protozoan parasites

5.1. *Entamoeba histolytica* and *Giardia lamblia*

Gastrointestinal diseases occur worldwide and are associated with poor sanitary conditions, overcrowding, poor water quality control, and low socioeconomic level. Different microorganisms can produce these symptoms; two of them are the protozoan parasites *E. histolytica* and *G. lamblia* (or *G. intestinalis* or *G. duodenalis*). *E. histolytica* is responsible for human amoebiasis. Trophozoites live and proliferate in the intestinal tract by eating bacteria and cellular debris. In some cases, parasites cross the epithelial wall to reach the bloodstream and spread throughout the body to invade other organs, mainly liver, as well as lungs, brain, or spleen. Trophozoites can also form cysts that are eliminated with feces. Most infected patients are asymptomatic; others present a wide range of symptoms including diarrhea, stomachache, and hemorrhagic colitis. The extraintestinal localization of trophozoites can produce fatal abscesses. Amoebiasis remains a major health problem, affecting more than 10% of the world's population, mainly in developing countries. Globally, it accounts for 50 million clinical cases and is responsible for approximately 110,000 deaths annually, which makes it the second-leading cause of death from a protozoan parasite after malaria [69–71]. Giardiasis, also called Beaver fever, is the other common intestinal infection associated with diarrhea, producing over 250 million symptomatic human infections per year worldwide, with a high prevalence in children in developing countries. The flagellated protozoan *G. lamblia* is the causal agent of giardiasis. Colonization of the small intestine produces acute or chronic diarrhea, mal absorption, excess gas, stomach or abdominal cramps, nausea, and failure to thrive. *Giardia* infection also alters child linear growth and psychomotor development, due to iron-deficiency anemia, micronutrient deficiencies and growth retardation associated with diarrhea and malabsorption syndrome [72]. Both *E. histolytica* and *G. lamblia* are transmitted by the fecal-oral route, through ingestion of food and water that have been contaminated by feces of an infected host.

Metronidazole and other 5-nitroimidazoles are the drugs of choice against *E. histolytica and G. lamblia*; however, there are some reports about their mutagenicity in bacteria and their carcinogenic effects in rodents. Additionally, metronidazole provokes several side effects, including headache, dry mouth, metallic taste, glossitis, and urticaria [73–75].

5.2. Relevant studies about Mexican plants with activity against *Entamoeba histolytica* and *Giardia lamblia*

Mexican native communities use a large number of plants to treat intestinal ailments. However, only few species have been scientifically evaluated to confirm their potential such as anti-*Giardia* or anti-*Entamoeba* treatments (**Table 1**). *Zanthoxylum liebmannianum*, commonly known as *Colopahtle*, is recommended for the treatment of stomachaches, amoebiasis, intestinal parasites, and as a local anesthetic agent. The crude ethanol extract from leaves of *Z. liebmannianum* exhibited an inhibitory effect on the proliferation of *E. histolytica* and *G. lamblia* trophozoites with IC50 values of 3.48 and 58.00 μg/ml, respectively. Asarinin, hyperin, β-sitosterol, and β-sitosterol glucoside were isolated from this extract. Among them, asarinin was the most active compound with IC50 values of 19.86 μg/ml for *E. histolytica* and 35.45 μg/ml for *G. lamblia* [76].

In 2003, Calzada et al. [77] reported the isolation and antiprotozoal activity of one coumaric acid derivative, named melilotoside, and the flavonoids pinocembrine, pinostrobin, chrysin, narcissin, and rutin from *Teloxys graveolens*, a medicinal plant traditionally used to control some gastrointestinal diseases. Melilotoside exhibited the most potent activity toward *E. histolytica* and *G. lamblia* with IC50 values of 12.5 and 16.8 μg/ml, respectively. Interestingly, narcissin showed selectivity against *E. histolytica* (IC50 = 17.2 μg/ml).

The same year, Alanís et al. [78] isolated (-)-epicatechin, (+)-catechin, hyperin, nigaichigoside F1, Β-sitosterol 3-O-β-D-glucopyranoside, gallic acid, and ellagic acid from *Rubus coriifolius*, a medicinal plant used by the Maya communities in southern Mexico to treat bloody diarrhea. These compounds had activity against *E. histolytica* and *G. lamblia* trophozoites, being (-)-epicatechin the most potent molecule with the IC50 values of 1.9 and 1.6 μg/ml, respectively. (-)-Epicatechin is also obtained from *Geranium mexicanum*, with the vernacular name *pata de leon*, an endemic Mexican species used as purgative, and as a remedy against tonsillitis, cough, whooping cough, urticaria, dysentery, and diarrhea. This flavonoid was active against *E. histolytica* and *G. lamblia* with IC50 values ranging from 1.9 to 79.2 μg/ml for *E. histolytica* and from 1.6 to 100.4 μg/ml for *G. lamblia*. In addition, *G. mexicanum* contains (+)-catechin, tyramine, and β-sitosterol 3-*O*-β-D-glucopyranoside, but they only had a moderate activity against these protozoan parasites [79].

In northeast Mexico, indigenous populations use infusion of leaves from *Artemisia ludoviciana* as an antidiarrheal treatment. Aqueous, methanolic, acetonic, and hexanic leaf extracts from plants collected in Monterrey City, Mexico, were found to be active *in vitro* against both

E. histolytica and *G. lamblia* trophozoites. Particularly, the acetonic (IC50 = 117.2 μg/ml) and hexanic (122.7 μg/ml) extracts showed an interesting activity against *E. histolytica*, while the hexanic extract had the highest effect upon *G. lamblia* (IC50 = 137.4 μg/ml) [80]. *A. ludoviciana* was also studied by Ramos-Guerra et al. [81], together with *M. vulgare*, *Mentha spicata*, and *Chenopodium ambrosioides* that are also popularly used against intestinal disorders. Surprisingly, *A. ludoviciana* was inactive against both protozoan species (IC50 >100 μg/mL) in this work. Acetonic and methanolic extracts from *M. vulgare* were very active against *G. lamblia* with an IC50 = 7 and 12 μg/ml, respectively, and slightly to moderately toxic to *E. histolytica* (IC50 = 90 and 34 μg/ml, respectively). Hexanic, acetonic, and methanolic extracts from *M. spicata* were also very potent against *G. lamblia* (IC50 = 17, 13, and 8 μg/ml, respectively) while only the acetonic extract was slightly active against *E. histolytica* (IC50 = 98 μg/ml). Hexanic and acetic *C. ambrosioides* extracts were moderately active against amoeba (IC50 = 57 and 58 μg/ml). The highest activity against both protozoan species was obtained with organic extract from *M. vulgare* and *M. spicata*, which require further studies to identify the active compounds.

Decachaeta incompta is a Mesoamerican flowering plant that has been traditionally used in Oaxaca, as well as in Chiapas, Colima, Guerrero, Michoacán, Mexico State, Jalisco, and Puebla, Mexico. Its antiprotozoal properties have been confirmed since the dichloromethane extract of leaves was effective against *E. histolytica* and *G. lamblia* trophozoites (IC50 values of 132.5 and 141.4 μg/ml, respectively). Bioassay-guided fractionation of crude extract resulted in the isolation of four sesquiterpene lactones named incomptines. Incomptine A, a sesquiterpene lactone of the heliangolide type, appeared to be the most potent antiamoebic and antigiardial compound with IC50 values of 2.6 μg/ml for *E. histolytica* and 18.1 μg/ml for *G. lamblia*. Its potency against *E. histolytica* was close to that of emetine (IC50 1.05 μg/ml) [82]. Recently, we used a proteomic approach based on two-dimensional gel electrophoresis and electrospray ionization tandem mass spectrometry (ESI-MS/MS) analysis to get insights into the molecular mechanisms involved in the antiamoebic activity of incomptine A. Our results evidenced the differential expression of 21 *E. histolytica* proteins in response to incomptine A treatment. Notably, three glycolytic enzymes, namely enolase, pyruvate:ferredoxin oxidoreductase and fructose-1,6-biphosphate aldolase, were downregulated. In addition, we observed an increased number of glycogen granules through ultrastructural analysis of trophozoites by electronic microscopy. Based on these data, we proposed that incomptine A could affect *E. histolytica* growth through alteration of energy metabolism [83].

Salvia polystachya Ort. (*Lamiaceae*), popularly known as *chia* is used in Mexican traditional medicine as a purgative, antigastralgic, antipyretic, and to treat dysentery. In 2010, Calzada et al. [84] evaluated the possible antiprotozoal *in vitro* activity of the crude extract and four neo-clerodane diterpenoids from *S. polystachya*. They found that linearolactone was the most potent antiamoebic and antigiardial compound with IC50 values of 22.9 and 28.2 μM, respectively. Polystachynes A, B, and D showed moderate antiprotozoal activity with IC50 values ranging from 117.0 to 160.6 μM for *E. histolytica* and from 107.5 to 134.7 μM for *G. lamblia*.

Since amoebiasis and giardiasis share intestinal symptoms, several groups of investigation used a screening approach to simultaneously evaluate the antiamoebic and antigiardial effects of a large number of Mexican medicinal plants that are recommended for gastrointestinal diseases. In 2006, Calzada et al. [85] studied 26 plants and found that methanolic extract obtained from *Chiranthodendron pentadactylon, Annona cherimola,* and *Punica granatum* was the most effective on *E. histolytica* with IC50 < 30 μg/ml. Interestingly, *C. pentadactylon* had an IC50 value of 2.5 μg/ml, which is close to the IC50 value of emetine, but far less than metronidazole used as control drugs. On the other hand, extracts of *Dorstenia contrajerva, Senna villosa,* and *R. chalepensis* were the most active toward *G. lamblia* with IC50 < 38 μg/ml. Recently, Camacho-Corona et al. [86] showed that the dichloromethane/methanol extract of *Larrea tridentata,* also known as *gobernadora* (governess) and *hediondilla* (little smelly one) in Mexico, exhibits a moderate inhibitory activity against *E. histolytica* (IC50 = 100 μg/ml). The extract of *Hyptis albida* was the most active against *G. lamblia* with an IC50 value of 16.11 μg/ml. Extracts of *Crataegus mexicana, Ocimun basilicum,* and *L. tridentata* exhibited a moderate activity against *G. lamblia* with IC50 values of 153 and 116 μg/ml, respectively.

5.3. Relevant studies about Mexican plant with activity against *Entamoeba histolytica*

Although amoebiasis and giardiasis share several symptoms, the protozoan parasites that are responsible for these infectious diseases are quite different. Therefore, several investigators focused their research on *Entamoeba* or *Giardia* to confirm the ethnobotanical properties of Mexican medicinal plants used to treat intestinal diseases and identify the phytochemicals that are responsible for their activity against these endemic pathogens (**Table 1**). Thus, Calzada et al. [87] reported scientific findings that support the ethnomedical use of roots of *Lepidium virginicum,* a herb of the highlands of Chiapas, Mexico, which is recommended for the treatment of diarrhea and dysentery. The crude extract of *L. virginicum* roots exhibited *in vitro* activity against *E. histolytica* trophozoites (IC50 = 100.1 μg/ml). Extract fractionation revealed that benzyl glucosinolate is responsible for this activity with an IC50 of 20.4 μg/ml. Later, Quintanilla-Licea et al. [88] performed an antiamoebic screening among methanolic extracts of 32 plants used in northeast Mexican traditional medicine. Six extracts induced more than 80% growth inhibition at a concentration of 150 μg/ml. *L. graveolens* Kunth and *R. chalepensis* Pers. showed the most significant antiprotozoal activity (91.54 and 90.50% growth inhibition at a concentration of 150 μg/ml with IC50 values of 59.14 and 60.07 μg/ml, respectively). Bioassay-guided fractionation of the methanolic extracts afforded carvacrol (IC50 = 44.3 μg/ml) and chalepensin (IC50 = 45.95 μg/ml), respectively, as bioactive compounds. Recently, Herrera-Martínez et al. [89] reported that ethyl acetate extract of *Adenophyllum aurantium* root exhibits antiamoebic activity *in vitro* with an IC50 of 230 μg/ml. This extract was also able to inhibit the encystation process of *E. invadens,* the protozoan parasite of reptiles. Interestingly, this extract affected virulence properties of amoeba, since the intraperitoneal administration (2.5 or 5 mg) to *E. histolytica*-infected hamsters prevented the development of amoebic liver abscesses in 48.5 or 89.0% of the animals, respectively. Moreover, adhesion and erythrophagocytosis were 28.7 and 37.5% inhibited, respectively. These effects were associated with alterations in trophozoite organization, namely a reduced number of vacuoles and alterations in the actin cytoskeleton. Thiophenes were identified as the major components by carbon-13 nuclear magnetic resonance (^{13}C-NMR) analysis; however, their relevance for antiamoebic activity remains to be confirmed.

5.4. Relevant studies about Mexican plant with activity against *Giardia lamblia*

In an attempt to characterize the *in vitro* activity against *Giardia*, Ponce-Macotela et al. [90] evaluated 14 medicinal plants commonly used as antidiarrheic and antiparasitic treatment in Mexico. Nine species presented a clear antigiardial effect when they were used at the concentrations traditionally recommended. Notably, *Justicia spicigera, Lipia beriandieri,* and *Psidium guajava* produced a higher mortality (91 ± 0.5%, 90 ± 0.6%, and 87 ± 1.0%, respectively) than tinidazole used as reference drug (79 ± 1.9%). Later, the same group of investigation reported that trophozoites exposed to *J. spicigera* extract have significant changes in ultrastructure, mainly modification in size and shape, as well as damage in nucleus structure, which may be due to alterations in the pattern of nucleoskeleton proteins as a result of the effects of plant phytochemicals [91, 92].

The state of Yucatan, Mexico, is a rich source of Mayan medicinal plants for treatment of dysentery, gastritis, gastric ulcers, and other intestinal problems. In 2002, Ankli et al. [49] confirmed that six species have activity against *G. lamblia* with IC50 values less than 100 μg/ml, three of them with minimum inhibitory concentration (MIC) values less than 100 μg/ml. The most active extract was the nonpolar extract A of *Crossopetalum gaumeri* (MIC = 6.3 μg/ml), whereas the polar extract B showed a very weak antiprotozoal activity. The nonpolar and polar extracts of *Psidium sartorianum, Piscidia piscipula, Bidens squarrosa* and *Casimiroa tetrameria* and the nonpolar fraction of *Bauhinia divaricata* showed weak activity with IC50 values between 20 and 90 μg/ml. Later, Peraza-Sánchez et al. [93] demonstrated the *in vitro* antigiardial activity of another set of 10 native plants from Yucatan, Mexico: *Byrsonima crassifolia* (L.) Kunth, *Cupania dentata* DC., *Diphysa carthagenensis* Jacq., *Dorstenia contrajerva L., Gliricidia sepium* (Jacq.) Kunth ex Walp., *Justicia spicigera* Schldl., *Pluchea odorata* (L.) Cass., *Spigelia anthelmia* L., *Tridax procumbens* L., and *Triumfetta semitriloba* Jacq. The extract obtained from *T. procumbens* was the most active (IC50 = 6.34 μg/ml), followed by *C. dentata* (IC50 = 7.59 μg/ml), *D. carthagenensis* (IC50 = 11.53 μg/ml), and *B. crassifolia* (IC50 = 15.55 μg/ml). *G. sepium, J. spicigera, P. odorata, S. anthelmia,* and *T. semitriloba* were active in the range from 46.41 to 117.41 μg/ml. *Hippocratea excelsa* is another Mayan medicinal plant with a confirmed anti-*Giardia* activity. From the different triterpenoids that have been isolated from the root bark of *H. excelsa*, pristimerine and tingenone were the most active compounds with IC50 values of 0.11 and 0.74 μM, respectively [94].

Barbosa et al. [95] isolated the flavonoids kaempferol, tiliroside and (−)-epicatechin from *G. mexicanum, Cuphea pinetorum, Helianthemum glomeratum,* and *Rubus coriifolius,* which are medicinal plants used for the treatment of gastrointestinal disorders in Mexico, and evaluated their antiprotozoal activity in suckling females CD-1 mice infected with *G. lamblia.* The most active flavonoid was (−)-epicatechin (ED50 = 0.072 μmol/kg); its activity was even stronger than that of metronidazole and emetine used as reference drugs. In the case of kaempferol and tiliroside, their potency was close to that of metronidazole, but far less than emetine (ED50=2.057 and 1.429 μmol/kg, respectively).

C. dentata (Sapindaceae family) is traditionally used against inflammation in Veracruz, Mexico and pain in Quintana Roo, Mexico. Hernández-Chávez et al. [96] showed that methanolic, hexanic, dichloromethane, ethyl acetate and butanolic extracts of *C. dentata* are able to inhibit

http://dx.doi.org/10.5772/67259

the proliferation of *Giardia* trophozoites (IC50 = 8.17, 4.42, 2.12, 9.52 and 6.5 μg/ml, respectively). The phytochemical study of fractions resulted in the isolation of taraxerone, taraxerol, scopoletin, and two mixtures of steroidal compounds. Among them, taraxerone was the metabolite with the highest giardicidal activity (IC50 = 11.33 μg/ml).

6. Mexican medicinal plants against *Trichomonas vaginalis*

6.1. *Trichomonas vaginalis* and trichomoniasis

T. vaginalis is an anaerobic flagellated protozoan that lives and replicates by binary fission in the urogenital tract of humans, namely vulva, vagina, or urethra, in women, and urethra, prostate and epididymis in men. The "pear" shaped trophozoite (10–20 μm in length) is the unique morphological stage for this monoxen parasite for which human is the only host. Trichomoniasis represents the most prevalent nonviral sexually transmitted infection in the world, affecting around 250 million people annually [97]. In Mexico, a recent report revealed that trichomoniasis is at the 12th place among the 20 principal causes of infectious diseases with a rate of 104.23 cases per 100,000 individuals. Women are more affected than men at a ratio of 36:1 and women aged 25–44 years represent the mayor number of cases (almost 60,000 infected women in 2011) [98]. At least 50% of infected individuals are asymptomatic; they are neither detected nor treated, which makes trichomoniasis a neglected parasitic infection that can silently spread worldwide [99]. Symptomatic women develop vaginitis, cervicitis, urethritis, a malodourous seropurulent vaginal discharge and infertility. Moreover, *Trichomonas* infection has been linked to bad pregnancy outcomes (preterm birth, low birth weight, and respiratory infections in the newborn). Importantly, trichomoniasis is an enhanced risk factor of getting or spreading other sexually transmitted infections, such as human immunodeficiency virus (HIV), papilloma virus (HPV) and herpes simplex virus II (HSV-2) [100–102]. Men usually represent the short-term reservoir of *T. vaginalis*, but they may also suffer from urethritis [103]. In addition, an association with worse prostate cancer prognosis has been reported [104].

Since the early 60s, the drug of choice for treating trichomoniasis is metronidazole and its derivatives (tinidazole and secnidazole) [105]. As in the case of other anaerobic protozoan pathogens, important side effects have been reported, including headache, nausea, gastrointestinal disturbance, and anorexia, as well as cytotoxic effects, which limit the efficacy of the treatment [106, 107]. However, the main cause of treatment failure is the resistance of parasite to 5-nitroimidazole derivatives. MTZ resistance has been observed in 5–20% of patients [108] and around 10% of clinical isolates are 5-nitroimidazoles resistant *in vitro* [109]. In this context, new treatments for trichomoniasis are necessary.

6.2. Relevant studies about Mexican plant with activity against *Trichomonas vaginalis*

With the purpose of searching for new drugs for the control of trichomoniasis, several groups performed *in vitro* susceptibility assays to identify the anti-*Trichomonas* activity of Mexican plants that were selected on the basis of chemotaxonomical criteria, as well as ethnobotanical and ethnopharmacological uses for the treatment of clinical signs associated with trichomoniasis, such as abdominal pain, colic, and vaginal discharge (**Table 1**).

In 2007, Calzada et al. [110] reported the antitrichomonal effect of methanol extracts of *Carica papaya* and *Cocos nucifera* (IC50 values of 5.6 and 5.8 μg/ml, respectively), as well as *Bocconia frutescens, G. mexicanum,* and *Lygodium venustum* (IC50 values ranging from 30.9 to 60.9 μg/ml) collected in six states of the country, namely Mexico City, State of Mexico, Hidalgo, Guanajuato, Sinaloa, and Yucatan, Mexico. The genotoxicity of the sanguinarine alkaloid present in *B. frutescens* could explain the antiprotozoal activity of the extract.

In another study, Moo-Puc et al. [111] evaluated dichloromethane:methanol extracts of 25 tropical seaweeds (12 *Rhodophyta,* 5 *Phaeophyta,* and 8 *Chlorophyta*) from the coast of Gulf of Mexico and Caribbean in Yucatan, Mexico. The most active algal extracts were from *Lobophora variegata* (*Phaeophyta*) and *Udotea conglutinata* (*Chlorophyta*), with IC50 values of 1.3 ± 0.7 and 1.6 ± 0.1 μg/ml, respectively. Although their investigation did not involve structure elucidation, the authors suggested that this effect could be due to the presence of terpenes and polyphenols that are known antiprotozoal compounds [112]. Interestingly, extracts were not toxic for Madin-Darby canine kidney (MDCK) cells. The further characterization of the brown alga *L. variegata* revealed its antioxidant activity [113]. Fractionation using different solvents and isolation of antiprotozoal constituents indicated that the chloroformic fraction was the most effective against *T. vaginalis* due to the presence of sulfoquinovosyl-diacylglycerols 1–3 (SQDGs 1–3) according to chromatographic fractionation on Sephadex LH-20, chemical and enzymatic hydrolysis, as well as analysis of fast atom-mass spectrometry (FAB-MS) and NMR spectroscopic data. The mixture of SQDGs 1–3 only had a moderate activity against *T. vaginalis* trophozoites (IC50 = 8 μg/ml), being less effective than the whole extract. The authors concluded that crude extract and nonpolar fractions from *L. variegate,* mainly the ethyl acetate fraction, should contain the major inhibitory compounds [114].

In addition to their hypolipemic [115] and hypoglycemic [116] effects in animal models, extract obtained from *P. americana* seeds has activity against several fungi [117], bacteria [118], and protozoan parasites [90]. Notably, Jiménez-Arellanes et al. [119] showed that chloroformic and ethanolic extracts of *P. americana* seeds obtained from the town of Ario de Rosales in the state of Michoacan, Mexico, displayed significant activity against *T. vaginalis* (IC50 = 0.524 and 0.533 μg/ml, respectively). According to a preliminary analysis, these extracts contain β-sitosterol, phytol and palmitic acid, and catechin and epicatechin, respectively, which could be responsible for the antiprotozoal activity.

7. Conclusion

It is clear that antiparasitic drugs currently available have been essential to control, at least partially, the spread and illnesses related to malaria, trypanosomiasis, leishmaniasis, amoebiasis, giardiasis, and trichomoniasis. However, besides the existence of this chemotherapeutic arsenal, these infections still represent a huge threat for human health worldwide, particularly in developing countries. Failure in parasite elimination is mainly due to drug toxicity and

http://dx.doi.org/10.5772/67259

emergence of drug resistance in both parasites and vectors. Thus, one of the main contemporary challenges in global health is to find new, efficient and safe alternatives to prevent the establishment of drug resistance strains. Mexican medicinal plants are recognized as important sources of therapeutic compounds. Particularly, the present review supports the popular uses of plants from different regions of Mexico for the treatment of some of the most prevalent parasitic infections (**Figure 1**). In addition, it clearly highlights their potential for the isolation and identification of new antiparasitic molecules. Unfortunately, it is worth noting that most extracts, fractions, or isolated molecules tested were less or as efficient as the drug of choice for each pathogen. This could be resolved by chemical modifications of the initial structure to improve the stability of the molecule and its antiparasitic activity. The identification of the biochemical targets could also allow the design of more active molecules through bioinformatics screening and docking studies. On the other hand, prospective studies aimed to improve delivery systems *in vivo* should help to circumvent the drawbacks related to stability, bioavailability, and integrity of natural compounds. Some of these techniques currently used with phytochemicals include nano- and microencapsulation in polymers of natural or synthetic origin, or lipids. Another important point is the necessity of toxicity and mutagenicity tests to confirm the safety of the most promising molecules.

Abbreviations

^{13}C-NMR	Carbon-13 nuclear magnetic resonance
ACT	Artemisinin-based combination therapy
ADQ	Amodiaquine
AS	Artesunate
ATM	Artemether
CE	Chloroform extract
DHA	Dihydroartemisinin
ED50	Effective dose 50
ESI-MS/MS	Electrospray ionization tandem mass spectrometry
FAB-MS	Fast atom bombardment-mass spectrometry
HE	Hexane extract
IC50	Half maximal inhibitory concentration
LD50	Median lethal dose
LMF	Lumefantrine
MC100	Concentration inducing 100% of the maximum response
ME	Methanol extract
MeOHe	Methanolic extract
MFQ	Mefloquine
MIC	Minimum inhibitory concentration
MTZ	Metronidazole
PPQ	Piperaquine
SM50	Security margin 50
WHO	World Health Organization

Author details

Esther Ramirez-Moreno[1], Jacqueline Soto-Sanchez[1], Gildardo Rivera[2] and Laurence A. Marchat[1]*

*Address all correspondence to: lmarchat@gmail.com

1 ENMH, National Polytechnic Institute (Instituto Politécnico Nacional), Mexico City, Mexico

2 Genomic Biotechnology Center, National Polytechnic Institute (Instituto Politécnico Nacional), Reynosa, Mexico

References

[1] WHO. World Malaria report 2011 [Internet]. 2011. Available from: http://www.who.int/iris/handle/10665/44792 [Accessed: 2016-09-02]

[2] Teixeira SM, de Paiva RM, Kangussu-Marcolino MM, Darocha WD. Trypanosomatid comparative genomics: contributions to the study of parasite biology and different parasitic diseases. Genetics and Molecular Biology. 2012;**35**:1–17.

[3] Jackson TF. Epidemiology. In: Ravdin JI, editor. Amoebiasis. London: Imperial College Press; 2000. pp. 47–63.

[4] Feng Y, Xiao L. Zoonotic potential and molecular epidemiology of Giardia species and giardiasis. Clinical Microbiology Reviews. 2011;**24**:110–140. DOI: 10.1128/CMR.00033-10

[5] WHO. Global incidence and prevalence of selected curable sexually transmitted infections—2008 [Internet]. 2012. Available from: http://www.who.int/reproductivehealth/publications/rtis/stisestimates/en/[Accessed: 2016-10-03]

[6] Campbell WC, Rew RS. Chemotherapy of Parasitic Diseases. New York and London: Plenum Press; 2013. 684 p. DOI: 10.1007/978-1-4684-1233-8

[7] González U, Pinart M, Sinclair D, Firooz A, Enk C, Vélez ID, Esterhuizen TM, Tristan M, Alvar J. Vector and reservoir control for preventing leishmaniasis. The Cochrane Database of Systematic Reviews. 2015;(8):CD008736. DOI: 10.1002/14651858.CD008736.pub2

[8] Steinmann P, Stone CM, Sutherland CS, Tanner M, Tediosi F. Contemporary and emerging strategies for eliminating human African trypanosomiasis due to *Trypanosoma brucei* gambiense: review. Tropical Medicine & International Health. 2015;**20**(6):707–18. DOI: 10.1111/tmi.12483

[9] Benelli G, Mehlhorn, H. Declining malaria, rising of dengue and Zika virus: insights for mosquito vector control. Parasitology Research. 2016; **115**(5), 1747–1754. DOI: 10.1007/s00436-016-4971-z

[10] Sarjapuram N, Mekala N, Singh M, Tatu U. The potential of *Lactobacillus casei* and *Enterococcus faecium* combination as a preventive probiotic against Entamoeba. Probiotics and Antimicrobial Proteins. 2016. In press. DOI:10.1007/s12602-016-9232z

[11] Travers MA, Sow C, Zirah S, Deregnaucourt C, Chaouch S, Queiroz RM, Charneau S, Allain T, Florent I, Grellier P. Deconjugated bile salts produced by extracellular bile-salt hydrolase-like activities from the probiotic *Lactobacillus johnsonii* La1 inhibit giardia duodenalis in vitro growth. Frontiers in Microbiology. 2016;**7**:1453.

[12] Gressler LT, Da Silva AS, Machado G, Dalla Rosa L, Dorneles F, Gressler LT, Oliveira MS, Zanette RA, de Vargas AC, Monteiro SG. Susceptibility of Trypanosoma evansi to propolis extract in vitro and in experimentally infected rats. Research in Veterinary Science. 2012;**93**(3):1314–1317. DOI: 10.1016/j.rvsc.2012.02.007

[13] Higashi KO, de Castro SL. Propolis extracts are effective against Trypanosoma cruzi and have an impact on its interaction with host cells. Journal of Ethnopharmacology. 1994;**43** (2):149–155.

[14] García-Montoya IA, Cendón TS, Arévalo-Gallegos S, Rascón-Cruz Q. Lactoferrin a multiple bioactive protein: an overview. Biochimica et Biophysica Acta. 2012;**1820** (3) 226–236. DOI: 10.1016/j.bbagen.2011.06.018

[15] Khater HF. Prospects of botanical biopesticides in insect pest management. Pharmacologia. 2012;**3**: 641–656. DOI: 10.5567/pharmacologia.2012.641.656

[16] Khater HF. Bioactivity of essential oils as green biopesticides: recent global scenario. In: Govil JN, Bhattacharya S, editors. Recent Progress in Medicinal Plants, Vol. 37: Essentials Oils II. USA: Studium Press; 2013. pp. 151–218.

[17] Govindarajan M, Kadaikunnan S, Alharbi NS, Benelli G. Single-step biological fabrication of colloidal silver nanoparticles using Hugonia mystax: larvicidal potential against Zika virus, dengue, and malaria vector mosquitoes. Artificial Cells, Nanomedicine, and Biotechnology. 2016:1–9. DOI: 10.1080/21691401.1228664

[18] Govindarajan M, Vijayan P, Kadaikunnan S, Alharbi NS, Benelli G. One-pot biogenic fabrication of silver nanocrystals using Quisqualis indica: effectiveness on malaria and Zika virus mosquito vectors, and impact on non-target aquatic organisms. Journal of Photochemistry and Photobiology B. 2016;**162**:646–655. DOI: 10.1016/j.jphotobiol.2016.07.036

[19] Govindarajan M, Khater HF, Panneerselvam C, Benelli G. One-pot fabrication of silver nanocrystals using Nicandra physalodes: a novel route for mosquito vector control with moderate toxicity on non-target water bugs. Research in Veterinary Science. 2016;**107**:95–101. DOI: 10.1016/j.rvsc.2016.05.017

[20] Murugan K, Priyanka V, Dinesh D et al. Predation by Asian bullfrog tadpoles, Hoplobatrachus tigerinus, against the dengue vector, Aedes aegypti, in an aquatic environment treated with mosquitocidal nanoparticles. Parasitology Research. 2015;**114**:3601–3610. DOI:10.1007/s00436-015-4582-0

[21] Roni M, Murugan K, Panneerselvam C, Subramaniam J, Nicoletti M, Madhiyazhagan P, Dinesh D, Suresh U, Khater HF, Wei H, Canale A, Alarfaj AA, Munusamy MA, Higuchi A, Benelli G. Characterization and biotoxicity of Hypnea musciformis-synthesized silver nanoparticles as potential eco-friendly control tool against Aedes aegypti and Plutella xylostella. Ecotoxicology and Environmental Safety. 2015;**121**:31–38. DOI: 10.1016/j.ecoenv.2015.07.005

[22] Grimberg BT, Mehlotra RK. Expanding the Antimalarial Drug Arsenal-Now, But How? Pharmaceuticals. 201; **4**:681−712.

[23] Ogungbe IV, Setzer WN. The potential of secondary metabolites from plants as drugs or leads against protozoan neglected diseases—Part III: in-silico molecular docking investigations. Molecules. 2016;**21**(10). E1389.

[24] Demain AL, Fang A. The natural functions of secondary metabolites. Advances in Biochemical Engineering/Biotechnology. 2000;**69**:1–39.

[25] Callaway E, Cyranoski D. Anti-parasite drugs sweep Nobel prize in medicine 2015. Nature. 2015;**526**(7572):174–175. DOI: 10.1038/nature.2015.18507

[26] Argueta-Villamar A, Cano-Asseleih LM, Rodarte ML. Atlas de las plantas de la medicina tradicional Mexicana (Atlas of plants of traditional Mexican medicine). Mexico: Instituto Nacional Indigenista; 1994. 1786 p.

[27] Heinrich M, Frei Haller B, Leonti M. A perspective on natural products research and ethnopharmacology in Mexico: the eagle and the serpent on the prickly pear cactus. Journal of Natural Products. 2014;**77**(3):678–89. DOI: 10.1021/np4009927

[28] WHO. Fact Sheet: World Malaria Report 2015 [Internet]. 2015. Available from: http://www.who.int/malaria/media/world-malaria-report-2015/en/[Accessed: 2016-10-10]

[29] White NJ. Declining malaria transmission and pregnancy outcomes in Southern Mozambique. The New England Journal of Medicine. 2015;**373**:1670–1671. DOI: 10.1056/NEJMe1511278

[30] Cibulskis RE, Alonso P, Aponte J, Aregawi M, Barrette A, Bergeron L, et al. Malaria: global progress 2000–2015 and future challenges. Infectious Diseases of Poverty. 2016;**5**:61. DOI: 10.1186/s40249-016-0151-8

[31] Ngoubangoye B, Boundenga L, Arnathau C, Mombo IM, Durand P, Tsoumbou TA, et al. The host specificity of ape malaria parasites can be broken in confined environments. International Journal for Parasitology. 2016;**46**(11):737–744. DOI: 10.1016/j.ijpara.2016.06.004

[32] Molina-Cruz A, Canepa GE, Kamath N, Pavlovic NV, Mu J, Ramphul U N, Ramirez JL, et al. Plasmodium evasion of mosquito immunity and global malaria transmission: the lock-and-key theory. Proceedings of the National Academy of Sciences of the United States of America. 2015;**112**(49):15178–15183. DOI: 10.1073/pnas.1520426112

[33] Negi AS, Gupta A, Hamid AA. Combating malaria with plant molecules: a brief update. Current Medicinal Chemistry. 2014;**21**(4):458–500.

[34] Wallqvist A, Fang X, Tewari SG, Ye P, Reifman J. Metabolic host responses to malarial infection during the intraerythrocytic developmental cycle. BMC Systems Biology. 2016;**10**:58. DOI: 10.1186/s12918-016-0291-2

[35] Vangapandu S, Jain M, Kaur K, Patil P, Patel SR, Jain R. Recent advances in antimalarial drug development. Medicinal Research Reviews. 2007;**27**(1):65–107.

[36] Ashley EA, Dhorda M, Fairhurst RM, Amaratunga C, Lim P, Suon S, Sreng S, Tracking Resistance to Artemisinin Collaboration (TRAC). Spread of artemisinin resistance in plasmodium falciparum malaria. The New England Journal of Medicine. 2014;**371**:411–423. DOI: 10.1056/NEJMoa1314981

[37] Njokah MJ, Kang'ethe JN, Kinyua J, Kariuki D, Kimani FT. In vitro selection of *Plasmodium falciparum* Pfcrt and Pfmdr1 variants by artemisinin. Malaria Journal. 2016;**15** (1):381. DOI: 10.1186/s12936-016-1443-y

[38] Veiga MI, Dhingra SK, Henrich PP, Straimer J, Gnädig N, Uhlemann AC, Martin RE, et al. Globally prevalent PfMDR1 mutations modulate Plasmodium falciparum susceptibility to artemisinin-based combination therapies. Nature Communications. 2016;**7**:11553.

[39] Cohen J, Benns S, Vekemans J, Leach A, Schnermann L. Development of the RTS, S/AS vaccine candidate from concept to phase III. In: Mehlhorn H, editor. Progress in Parasitology. Parasitology Research Monographs: Springer; 2011. Vol. 2, pp. 121–133.

[40] WHO. Background paper: malaria vaccine RTS, S/AS01 [Internet]. 2015. Available from: http://www.who.int/immunization/sage/meetings/2015/october/1_Final_malaria_vaccine_background_paper_v2015_09_30.pdf [Accessed: 2016-09-15]

[41] Long CA, Zavala F. Malaria vaccines and human immune responses. Current Opinion in Microbiology. 2016;**32**:96–102. DOI: 10.1016/j.mib.2016.04.006

[42] Schmidt TJ, Khalid SA, Romanha AJ, Alves TMA, Biavatti MW, Brun R, Da Costa FB, et al. The potential of secondary metabolites from plants as drugs or leads against protozoan neglected diseases—part I. Current Medicinal Chemistry. 2012;**19**:2128–2175.

[43] Schmidt TJ, Khalid SA, Romanha AJ, Alves TMA, Biavatti MW, Brun R, et al. The potential of secondary metabolites from plants as drugs or leads against protozoan neglected diseases—part II. Current Medicinal Chemistry. 2012;**19**:2176–2228.

[44] Noster S, Kraus LJ. In vitro antimalarial activity of Coutarea latiflora and Exostema caribaeum extracts on Plasmodium falciparum. Planta Medica. 1990;56(1):63–65.

[45] Köhler I, Jenett-Siems K, Mockenhaupt FP, Siems K, Jakupovic J, González JC, Hernández MA, et al. In vitro antiplasmodial activity of 4-phenylcoumarins from Exostema mexicanum. Planta Medica. 2001;**67**(1):89–91.

[46] Argotte-Ramos R, Ramírez-Avila G, Rodríguez-Gutiérrez MC, Ovilla-Muñoz M, Lanz-Mendoza H, Rodríguez MH, Gonzalez-Cortazar M, et al. Antimalarial 4-phenylcoumarins from the stem bark of Hintonia latiflora. Journal of Natural Products. 2006;**69**(10):1442–1444.

[47] Rivera N, López PY, Rojas M, Fortoul TI, Reynada DY, Reyes AJ, Rivera E, et al. Antimalarial efficacy, cytotoxicity, and genotoxicity of methanolic stem bark extract from Hintonia latiflora in a *Plasmodium yoelii yoelii* lethal murine malaria model. Parasitology Research. 2014;**113**(4):1529–1536. DOI: 10.1007/s00436-014-3797-9

[48] Malagon, F, Vazquez, J, Delgado, G, Ruiz A. Antimalaric effect of an alcoholic extract of Artemisia ludoviciana mexicana in a rodent malaria model. Parassitologia. 1997;**39** (1):3–7.

[49] Ankli A, Heinrich M, Bork P, Wolfram L, Bauerfeind P, Brun, R. Schmid C, et al. Yucatec Mayan medicinal plants: evaluation based on indigenous uses. Journal of Ethnopharmacology. 2002;**79**(1):43–52.

[50] WHO. Chagas Disease (American Trypanosomiasis) [Internet]. 2016. Available from: http://www.who.int/mediacentre/factsheets/fs340/en/[Accessed: 2016-09-22]

[51] Hotez PJ, Dumonteil E, Cravioto MB, Bottazzi ME, Tapia-Conyer R, Meymandi S, Karunakara U, et al. An unfolding tragedy of chagas disease in North America. PLoS Neglected Tropical Diseases. 2013;**7**(10):e2300. DOI:10.1371/journal.pntd.0002300

[52] Vilar-Pereira G, Ruivo LA de S, Lannes-Vieira J. Behavioural alterations are independent of sickness behaviour in chronic experimental Chagas disease. Memórias do Instituto Oswaldo Cruz. 2015;**110**(8):1042-1050. DOI: 10.1590/0074-02760150300

[53] Porcal W, Hernández P, Boiani L, Boiani M, Ferreira A, Chidichimo A, Cazzulo JJ, et al. New trypanocidal hybrid compounds from the association of hydrazone moieties and benzofuroxan heterocycle. Bioorganic and Medicinal Chemistry. 2008;**16**(14):6995–7004. DOI: 10.1016/j.bmc.2008.05.038

[54] Abe F, Nagafuji S, Yamauchi T, Okabe H, Maki J, Higo H, Akahane H, et al. Trypanocidal constituents in plants 1. Evaluation of some Mexican plants for their trypanocidal activity and active constituents in Guaco, roots of *Aristolochia taliscana*. Biological & Pharmaceutical Bulletin. 2002;**25**(9):1188–1191.

[55] Abe F, Nagafuji S, Okawa M, Kinjo J, Akahane H, Ogura T, Martinez-Alfaro MA, et al. Trypanocidal constituents in plants 5. Evaluation of some Mexican plants for their trypanocidal activity and active constituents in the seeds of *Persea americana*. Biological & Pharmaceutical Bulletin. 2005;**28**(7):1314–1317.

[56] Jimenez-Coello M, Acosta-Viana KY, Guzman-Marin E, Perez GC, Perez GMS. Antitrypanosomal activity of (8-hydroxymethylen)-trieicosanyl acetate against infective forms of Trypanosoma cruzi. Pharmaceutical Biology. 2010;**48**:666–671. DOI: 10.3109/13880200903241853

[57] Jimenez-Coello M, Guzman-Marin E, Perez-Gutierrez S, Polanco-Hernandez GM, Acosta-Viana KY. Antitrypanosomal activity of Senna villosa in infected BALB/c mice with Trypanosoma cruzi during the subacute phase of infection. African Journal of Traditional, Complementary, and Alternative Medicines. 2011;**8**(5 Suppl):164–169. DOI: 10.4314/ajtcam.v8i5S.21

[58] Molina-Garza ZJ, Bazaldúa-Rodríguez AF, Quintanilla-Licea R, Galaviz-Silva L. Anti-Trypanosoma cruzi activity of 10 medicinal plants used in northeast Mexico. Acta Tropica. 2014;**136**:14–18. DOI: 10.1016/j.actatropica.2014.04.006

[59] Pérez-Treviño KC, Molina-Garza ZJ, Galaviz-Silva L. Evaluación de la actividad antitrypanosomal de extractos metanólicos de plantas con uso medicinal (Evaluation of antitrypanosomal activity of methanol extract from medicinal plants). Entomología Mexicana. 2016;**3**:656–659.

[60] Jimenez-Coello M, Acosta-Viana KY, Ortega-Pacheco A, Perez-Gutierrez S, Guzman-Marin E. In vivo antiprotozoal activity of the chloroform extract from *Carica papaya* seeds against amastigote stage of trypanosoma cruzi during indeterminate and chronic phase of infection. Evidence-based Complementary and Alternative Medicine: eCAM. 2014;**2014**:458263. DOI: 10.1155/2014/458263

[61] Murray HW, Berman JD, Davies CR, Saravia NG. Advances in leishmaniasis. Lancet. 2005;**366**(9496):1561–1577.

[62] Dey A, Singh S. Transfusion transmitted leishmaniasis: a case report and review of literature. Indian Journal of Medical Microbiology. 2006;**24**(3):165–170.

[63] Von Stebut, E. Leishmaniasis. Journal der Deutschen Dermatologischen Gesellschaft. 2015;**13** (3):191–201. DOI: 10.1111/ddg.12595

[64] WHO. Leishmaniasis [Internet]. 2016. Available from: http://www.who.int/leishmaniasis/en/[Accessed: 2016-09-11]

[65] Lezama-Davila CM, Isaac-Márquez AP, Zamora-Crescencio P, Uc-Encalada Mdel R, Justiniano-Apolinar SY, del Angel-Robles L, Satoskar A, et al. Leishmanicidal activity of Pentalinon andrieuxii. Fitoterapia. 2007;**78**(3):255–257.

[66] Pan L, Lezama-Davila CM, Isaac-Marquez AP, Calomeni EP, Fuchs JR, Satoskar AR, Kinghorn AD. Sterols with antileishmanial activity isolated from the roots of Pentalinon andrieuxii. Phytochemistry. 2012; **82**:128–135. DOI: 10.1016/j.phytochem.2012.06.012

[67] Martínez Ruiz MG, Richard-Greenblatt M, Juárez ZN, Av-Gay Y, Bach H, Hernández LR. Antimicrobial, anti-inflammatory, antiparasitic, and cytotoxic activities of Laennecia confusa. The Scientific World Journal. 2012;**2012**:263572. DOI: 10.1100/2012/263572

[68] Cruz-Paredes C, Bolívar Balbás P, Gómez-Velasco A, Juárez ZN, Sánchez Arreola E, Hernández LR, Bach H. Antimicrobial, antiparasitic, anti-Inflammatory, and cytotoxic activities of Lopezia racemosa. The Scientific World Journal. 2013; **2013**, 237438. DOI: 10.1155/2013/237438

[69] Haque R, Ali IK, Akther S, Petri WA Jr. Comparison of PCR, isoenzyme analysis, and antigen detection for diagnosis of Entamoeba histolytica infection. Journal of Clinical Microbiology. 1998;**36**(2):449–452.

[70] Stanley SL. Pathophysiology of amoebiasis. Trends in Parasitology. 2001;**17**(6):280–285.

[71] Ackers JP, Mirelman D. Progress in research on *Entamoeba histolytica* pathogenesis. Current Opinion in Microbiology. 2006;**9**:367–373.

[72] Thompson SC. Giardia lamblia in children and the child care setting: a review of the literature. Journal of Paediatrics and Child Health. 1994;**30**: 202–209.

[73] Aguirre-Cruz ML, Valadez-Salazar A, Muñoz O. In vitro sensitivity of *Entamoeba histolytica* to metronidazole. Archivos de Investigación Médica. 1990;**1**:23–26.

[74] Oxberry ME, Thompson RCA, Reynolds JA. Evaluation of the effects of albendazole and metronidazole on the ultrastructure of *Giardia duodenalis, Trichomonas vaginalis* and *Spironucleus muris* using transmission electron microscopy. International Journal for Parasitology. 1994; **24**:695–703.

[75] Kapoor K, Chandra M, Nag D, Paliwal JK, Gupta RC, Saxena RC. Evaluation of metronidazole toxicity: a prospective study. International Journal of Clinical Pharmacology Research. 1999;**19**:83–88.

[76] Arrieta J, Reyes B, Calzada F, Cedillo-Rivera R, Navarrete A. Amoebicidal and giardicidal compounds from the leaves of *Zanthoxylum Liebmannianun*. Fitoterapia. 2001;**72**: 295–297.

[77] Calzada F, Velázquez C, Cedillo-Rivera R, Esquivel B. Antiprotozoal activity of the constituents of Teloxys graveolens. Phytotherapy Research. 2003;**17**(7):731–732.

[78] Alanís AD, Calzada F, Cedillo-Rivera R, Meckes M. Antiprotozoal activity of the constituents of Rubus coriifolius. Phytotherapy Research. 2003;**17**(6):681–682.

[79] Calzada F, Cervantes-Martínez JA, Yépez-Mulia L. In vitro antiprotozoal activity from the roots of *Geranium mexicanum* and its constituents on Entamoeba histolytica and Giardia lamblia. Journal of Ethnopharmacology 2005;**98**(1–2):191–193.

[80] Said FS, Ramos GMC, Mata CBD, Vargas VJ, Villarreal TL. In vitro antiprotozoal activity of the leaves of Artemisia ludoviciana. Fitoterapia. 2005;**76**(5):466–468.

[81] Ramos-Guerra MC, Mata-Cárdenas BD, Vargas-Villarreal J, Sampayo-Reyes A, González-Salazar F, Morales-Vallarta M, Said-Fernández S. In vitro activity of organic leaf/stem extracts from *Marrubium vulgare and Mentha spicata* against *Entamoeba histolytica* and *Giardia lamblia*. Pharmacology online. 2007;**1**:108–112.

[82] Calzada F, Yepez-Mulia L, Tapia-Contreras A, Ortega A. Antiprotozoal and antibacterial properties of Decachaeta incompta. Revista Latinoamericana de Química. 2009;**37**: 97–103.

[83] Velázquez-Domínguez J, Marchat LA, López-Camarillo C, Mendoza-Hernández G, Sánchez-Espíndola E, Calzada F, Ortega-Hernández A, et al. Effect of the sesquiterpene lactone incomptine A in the energy metabolism of Entamoeba histolytica. Experimental Parasitology. 2013;**135**(3):503–510. DOI: 10.1016/j.exppara.2013.08.015

[84] Calzada F, Yepez-Mulia L, Tapia-Contreras A, Bautista E, Maldonado E, Ortega A. Evaluation of the antiprotozoal activity of neo-clerodane type diterpenes from Salvia polystachya against Entamoeba histolytica and Giardia lamblia. Phytotherapy Research. 2010;**24**(5):662–665. DOI: 10.1002/ptr.2938

[85] Calzada F, Yépez-Mulia L, Aguilar A. In vitro susceptibility of Entamoeba histolytica and Giardia lamblia to plants used in Mexican traditional medicine for the treatment of gastrointestinal disorders. Journal of Ethnopharmacology. 2006;**108**(3):367–370.

[86] Camacho-Corona MR, García A, Mata-Cárdenas BD, Garza-González E, Ibarra-Alvarado C, Rojas-Molina A, Rojas-Molina I, et al. Screening for antibacterial and antiprotozoal activities of crude extracts derived from Mexican medicinal plants. The African Journal of Traditional, Complementary and Alternative Medicines. 2015;**12** (3):104–112.

[87] Calzada F, Barbosa E, Cedillo-Rivera R. Antiamoebic activity of benzyl glucosinolate from *Lepidium virginicum*. Phytotherapy Research. 2003;**17**(6):618–619.

[88] Quintanilla-Licea R, Mata-Cárdenas BD, Vargas-Villarreal J, Bazaldúa-Rodríguez AF, Kavimngeles-Hernández I, Garza-González JN, Hernández-García ME.· Antiprotozoal activity against Entamoeba histolytica of plants used in northeast Mexican traditional medicine. Bioactive compounds from *Lippia graveolens* and *Ruta chalepensis*. Molecules. 2014;**19**(12):21044–21065. DOI: 10.3390/molecules191221044

[89] Herrera-Martínez M, Hernández-Ramírez VI, Hernández-Carlos B, Chávez-Munguía B, Calderón-Oropeza MA, Talamás-Rohana P. Antiamoebic activity of Adenophyllum aurantium (L.) Strother and its effect on the actin cytoskeleton of Entamoeba histolytica. Frontiers in Pharmacology. 2016;**7**:169. DOI: 10.3389/fphar.2016.00169

[90] Ponce-Macotela M, Navarro-Alegría I, Martínez-Gordillo MN, Alvarez C. Efecto antigiardiásico in vitro de 14 extractos de plantas (In vitro anti-Giardia effect of 14 plants extracts). Revista de Investigación Clínica. 1994;**46**:343–347.

[91] Ponce-Macotela M, Rufino-González Y, Mora-de-la-Mora JI, González MA, Reynoso-Robles R, Martinez-Gordillo M. Mortality and morphological changes in *Giardia duodenalis* induced by exposure to ethanolic extracts of *Justicia spicigera*. Proceedings of the Western Pharmacology Society. 2001;**44**:151–152.

[92] Ponce-Macotela M, Rufino-Gonzáles Y, Gonzáles-Maciel A, Reynoso-Robles R, Martinez-Gordilho MN. Orégano (*Lippia* spp.) kills *Giardia duodenalis* trophozoites *in vitro*: antigiardasic and ultrastructural damage. Parasitology Research. 2006;**98**: 557–569.

[93] Peraza-Sánchez S, Poot-Kantún S, Torres-Tapia LW, May-Pat F, Simá-Polanco P, Cedillo-Rivera R. Screening of native plants from Yucatan for anti-*Giardia lamblia* activity. Pharmaceutical Biology.2005; **43**:594–598.

[94] Mena-Rejón GJ, Pérez-Espadas AR, Moo-Puc RE, Cedillo-Rivera R, Bazzocchi IL, Jiménez-Diaz IA, Quijano L. Antigiardial activity of triterpenoids from root bark of Hippocratea excelsa. Journal of Natural Products. 2007;**70**(5):863–865.

[95] Barbosa E, Calzada F, Campos R. In vivo antigiardial activity of three flavonoids isolated of some medicinal plants used in Mexican traditional medicine for the treatment of diarrhea. Journal of Ethnopharmacology. 2007;**109**(3):552–554.

[96] Hernández-Chávez I, Torres-Tapia LW, Simá-Polanco P, Cedillo-Rivera R, Moo-Puc P, Peraza-Sánchez SR. Antigiardial activity of Cupania dentata bark and its constituents. Journal of Mexican Chemical Society. 2012;**56**(2):105–108.

[97] WHO. Global incidence and prevalence of selected curable sexually transmitted infections—2008 [Internet]. 2012. Available from: http://www.who.int/reproductivehealth/publications/rtis/stisestimates/en/[Accessed: 2016-10-10]

[98] Secretaría de Salud. SUIVE/DGE/SALUD/Información Epidemiológica de Morbilidad, Anuario 2011 (SUIVE/DGE/SALUD/ Epidemiológic Information on Morbility, Yearbook 2011). Versión Ejecutiva [Internet]. 2012. Available from: http://www.epidemiologia.salud.gob.mx/doctos/infoepid/publicaciones/2012/ver_ejecutiva_2011.pdf [Accessed: 2016-09-10]

[99] Carlton JM, Hirt RP, Silva JC, Delcher AL, Schatz M, Zhao Q, Wortman JR, et al. Draft genome sequence of the sexually transmitted pathogen *Trichomonas vaginalis*. Science. 2007;**315**(5809):207–212.

[100] Cotch MF, Pastorek JG 2nd, Nugent RP, Hillier SL, Gibbs RS, Martin DH, Eschenbach DA, et al. *Trichomonas vaginalis* associated with low birth weight and preterm delivery. The Vaginal Infections and Prematurity Study Group. Sexually Transmitted Diseases. 1997;**24**:353–360.

[101] Sorvillo F, Kerndt P. *Trichomonas vaginalis* and amplification of HIV-1 transmission. Lancet. 1998;**351**:213–214.

[102] Boselli F, Chiossi G, Bortolamasi M, Gallinelli A. Prevalence and determinants of genital shedding of herpes simplex virus among women attending Italian colposcopy clinics. European Journal of Obstetrics, Gynecology, and Reproductive Biology. 2005;**118**(1):86–90.

[103] Sena AC, Lensing S, Rompalo A, Taylor SN, Martin DH, Lopez LM, Lee JY, et al. Chlamydia trachomatis, Mycoplasma genitalium, and *Trichomonas vaginalis* infections in men with nongonococcal urethritis: predictors and persistence after therapy. The Journal of Infectious Diseases. 2012;**206**:357–365. DOI: 10.1093/infdis/jis356

[104] Sutcliffe S, Neace C, Magnuson NS, Reeves R, Alderete JF. Trichomonosis, a common curable STI, and prostate carcinogenesis - a proposed molecular mechanism. PLoS Pathogens. 2012;**8**:e1002801. DOI: 10.1371/journal.ppat.1002801

[105] Wendel KA, Workowski KA. Trichomoniasis: challenges to appropriate management. Clinical Infectious Diseases. 2007;**44** Suppl. 3:S123–129.

[106] Müller M, Lossick JG, Gorell TE. In vitro susceptibility of *Trichomonas vaginalis* to metronidazole and treatment outcome in vaginal trichomoniasis. Sexually Transmitted Diseases. 1988;**15**:17e249.

[107] Upcroft JA, Dunn LA, Wright JM, Benakli K, Upcroft P, Vanelle P. 5-Nitroimidazole drugs effective against metronidazole-resistant *Trichomonas vaginalis* and Giardia duodenalis spp. Antimicrobial Agents and Chemotherapy. 2006;**50**:344–347.

[108] Krashin JW, Koumans EH, Bradshaw-Sydnor AC, Braxton JR, Evan Secor W, Sawyer MK, Markowitz LE. *Trichomonas vaginalis* prevalence, incidence, risk factors and antibiotic-resistance in an adolescent population. Sexually Transmitted Diseases. 2010;**37**(7):440–444. DOI: 10.1097/OLQ.0b013e3181cfcd8c

[109] Schwebke JR, Barrientes FJ. Prevalence of *Trichomonas vaginalis* isolates with resistance to metronidazole and tinidazole. Antimicrobial Agents and Chemotherapy. 2006;**50**:4209–4210.

[110] Calzada F, Yépez-Mulia L, Tapia-Contreras A. Effect of Mexican medicinal plant used to treat trichomoniasis on *Trichomonas vaginalis* trophozoites. Journal of Ethnopharmacology. 2007;**113**(2):248–251.

[111] Moo-Puc R, Robledo D, Freile-Pelegrin Y. Evaluation of selected tropical seaweeds for in vitro anti-trichomonal activity. Journal of Ethnopharmacology. 2008;**120**(1):92–97.

[112] Chan-Bacab MJ, Pena-Rodríguez LM. Plant natural products with leishmanicidal activity. Natural Product Reports. 2001;**18**:674–688.

[113] Zubia M, Robledo D, Freile-Pelegrin Y. Antioxidant activities in tropical marine macroalgae from the Yucatan Peninsula, Mexico. Journal of Applied Phycology. 2007;**19**:449–458.

[114] Cantillo-Ciau Z, Moo-Puc R, Quijano L, Freile-Pelegrín Y. The tropical brown alga Lobophora variegata: a source of antiprotozoal compounds. Marine Drugs. 2010;**8**(4):1292–1304. DOI: 10.3390/md8041292

[115] Asaolu MF, Asaolu SS, Oyeyemi AO, Aluko BT. Hypolipemic effects of methanolic extract of *Persea americana* seeds in hypercholesterolemic rats. Journal of Medicine and Medical Sciences. 2010;**1**(4):126–128.

[116] Edem D, Ekanem I, Ebong P. Effect of aqueous extracts of alligator pear seed (*Persea americana* Mill.) on blood glucose and histopathology of pancreas in alloxan-induced diabetic rats. Pakistan Journal of Pharmaceutical Sciences. 2009;**22**(3):272–276.

[117] Giffoni LJ, Salles EH, Aguiar R, Nogueira RS, Costa JJ, Medeiros SL, De Morais S, et al. Chemical composition, toxicity and larvicity and antifungal activities of *Persea americana* (avocado) seed extracts. Revista da Sociedade Brasileira de Medicina Tropical. 2009;**42**:110–113.

[118] Raymond Chia TW, Dykes GA. Antimicrobial activity of crude epicarp and seed extracts from mature avocado fruit (*Persea americana*) of three cultivars. Pharmaceutical Biology. 2011;**48**(7):753–756.

[119] Jiménez-Arellanes A, Luna-Herrera J, Ruiz-Nicolás R, Cornejo-Garrido J, Tapia A, Yépez-Mulia L. Antiprotozoal and antimycobacterial activities of *Persea americana* seeds. BMC Complementary and Alternative Medicine. 2013;**13**:109. DOI: 10.1186/1472–6882-13-109

Chapter 4

Can the Cure for Chagas' Disease be Found in Nature?

Nelissa Pacheco Vaz

Additional information is available at the end of the chapter

http://dx.doi.org/10.5772/67225

Abstract

Nature is a skilled factory that produces a wide variety of secondary metabolites known as natural products. Those compounds synthesized by living organisms are usually related to their vital processes. Many drugs used nowadays, had its origins in medicinal plants and other organisms such as herbs, fungi and sponges. Hence, those sources constitute a viable alternative to conventional medicine in many developing countries. In other hand, protozoan diseases like Chagas, represent a health threat causing mortality to populations around the world. The classic treatment for Chagas' disease is chemotherapic and includes benznidazole and nifurtimox, although, the search for new drugs still remains. Triatomines that may spread Chagas can also be controlled making use of the insecticide property of certain plants. After literature survey it was found, classes of natural products, plant extracts, essential oils, and other natural sources that have shown activity against *T. cruzi*. In this context, many substances were tested *in vitro* and *in vivo* assays to verify trypanocidal efficacy. Promising results were published regarding to compounds arising from plants and sponges that showed high toxicity on different forms of the parasite with low toxicity on mammalian cells, although few were clinically tested on Chagas' disease.

Keywords: medicinal plants, natural products chemistry, Chagas' disease, *Trypanosoma cruzi*

1. Introduction

Plants have been used for many centuries with the purpose of feeding populations worldwide and to establish or bring back health, well-being, and the cure for several illnesses. The use of medicinal plants is very advantageous in terms of resource on chemical and biological research in natural products area. The plant secondary metabolism yields a wide range of chemical compounds, most of them highly bioactive and whose structural diversity is continuously evolving together with plants [1]. In vegetables, these compounds are the main responsible for chemical defence against fungi, phytopathogens, birds, and other natural predators, being also used by plants to attract pollinators as well, being indispensable to guarantee plant's survival and its spreading through the globe. However, human population takes advantage of these remarkable properties and uses some compounds produced by diverse organisms including plants, fungi, and sponges to develop new medicines. Those metabolites coming from natural sources will promote the desirable healing action, bringing fewer side effects to the users.

In addition to teas, infusions, plasters, and herbal medicines, many traditional "western drugs" that are widely used nowadays had its origins on medicinal plants, such as (1) aspirin (acetylsalicylic acid—*Spiraea* spp.), (2) artemisinin (sweet wormwood—*Artemisia annua*), and more recently, (3) taxol (or paclitaxel from Pacific yew—*Taxus brevifolia*) on **Figure 1** can exemplify [2]. Therefore, nature is an endless source of bioactive substances, as plants can convert just carbon dioxide and water through photosynthesis to produce highly complex organic molecules that could be very useful in human health.

Medicinal plant species constitute a valuable alternative to conventional medicine in many developing countries; especially in poor communities that inhabit rural areas, lacking access to health services. Several of them use plants as the primary health care, as teas, plasters, infusions, and ointments among others. The traditional use of medicinal plants and natural remedies with no established efficacy and safety is a widespread in many countries around the world. Accordingly, all the information about ethnobotany is of utmost importance: this kind of millenary knowledge built during centuries usually combines information from native indigenous culture, together with acquirements brought by the Europeans and the Africans and provides a more rational use for the local biodiversity.

In other hand, protozoan diseases represent an important health threat in countries of tropical and subtropical regions, causing mortality to their populations [3]. Many neglected tropical diseases (NTDs) transmitted by parasites are reported to have life cycles including man as a secondary host, in which they cause disease. About 37 million individuals are presently

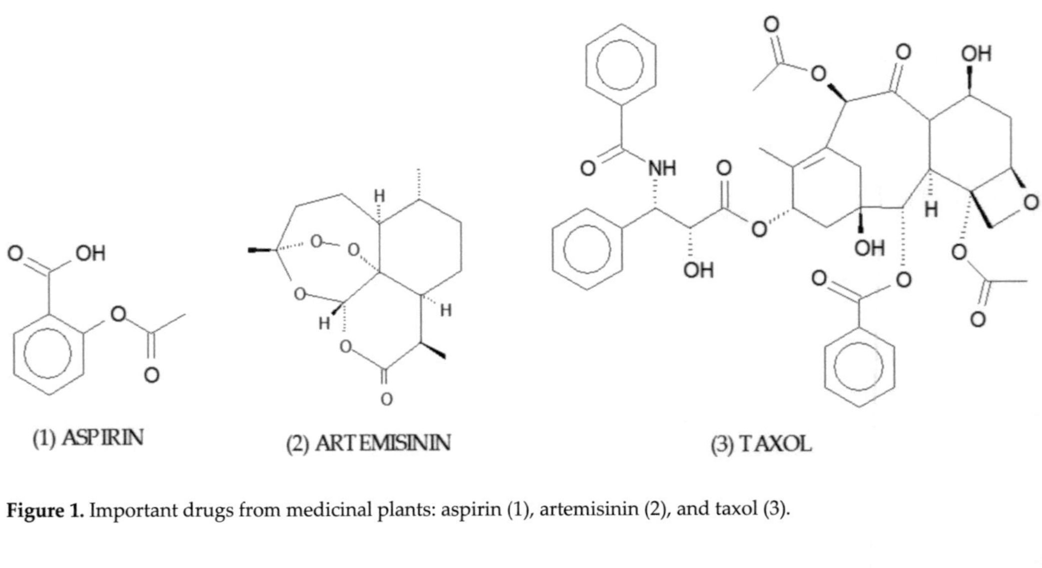

(1) ASPIRIN (2) ARTEMISININ (3) TAXOL

Figure 1. Important drugs from medicinal plants: aspirin (1), artemisinin (2), and taxol (3).

infected by parasites around the world. Together with malaria and amoebiasis, the parasitic illnesses are the main cause of thereabout one million deaths per year. Infections caused by protozoan species such as *Trypanosoma, Plasmodium,* and *Leishmania* are a major worldwide health problem causing significant morbidity and mortality in the poorest countries like Africa, Asia, and Latin America for instance.

Leishmaniasis, Chagas' disease, and human African trypanosomiasis (HAT) are among the most important protozoan parasitic illnesses caused by trypanosomatids. Chagas' disease, also known as American trypanosomiasis, is a widespread disease, caused by the kinetoplastid protozoan Tripanosome—*Trypanosoma cruzi.* It is estimated that about 8 million in America are currently infected. However, this disease is expanding worldwide due to migration phenomena. The parasites that have a kinetoplast and a single flagellum are characterized as *Trypanosomatids* [3].

That's why Chagas is recognized as one of the most devastating diseases caused by the parasites of the *Trypanosomatidae* family. The most epidemiologically important form of transmission is through the bite of vector, triatomine hematophagous insects such as *Triatoma infestans* (kissing bug or barbeiro in Brazil). Nevertheless, congenital and transfusion are also relevant for the transmission cycle, since they are responsible for the advancement of this disease in nonendemic areas [4]. These diseases represent significant health problems in endemic countries, and this situation is aggravated by the increasing on treatment failures with available drugs as we will discuss in detail later.

This chapter is therefore aimed to review the great potential of natural products that are available in nature (mainly plants and sponges) regarding to the prevention and treatment of Chagas' disease and the combat of triatomine bugs.

2. Neglected tropical diseases

Neglected tropical diseases (NTDs) are often chronic and debilitating illnesses that currently affect over one billion people worldwide. NTDs are a diverse group of infectious diseases that affect primarily rural and low-income populations residing in tropical and subtropical regions worldwide. The World Health Organization (WHO) officially recognized nowadays 17 NTDs, comprising a highly diverse group of bacterial, protozoan, and helminth infections, transmitted via insects, contaminated food, water, and soil, and/or through human-to-human contact. These diseases cause easily over 200,000 deaths per year affecting many millions more around the globe, although the number of new infections appears to be dwindling. NTDs include the three major protozoan diseases: human African trypanosomiasis (HAT or "sleeping sickness"), Chagas' disease, and leishmaniasis [5]. Dengue, foodborne trematodiases, leprosy, lymphatic filariasis, schistosomiasis, soil transmitted helminthiasis, and trachoma [6] are also classified as NTDs.

The socioeconomic impact of NTDs in the developing countries surpasses that of any other infectious disease (with exception of HIV/AIDS) and perhaps may have permanent socioeconomic effects on many nations. It is such a waste that billions of dollars of productivity are lost to NTDs every year in treatment and prevention costs, besides bearing 149 countries plus the information that the threat of NTDs is no longer confined to nations where these diseases are endemic. Due to globalization and the increasing social, financial, and technological connectedness, the burden to carry NTDs has become global issues.

Massive efforts of community activists, health care workers, scientists, politicians, and economists are required to reduce significantly the significance of public health liability that NTDs oblige. The most effective approach for reducing these diseases is still prevention, due to the absence of affordable or effective curative therapies and the deficiency of preventive vaccines. Between such relevant public health issues and many lives directly or indirectly affected by NTDs, there is education that offers a solution to connect NTD prevention to treatment efforts [7].

2.1. Chagas' disease

Trypanosomiasis is a group of parasitic diseases caused by protozoan from *Trypanosoma* genus. It is caused by trypanosomes of the species *Trypanosoma brucei*. There are two types that infect humans, *Trypanosoma brucei gambiense* (Tbg) and *Trypanosoma brucei rhodesiense* (Tbr). Tbg causes over 98% of reported cases. Both are usually transmitted by the bite of an infected tsetse fly and are most common in rural areas. African trypanosomiasis is a major cause of death in sub-Saharan Africa and poses a major health and economic burden in these regions with an estimated 60 million people at risk of contracting this disease, which is fatal if left untreated [8].

In 1909, the Brazilian physician and researcher Carlos Chagas discovered the etiologic agent of American trypanosomiasis *Trypanosoma cruzi* for which the name was given in honor to his friend Oswaldo Cruz. Since then, this illness received his name and is known worldwide as Chagas' disease [9]. It affects mainly heart and gastrointestinal systems many times being fatal to the bearer. The geographical distribution of reservoirs and vectors of Chagas' infection extends from the Southern USA to Southern Argentina and Chile. Nowadays, it is estimated that 8 million people in Latin America are infected with this pathogen, and 100,000 people are at risk of contracting it each year. Chagas' is also spreading to the USA, Canada, and many parts of Europe and the Western Pacific mainly due migratory flows [10]. There is an estimative that more than 400,000 individuals are currently infected in nonendemic areas like in USA and European countries [11]. These parasites are primarily transmitted by the bite of triatomine bugs from *Triatoma, Rhodnius,* and *Panstrongylus* genus [12].

Fever, headache, enlarged lymph glands, and swelling of the eyelid, close to the site of the bite of the insect, are some of the more common mild symptoms of the initial American trypanosomiasis acute phase. This infection is characterized by two distinct clinical stages: the acute phase, with high parasitemia, commonly progresses to a subsequent state of latency, and the chronic phase, with clinical manifestations in various organs. The most common symptoms characteristic of the chronic phase are enlargement of heart ventricles

http://dx.doi.org/10.5772/67225

and enlarged esophagus or colon [13], and these manifestations are occasionally life threatening [14].

2.1.1. *Trypanosoma cruzi—life cycle and transmission*

Chagas' infection has a wild cycle in nature that exists for millions of years. It is believed that some accidental cases involving humans might have happened at the time, similarly as they occur nowadays: when mankind invades vectors' wild ecotope or when triatomine bugs invade human domiciles. However, *T. cruzi* has been identified infecting human mummies only between 4000 and 9000 years ago. [9, 15].

Triatomines have been known since the sixteenth century but they have only settled down on human households with the beginning of the agricultural cycle. The increasing deforestation through the centuries that marked the livestock cycle leads to the removal of the native animals that once were the main sources of nourishment for the triatomines. Hence, these bugs have adapted progressively to inhabit areas surrounding human residences and the interiors of these dwellings. When humans invaded wild ecotopes and became infected, the transmission of Chagas' disease ceased to be treated as an enzootic disease of wild animals and is so called anthropozoonosis [15].

It is reported for *T. cruzi* to have wild, peridomestic, and domestic life cycles in nature: the wild cycle is merely enzootic and involves triatomine bugs and wild animals, such as rats and common opossum—*Didelphis marsupialis* for example. Meanwhile, the peridomestic cycle is derived from the wild cycle, keeping the infection among domestic animals in areas circumjacent of human residences, through the action of peridomestic triatomines and eventually through interchanges with the wild cycle (like dogs or cats hunting wild animals and wild animals invading areas surrounding human dwellings) [9]. The domestic cycle is characterized by enfold domesticated triatomines that are involved on the transmission of the infection from domestic animals to humans and between humans as well.

In this way, it is possible to perceive that *Trypanosoma cruzi* has a very complex biological cycle, involving several species of triatomines, Trypanosomatids in different stages of growth, wild and domestic mammals, and humans [16]. There are different forms of the *T. cruzi* parasite related to their stage of development: trypomastigote, epimastigote, and amastigote (**Figure 2**).

After triatomines bite an infected mammalian, they ingest the trypomastigotes form of *T. cruzi* from animal bloodstream. Inside the posterior intestine of the triatomine, the trypomastigotes transform into epimastigotes, which are able to proliferate and differentiate into metacyclic forms [17]. These parasitic forms are eliminated by triatomines through the feces, being able to invade new vertebrate cells, where they infect mainly macrophages or cardiac and smooth muscle fibers. Inside the mammalians, they undergo another round of differentiation into the proliferative intracellular amastigote forms. The amastigotes proliferate inside the host cell and give origin to new trypomastigotes when they reach the host's bloodstream. After trypomastigotes arrive at the circulatory system, the infection is disseminated [5].

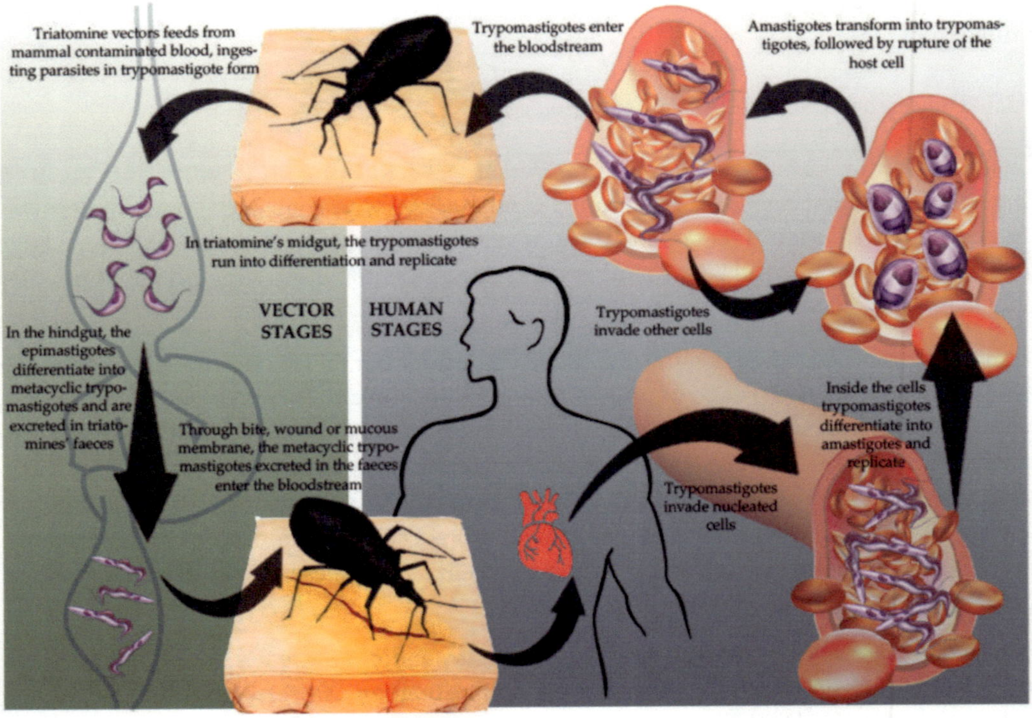

Figure 2. Life cycle of *Trypanosoma cruzi* parasite in triatomine insects and humans.

It is reported that the transmission mechanisms for Chagas' infection can be divided into two distinct groups [9]:

- Principal mechanisms: by means of triatomines (representing around 70% of the cases), blood transfusion (up to 20% of the cases), oral transmission, contaminated food, and placental or birth canal transmission;
- Secondary mechanisms: by means of management of infected animals, organ transplants, laboratory accidents, wounds, sexual transmission, contact with menstrual fluid, or sperm contaminated with parasites, and also, the hypothetic cases of purposeful criminal inoculation and contamination of food with *T. cruzi*.

2.1.2. Traditional Chagas' treatment

The challenge on searching for new Chagas' disease drugs remains for decades. Nowadays, the usual recommended traditional treatment is chemotherapic including either one of the two nitro-aromatic heterocyclic compounds (**Figure 3**) benznidazole (4) and nifurtimox (5).

As cited previously, this infection is clinically characterized by two distinct stages: the acute usually asymptomatic phase, defined by high parasitemia, and a long chronic and progressive phase in which symptoms can manifest after some years. When the patient is in the acute phase of the infection, the treatment with these drugs can cure up to 80% of the cases.

http://dx.doi.org/10.5772/67225

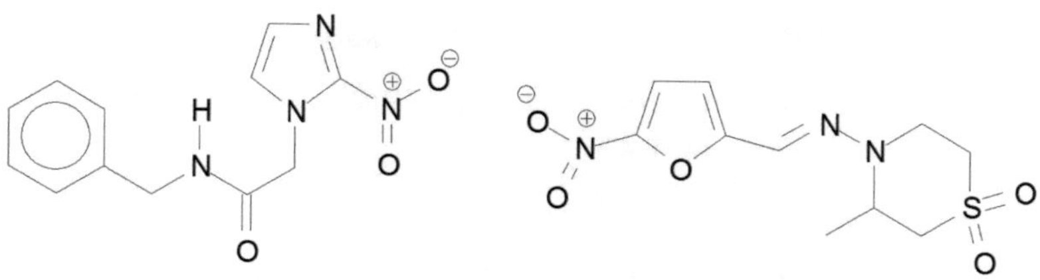

(4) BENZNIDAZOLE (5) NIFURTIMOX

Figure 3. Recommended chemotherapic drugs (4) and (5) used on treatment for Chagas' disease.

Depending on medical orientation, drugs benznidazole (4) and nifurtimox (5) can be administered either separately or simultaneously. However, on the treatment of patients in the chronic phase, drug efficacy decreases dramatically curing only 5–20% of the cases. In addition to this limited therapeutic potential, both compounds feature high toxicity [3].

There are many papers discussing the limitations of the conventional therapeutic approach [10, 12]:

- the high dosages of drugs used and the long duration of the treatment, both necessary to produce the desired medicinal effect;
- the ineffectiveness of such drugs against all the stages of the disease and all strains of the parasite;
- problems related to the lack of efficiency in drugs' production and distribution;
- several toxic effects carried out by these drugs on the patients;
- their limited effectiveness during the chronic stage;
- regional degrees of effectiveness due to drug resistance and;
- the presence of severe side effects leading to the immediate interruption of treatment in a high percentage of the patients.

All those reasons highlight the urgent need for research on new Chagas' drugs and/or safer alternative treatments.

3. Natural sources for Chagas' treatment

Through the last decades, many efforts have been made, aiming for an effective treatment for Chagas' disease without major prejudice to patients' health. There were meritorious advances regarding to molecular biology field and pathophysiology of Chagas' disease. However, according to Coura and Viñas [14], those efforts were yet unsuccessful due to:

- the usual lack of symptoms in the illness' acute phase;
- the occurrence of various parasites strains (with different drug resistance profile);

- the hardness to find a selective and more suitable drug for the parasites and;
- the inefficient fund distribution for research while most of investments are aimed to prevention and to develop diagnostic tests.

Most of the current knowledge about parasites' biology, the identification of potential molecular targets, together with the potential natural molecules from the plant kingdom, has encouraged researchers to keep searching sorely for new drugs against *T. cruzi* in nature [14].

3.1. Plant extracts

Nature is a skilled factory that produces a wide variety of chemical substances with broad structural patterns that researchers call as natural products. Most of them are secondary metabolites synthesized by plants that are directly or indirectly related to their vital processes from metabolism to chemical defense and every single way that vegetables relate to the environment.

Searching in the literature, it is possible to find many works about broad classes of secondary metabolites that have proven to be active against *T. cruzi* [16]. Usually, as part of preliminary investigation, medicinal plant extracts, fractions, isolated natural products, or pure compounds are subjected to chemical characterization tests and *in vitro* assays for screening their biological activity. Based on the evaluated biological response, it is possible to infer which chemical classes may be present in each case [1] and decide if it is suitable for advise them in a treatment or not. Historically, plant produces many active classes of natural compounds, such as alkaloids, terpenoids, flavonoids, and quinones and many of them widely reported as promising sources of antiparasitic agents.

Bioactive natural compounds despite being very attractive sources for new drugs in their original form can also be subjected to derivatization reactions or via synthetic steps, aiming to change chemically functional groups to magnify their bioactivity [14]. In this way, many classes of secondary metabolites, pure compounds, and its derivatives have been specifically tested *in vitro* and *in vivo* assays to verify their trypanocidal efficacy. More recently, promising results were published regarding to terpenes and sesquiterpene lactones arising from plant's leaves that presented high toxicity on different evolutional stages of parasites with low toxicity on mammalian cells. Some other substances even have showed strong activity *in vitro*, but only few of them were clinically tested on Chagas' disease yet.

Abdel-Sattar and co-workers [8] investigated the *in vitro* activity of the methanol extracts from 51 plants collected in Saudi Arabia. Among these, 15 exhibited pronounced activity against *T. cruzi* ($IC_{50} < 2$ μg ml^{-1}: *Hypoestes forskaolii* (white ribbon bush), *Capparis spinosa* (caper bush), *Kleinia odora, Psiadia punctulata, Cucumis prophetarum* (*concombre du prophète*), *Ricinus communis* (castor oil plant), the latex of *Euphorbia ammak* (candelabra spurge), *Euphorbia schimperiana* (dafeuina), *Marrubium vulgare* (horehound), *Commicarpus grandiflorus, Argemone ochroleuca* (chicalote), *Solanum villosum* (hairy nightshade), *Withania somnifera* (winter cherry), *Peganum harmala* (African hue), and *Tribulus macropterus* (Shershir).

A few other methanolic extracts showed moderate activity while 20 were considered to be inactive against *T. cruzi* ($IC_{50} > 15$ μg ml^{-1}). The methanolic extract of the Solanaceae

W. somnifera that showed potent activity for *T. cruzi*, parasites (IC_{50} of 1.93 μg ml^{-1}), after submitted to solvent-solvent partition, the chloroform fraction showed to be more potent with IC_{50} = 0.6 μg ml^{-1}, comparable to that of the standard Chagas' drug benznidazole (1) (IC_{50} of 0.52 μg ml^{-1}). The authors justify this as the chloroformic fraction concentrates the more active compounds, and this fact leads to the increasing on the biological activity of the considered fraction [8]. The chemical composition of this fraction still requires further investigation.

Another investigated Solanaceae is *Physalis angulata* L. (gooseberry), a widespread vegetable occurring mainly in tropical regions and used in folk medicine due to its active compounds and antiparasitic properties. The great medicinal potential of this species is often associated to the presence of physallins: *seco*-steroids (**Figure 4**) that have showed strong trypanocidal activity against different evolutive forms of *T. cruzi, Plasmodium falciparum,* and different *Leishmania* species as well.

Some results are very promising though one of the major problems faced by many research groups on natural products chemistry worldwide is related to the difficulty to obtain pure active secondary metabolites from natural sources. This fact could not be different for physalins: to isolate these compounds and obtain them in the pure form, it is quite difficult and time consuming, usually affording low yields at high costs. So economically, it can become very unattractive to treat any NTDs using pure isolated plant compounds like physalins for example.

On the other hand, the use of potential compounds from natural sources usually presents good alternative. Activity assays were performed on crude ethanolic extract of *P. angulata* that concentrates the active constituents and showed to be effective against different studied parasite species [11]. The extract was evaluated against epimastigotes and trypomastigotes forms of *T. cruzi,*

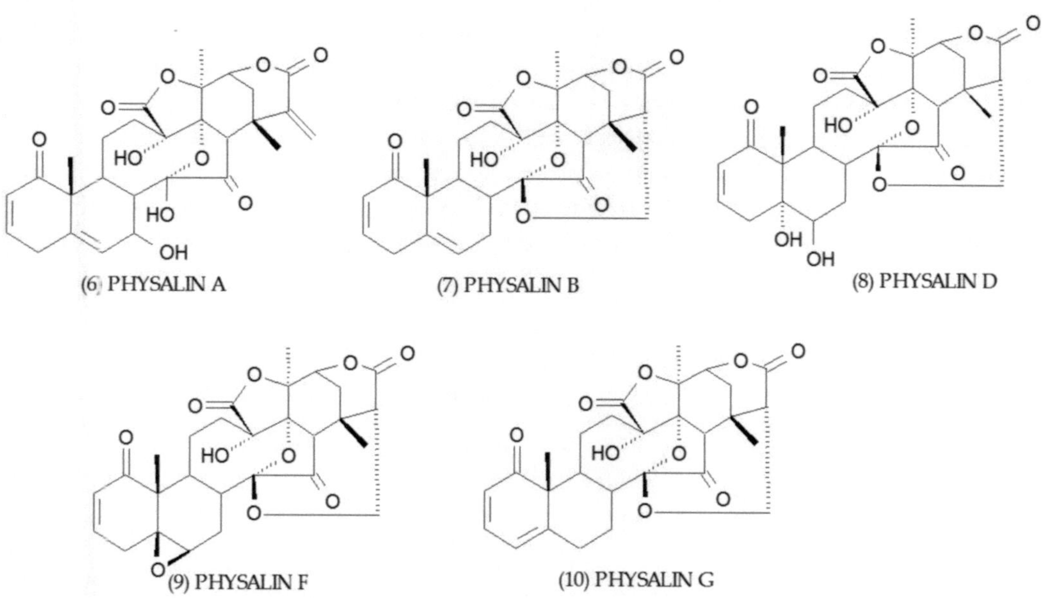

Figure 4. Physalins A (6), B (7), D (8), F (9), and G (10) isolated from *Physalis angulata*.

showing potent anti–*T. cruzi* activity, being able to inhibit the proliferation of the epimastigote forms and lyse of trypomastigotes. Beyond being active, the use of the crude plant extract has its advantages is easily obtained, nonmutagenic, and presented low toxicity in mice and high stability, which many times help to avoid degradation of the compounds of interest. Herein, it is evident that in an extract, a rich mixture of natural compounds, their chemical interactions can combine synergistically and thus alter the effect that each would have by itself.

Furthermore, the presence of phenolic compounds (**Figure 5**) like chlorogenic acid (11), rosmarinic acid (12), and coumarin (13) and flavonoids (**Figure 6**) luteolin (14), kaempferol (15), and vitexin (16) in low concentrations may have been responsible for the weak bioactivity of *L. paniculata* and *P. crucis* ethanolic extracts against *T. cruzi* [16].

In vivo studies were also performed by Meira and collaborators [11] to evaluate the effects of the same extracts against *T. cruzi* infection in mice on acute phase. The treatment reduced significantly blood parasitemia in mice when compared to those treated only with vehicle. The authors suggest that the potent activity of concentrated ethanolic extract from *P. angulata* on different strains of *T. cruzi* and *in vivo* on an acute model of infection is due to its richness in physalins (**Figure 4**).

3.1.1. *Steroidal alkaloids from Solanum genus*

In *Solanaceae* family, distributed in tropical and subtropical regions of Americas, Africa, and Australia, the genus *Solanum* is the most representative comprising about 1400 species [18]. The glycoalkaloids (**Figure 7**) solamargine (18) and solasonine (19) are the typical metabolites of *Solanum* genus; however, several other classes of compounds, such as flavonoids, phenolic acids, steroids, tannins, and triterpenes, were also recognized.

Several *Solanum* species have their biological activities intensively investigated, being proved the antiviral, diuretic, antifungi, antispasmodic, anti-inflammatory, and other pharmacodynamic properties. Recent studies evidenced that extracts of wolf apple, *Solanum lycocarpum* and its glycoalkaloids α-solamargine (18) and α-solasonine (19), were active against parasites, flagellated protozoa, *Trypanosoma cruzi*, *Leishmania infantum*, and *Leishmania amazonensis*, as well as against helminthes *Strongyloides stercoral* and *Schistosoma mansoni* [19]. In the light of chemical ecology, the antiparasitic effect of *S. lycocarpum* in the wild is evident: the largest canid of South America, the maned-wolf (*Chrysocyon brachyurus*), eats the ripen fruits

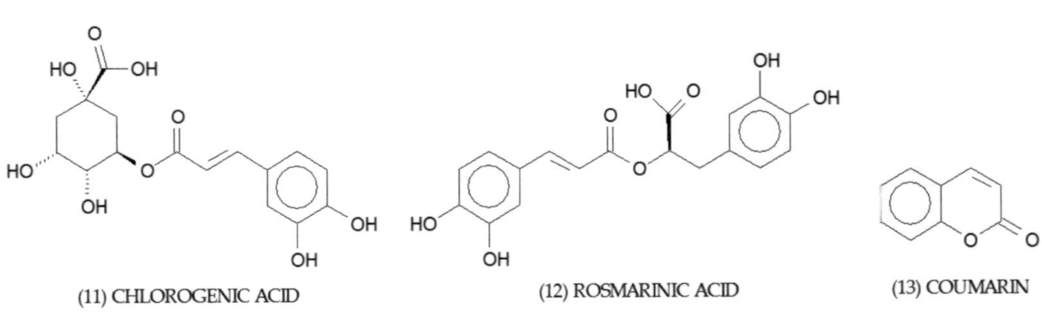

Figure 5. Active phenolic compounds (11), (12) and (13) from ethanol extracts of *L. paniculata* and *P. crucis*.

http://dx.doi.org/10.5772/67225

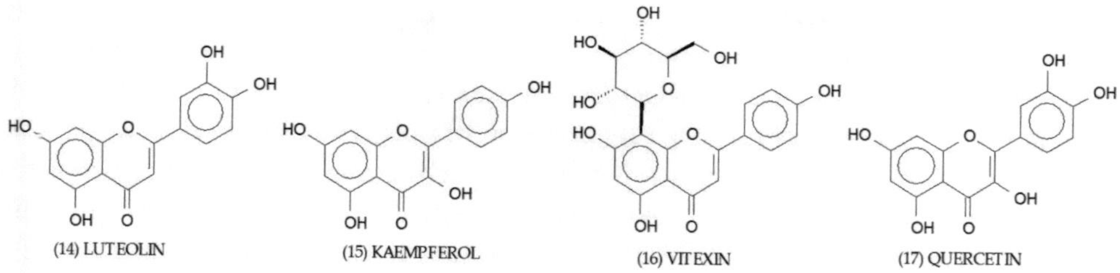

Figure 6. Active flavonoids (14), (15), (16) and (17) from ethanol extracts of *L. paniculata* and *P. crucis*.

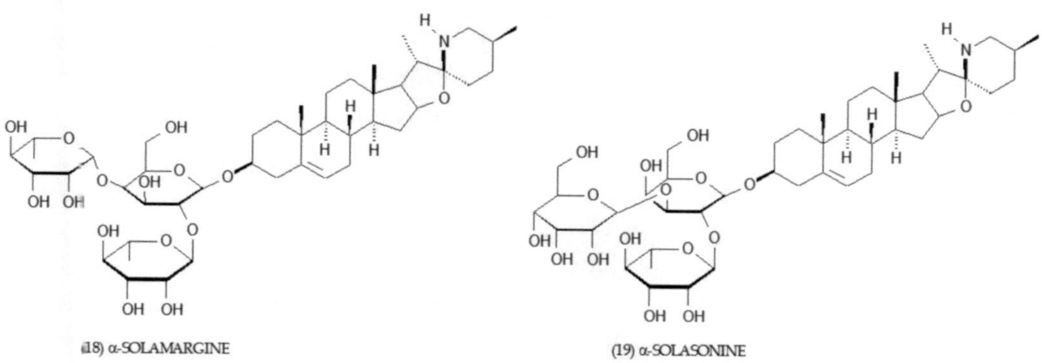

Figure 7. *Solanum* glycoalkaloids α-solamargine (18) and α-solasonine (19).

containing glycoalkaloids; this helps to control some parasitic diseases that affect it. At least that is believed by some authors [19].

The steroidal glycoalkaloid α-solamargine (18) was found on the ripe fruits of *Solanum palinacanthum* (*joá-bagudo*) as well and showed an IC_{50} of 15.3 μg ml^{-1} against *T. cruzi*, closely similar to benznidazole (1) with IC_{50} of 9.0 μg ml^{-1} [20]. Although the mechanism of action is not rightly understood, the authors speculated that the positioning of the terminal sugars in α-solamargine (18) binds more favorably with the parasites' mucin-rich cell surface when compared to α-solasonine (19). The glycoalkaloid α-solamargine (18) demonstrated to be active in the trypanocidal effect could be suitable as a candidate to prepare new therapeutic substance.

Solanum nudum Dunal (or zapata) has been used ethnopharmacologically to treat fevers. Extracts from leaves were reported to have antimalarial activity *in vitro* against asexual blood forms of protozoan *Plasmodium falciparum*. Based on this, Londoño and collaborators [12] evaluated the leishmanicidal, tripanocidal, antiplasmodial, and cytotoxic activity of eight extracts from *Solanum ovalifolium* (*cucubo*) and *Solanum arboreum* (*hoja hedionda*) obtained in different polarities, aiming to contribute to new therapeutic alternatives against protozoan diseases.

An early phytochemical analysis showed a very similar profile of secondary metabolites for both species extracts, revealing the presence of triterpenes, phenols, saponins, flavonoids, coumarins, and anthocyanosids on polar extracts. The authors found that biological activity of *S. ovalifolium* dichloromethane and hexane extracts was selective for *T. cruzi*, while the ethanol extract was selective for *T. cruzi* and *Leishmania panamensis*. Meanwhile, the ethanol and dichloromethane extracts from *S. arboreum* showed activity against all tested parasites: *L. panamensis, T. cruzi,* and *P. falciparum*. The ethanol extract activity was comparable to benznidazole (4), probably due to the identification of polar compounds, known to exhibit antiprotozoal activity such as saponins, flavonoids, and coumarins. In the dichloromethane extract was found the presence of steroids such as diosgenone, which can explain its activity [12]. The cytotoxicity is related to the cell type, although steroids of *Solanum* species are also important for their cytotoxicity.

Based on activity observed for dichloromethane and ethanol extracts of *S. arboreum* on intracellular amastigotes of *L. panamensis* and *T. cruzi* and total forms of *P. falciparum*, it suggests that these extracts could be considered as promising in the search for new antiprotozoal compounds. However, additional studies on toxicity using other cell lines are required in order to discriminate whether the toxicity shown by these extracts is against tumoral or nontumoral cells [12].

3.1.2. Terpenoids

More than 20,000 known compounds are triterpenoids produced by plants through squalene cyclization. The terpenes are considered to be the most representative group of phytochemicals [21] being the structural base for several classes of derivatives. Hence, compounds from these classes are very abundant in nature being an attractive group to be screened for biological activities of interest. Hundreds of new terpene-derived molecules exhibiting trypanocidal activity have been described on the past 10 years; some of them have already been assayed *in vitro* and *in vivo* against *T. cruzi* [14].

The diterpenoids with an abietane-type skeleton (**Figure 8**) present in many plants are known to possess a wide range of biological activities, including anti-inflammatory, antibacterial, antifungal, and antimalarial among others. For example, the phenolic abietane ferruginol (20), isolated from the roots of the herb *Craniolaria annua* (Martyniaceae) known locally as *escorzonera*, showed activity against trypomastigote and epimastigote forms of *T. cruzi*. Though, it also showed cytotoxic effects against fibroblastic Vero cells. *C. annua* is a perennial herb that grows in American tropical areas and is broadly used in traditional medicine. Previous examination of this plant has led to the isolation of montbretol derivative (22) which showed trypanocidal activity against trypomastigote (IC_{50} = 25 μM) and epimastigote (IC_{50} = 69 μM) forms of *T. cruzi* [18]. Some semi-synthetic abietane-type diterpenoids isolated from *Plectranthus barbatus* Andrews (*boldo de jardim*), *Dracocephalum komarovii* Lipsky, *Salvia cilicica* Boiss, and *Juniperus procera* Hochst. ex Endl. (African juniper) berries have shown promising trypanocidal activity together with a quinone derivative of dehydroabietic acid, 12-methoxycarnosic acid, and a few others [3]. A complete survey of abietane type terpenois and their biological activities is reviewed by Gonzalez [22], covering literature from 1980 up to 2014.

The triterpenes ursolic acid (23) and oleanolic acid (24) obtained in their pure form from *Miconia* species (Melastomataceae) were tested and shown to be active against the blood form of *T. cruzi*. Animals treated with both substances presented low parasitemia when compared to animals treated with benznidazole (4) [5]. It was also demonstrated that ursolic acid (23)

http://dx.doi.org/10.5772/67225

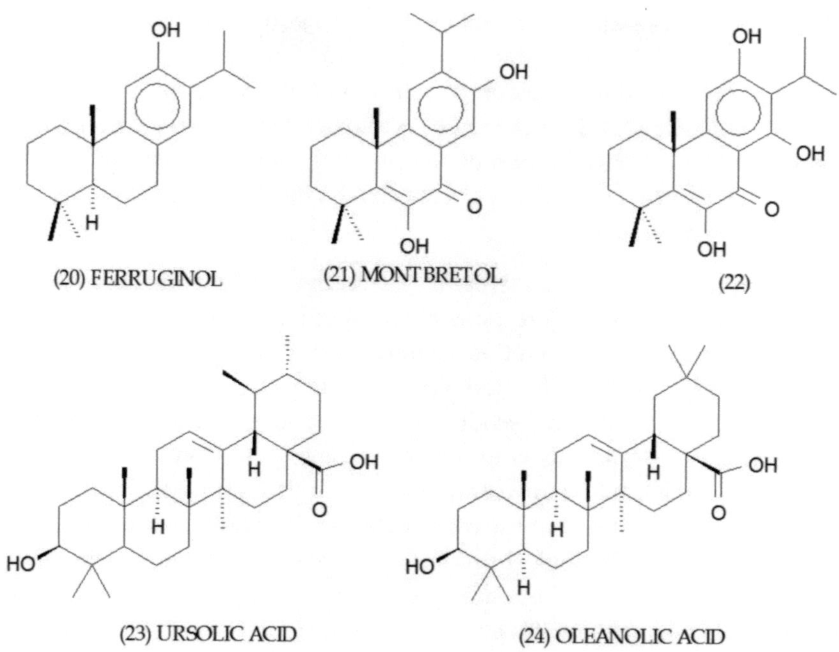

Figure 8. Active terpenoids (20, 21, and 22) and triterpenes (23 and 24) isolated from plants.

and oleanolic acid (24) were capable of controlling the peak of parasitemia in infected mice and, interestingly, treated mice did not show any alterations in their biochemical parameters, reinforcing the idea that these triterpenes are not toxic for animals. Considering the low or absent level of toxicity of triterpenes for mice, as well as their high trypanocidal activity, these results suggest that both compounds can be used for the development of new drugs against *T. cruzi* [21].

The sesquiterpene caryophyllene (25) and the phenylpropanoid eugenol (26) can be found in nature on many essential oils (**Figure 9**). Both were tested *in vitro* in their pure form against antiepimastigote and antipromastigote forms of parasites *L. brasiliensis* and *T. cruzi* [23]. The authors also tested the substances caryophyllene (25) and eugenol (26) regarding their cytotoxicity.

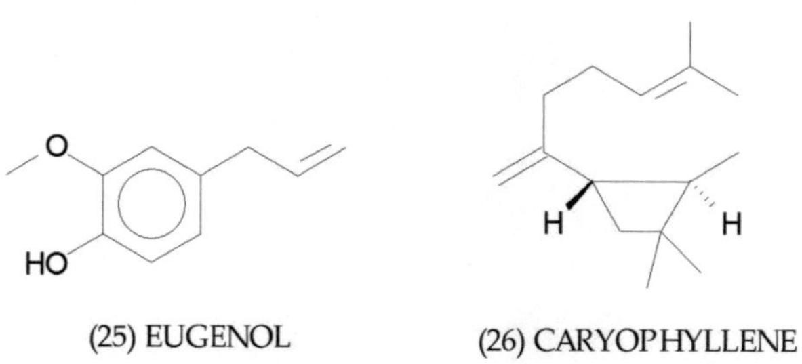

Figure 9. Structures of active compounds: caryophyllene (25) and eugenol (26).

Caryophyllene (25) showed higher percentage of parasite inhibition, being capable of eliminate 100% of *L. brasiliensis* in concentrations of 100 and 50 μg mL^{-1}. About *T. cruzi*, caryophyllene (25) inhibits 67% of the sample in concentration of 100 μg mL^{-1}, with an additional advantage: caryophyllene (25) did not exhibit cytotoxicity in concentration of 12.5 μg mL^{-1}. Similarly, eugenol (26) in concentration of 100 μg mL^{-1} showed percentage of inhibition of 17.34% and 40% for *T. cruzi* e *L. brasiliensis*, respectively. Eugenol (26) did not exhibit cytotoxicity in concentration of 50 μg mL^{-1}.

Sesquiterpene lactones (**Figure 10**) are terpenoid derivatives and usually have α,β-unsaturated carbonyl groups that are primarily responsible for mediate their wide spectrum of biological activities. Many compounds from this chemical class often show high activity against *T. cruzi* and have been isolated from the aerial parts of plants while their mechanism of action is currently under clarification. Some scholars in the area suspect that these compounds have the power to generate free radicals within trypanosomes [14]. Complementary ultra structural studies demonstrated that many compounds from this chemical class may affect mitochondrial function. It is known that the α-methylene-γ-lactone of sesquiterpene lactones is responsible for most of the biological properties of these compounds. Some authors have suggested that the interaction of the α-methylene portion from those lactones, with sulphydryl groups present in some parasites enzymes that are crucial for its survival, accounts the cytotoxicity of these compounds [14]. It is also practicable that these sequiterpene lactones may affect calcium metabolism, once they are similar to thapsigargin (28), a potent inhibitor of this ion. However, this hypothesis has not been tested yet.

Interestingly, some of these terpenic molecules are feasible to chemical modification in order to comprehend their mechanisms of action in such organisms or intended to optimize their effectiveness on elimination of parasites. It is possible to strategically perform chemical reactions on specific functional groups on some known natural products. This approach proved to be very effective, once with the increasing on lipophilicity of isolated diterpenes lead to a substantial improvement on their trypanocidal activity, for example. It is also reported that

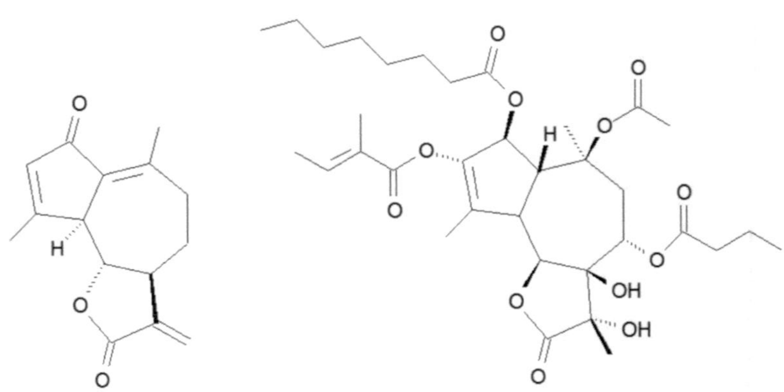

(27) DEHYDROLEUCODINE (28) THAPSIGARGIN

Figure 10. Sesquiterpene lactones: dehydroleucodine (27) and thapsigargin (28).

parasites have a rudimentary defence system highly sensitive to oxidative stress, being their main vulnerability [14].

3.1.3. *Flavonoids*

In addition to terpenoids, other group of natural products with very interesting bioactivity is the flavonoids (**Figures 6** and **11**). They are very abundant in nature being responsible for many interesting properties like antioxidant, anti-inflammatory, and free-radical scavengers. The ethanol leaf extract from the bay cedar, *Guazuma ulmifolia* Lam. (Malvaceae), was active *in vitro* against the tested parasite strains of *T. cruzi*, *L. brasiliensis*, and *L. infantum*, possibly due the presence of quercetin (17), a potent known leishmanicidal flavonoid from flavones group [16]. The cytotoxicity presented by the aforementioned extract reinforces the need for further tests, including *in vivo* trials, like antineoplastic activity in tumor cells, before considerate *G. ulmifolia* ethanol extracts as a potential alternative source of natural compounds against Chagas' disease.

Flavanones (**Figure 11**) naringenin (29), sakuranetin (30), and its methylated derivative sakuranetin-4′-methyl ether (31) have their antiparasital activity tested *in vitro* against four parasites from *Leishmania* spp. species and *T. cruzi* trypomastigotes and amastigotes [24].

In this study, the authors reported that sakuranetin (30) presented good activity against all tested *Leishmania* species and against *T. cruzi* trypomastigotes. Hence, sakuranetin (30) was chemically transformed thru methylation procedure furnishing sakuranetin-4′-methyl ether (31). This chemical modification yielded an inactive compound against the tested parasite species. However, this result is interestingly important once evidenced that the presence of hydroxyl group at C-4′ and of methoxyl group at C-7 in related flavanone are directly associated to the aforementioned activity. In conclusion, Grecco and collaborators [24] provided flavanone important structural information required for comprehension about anti-protozoan activity of these flavonoids. This kind of information could be very useful for the design of novel and more effective agents against Leishmaniasis and Chagas' disease for example.

3.1.4. *Lectins*

Lectin is the name given to a group containing all sugar-specific agglutinins of nonimmune origin. Those substances were found to be valuable because they could recognize and bind

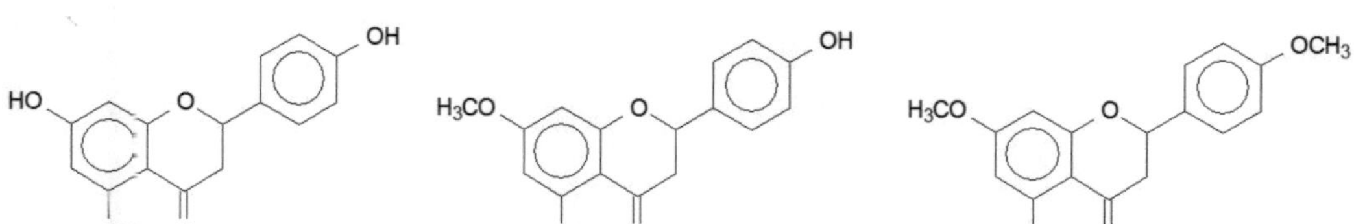

(29) NARINGENIN (30) SAKURANETIN (31) SAKURANETIN-4′-METHYL ETHER

Figure 11. Flavanones: naringenin (29), sakuranetin (30), and sakuranetin-4′-methyl ether (31).

carbohydrates specifically and reversibly. Hence, the lectins have great potential and value in the study of glycoproteins, helping to comprehend the mechanisms of many physiological and pathological processes [25]. The bonding between lectins and some protozoans' sugars is believed to cause interference in chemical or biological processes that eventually lead to the death of these parasites. Therefore, lectin isolated from triatomine insect *Rhodnius prolixus* (Reduviidae) showed to interfere on the life cycle of *Trypanosoma rangelii* effectively. Apparently, carbohydrates on the surface of *T. rangelii* and *T. cruzi* cells interact with lectins extracted from soy beans, *Glycine max* (Fabaceae), and castor-oil beans, *Ricinus communis* (Euphorbiaceae), suggesting that they could be helpful to determinate the presence of *T. cruzi* from the feces of *R. prolixus,* one of vectors of Chagas' parasite [26].

3.2. Essential oils

It is evident that many medicinal plants from *Artemisia* genus (Asteraceae) have ethnopharmacological importance. The classic example refers to *Artemisia annua* that furnished artemisinin (2) as aforementioned. Likewise, the species *Artemisia absinthium* L. (absinthe) had composition and biological effects of the essential oil and the extracts widely studied. Different researchers have demonstrated antimicrobial and antiprotozoal effects against *T. cruzi, Leishmania aethiopica, Leishmania donovani,* and *Leishmania infantum.*

Among the major constituents identified on *A. absinthium* essential oils, are (**Figure 12**) α-thujone (32), β-thujone (33), sabinene (34), β-pinene (35), myrcene (36), *trans*-sabinyl acetate (37), 1,8-cineole (38), linalool (39), *cis*-epoxyocimene (40), artemisiaketone (41), camphor (42), bornyl acetate (43), myrtenol (44), chrysanthenyl acetate (45) hydrocarbon monoterpenes, and sesquiterpene lactones, depending on the plant origin, mixtures of these components could be found in different ratio concentrations.

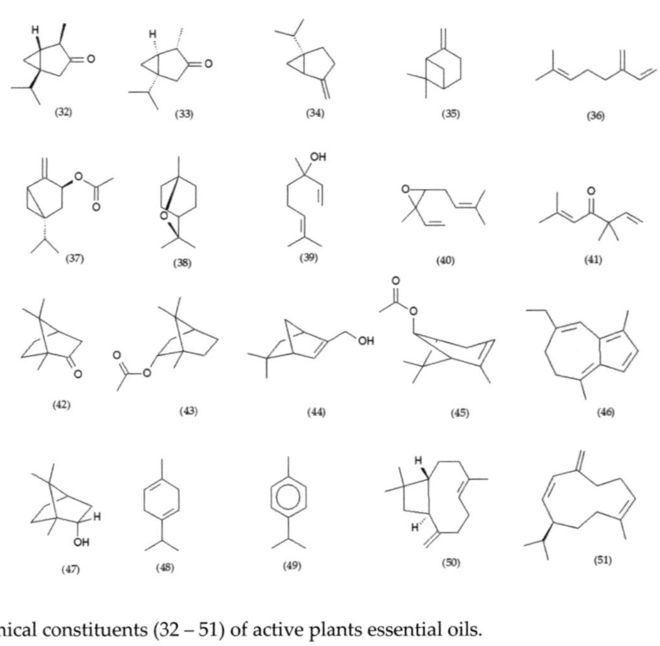

Figure 12. Some chemical constituents (32 – 51) of active plants essential oils.

Usually the collection of wild herbal populations can result in extracts and essential oils with variable compositions [10]. So, after *A. absinthium* essential oils chromatographic fractionation, the antiparasitic effects of some fractions revealed that compounds dihydrochamazulene (46) and *trans*-caryophyllene (50) (main compounds on their respective fractions) could be related to the observed activity.

Essential oils extracted from fresh leaves of velame, *Croton pedicellatus,* and sangre de drago, *Croton leptostachyus* (Euphorbiaceae), showed to be active against the extracellular forms of *T. cruzi in vitro*. The main compounds identified on crotons' oils were borneol (47), γ-terpinene (48), *p*-cymene (49), *trans*-caryophyllene (50), and germacrene D (51). The difference observed for the oils' activity could be related to the presence of these components in variable proportions or due to the existence of other minor components in volatile content. Unfortunately, despite of being active, Neira and co-workers [27] found out that these oils were toxic for Vero cells.

3.3. Marine organisms

3.3.1. Sponges

The crescent need for bioactive molecules that can be used as potential natural drugs, being able to cure diseases and reducing undesirable side effects at the same time, leads the researches all around the world to look to the sea. Many papers available in the literature report the search for new active compounds, and they have found that marine biodiversity is a promising source of natural products with remarkable biological activities. To the best of our knowledge, studies involving marine sponges yield close to 200 new pharmacologically active metabolites every year [28].

Being ancient organisms, some sponges contain diverse groups of metabolically active compounds. Hence, the investigation of biological activity is an important source to obtain extracts or compounds with potential biomedical action. So much that the effect of acetone extract from lyophilized Brazilian and Spanish marine sponges, *Chondrosia reniformis* (esponja de vidro—glass sponge), *Tethya rubra* (the red golfball sponge), *Tethya ignis* (esponja de fogo—fire sponge), *Mycale angulosa* (common sponge), and *Dysidea avara* (soft sponge), was evaluated on growth of *T. cruzi* forms. All the tested extracts showed activity against epimastigote forms of the parasite. The extracts of *D. avara* (IC_{50} = 23.4 μg ml^{-1}), *M. angulosa* (IC_{50} = 67.3 μg ml^{-1}), and *C. reniformes* (IC_{50} = 28.6 μg ml^{-1}) were the most active. Moreover, the extracts showed no toxic effects in normal cells ($LLCMK_2$) at concentrations that inhibited 50% of the parasites [28]. In this study, the marine sponges have some compounds identified by GC–MS (**Figure 13**): the steroids, stigmasterol (52), *β*-sitosterol (53), and brassicasterol (54) were found in larger quantities in sponges' organic extracts and show activity against *T. cruzi*.

The trypomastigotes were sensitive to the presence of different concentrations of marine sponge extracts as well. Although the action mechanism of steroids is unknown, it is accepted that these compounds may be initiated at the cell membrane but also via intracellular receptor binding. In addition, steroids may participate in growth regulation, proliferation and

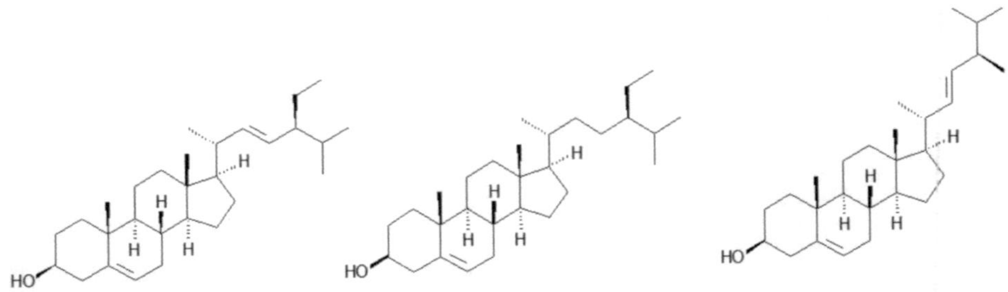

(52) STIGMASTEROL (53) β-SITOSTEROL (54) BRASSICASTEROL

Figure 13. Steroids stigmasterol (52), *β*-sitosterol (53), and brassicasterol (54) found in marine sponges.

cell death, and redox mechanisms [12]. These compounds could participate in a conjugated addition of nucleophilic amino acid residues present in target enzymes on *Leishmania*. This reaction occurs usually via Michael type mechanism that was also reported for other α,β-unsaturated compounds such as lactones and chromones [13].

3.4. Combating triatomine bed

As discussed through this chapter, triatomine bugs can affect human health acting as vectors transmitting Chagas' disease to many populations worldwide. The inappropriate use of synthetic insecticides, usually been used to control these insects, is closely linked to the development of resistance in pests, human diseases, and contamination of food and the environment. Resistance to the pyrethroid deltamethrin and other nonnatural insecticides, for example, has been reported in different areas of the Gran Chaco region of Argentina and Bolivia for *Triatoma infestans*, the major Chagas' disease vector in southern South America [29]. Nevertheless, the biological action of natural products and essential oils with insecticidal activity represents a very important alternative, which allows an environmental friendly management of pest insects without affecting people's health. Plants can produce a wide diversity of compounds that are involved in their chemical defense [30]. Those compounds are usually volatile and can be found concentrated on their essential oils [31]. Among these natural products, terpene compounds have been shown to have a significant potential for insect control [31] killing or at least repealing the insects away. However, little is known about the molecular properties related to their insecticidal activity.

For example, Nieto-Sanchez *et al.*, [32] have recently prospected in southern Ecuador for traditional Chagas' disease control strategies employed by general population. Among those actions they have found:

- the active search and elimination of triatomines;
- insecticide-based fumigation on infected places;
- educational activities managing population.

Those prevention methods are effective in short term for reducing triatomine infestation, although do not prevent reinfestation in the long run. Interestingly, they have also reported practices such as sweeping with brooms made from plants believed to have natural insecticide

http://dx.doi.org/10.5772/67225

properties by local residents: herbs such as porotillo (*Fallopia convolvulus*), moshquera (*Croton* spp.), florblanca (*Buddleja utilis* also known as monteramirez), and chamana (*Dodonaea viscosa*) are considered to be highly acidic plants by local populations; so they become a natural insecticide when turned into brooms. The natives described that sweeping more than once a day in and outside the domiciles using water to create less dust and to prevent the dirt to stick on the floor is the most common way.

Those findings suggest that multiple tasks are required to control bug recolonization, especially in poorly constructed houses. The usual use of synthetic chemical insecticides constitutes a fragile short-term solution for controlling Chagas' disease. There is a need to develop more sustainable long-lasting solutions for Chagas' disease transmission in areas that have high occurrence of triatomine infestation.

4. Final considerations

The studies reviewed briefly in this chapter along with many others that have been carried out since the 50s have brought valuable information aiming to contribute to the understanding about the parasite's life cycle and to highlight the crescent need to clarifying some biomolecular targets and enzymatic mechanisms that could be useful to the development of new natural drugs against *T. cruzi* and other parasites.

It is personally believed that the cure for Chagas' disease is hidden somewhere in nature; the scientists are currently working as explorers, prospecting this greatness in molecular levels, searching in every single bush for a viable solution that helps populations suffering for Chagas worldwide. Here in few lines, it was showed the great potential of natural products for the treatment of this parasitic disease. The plentiful Mother Nature furnishes material to the obtention of useful substances emerging from crude extracts, essential oils, and many fractions possessing very complex, variable, and rich composition. In this chapter, was portrayed, several groups of secondary metabolites, such as diterpenes, terpenes, triterpenes, sesquiterpenes, sesquiterpene lactones, steroids, flavonoids, polyketides, lectins, and many others.

Massive efforts of community activists, health care workers, politicians, and economists are also required to reduce significantly the significance of public health liability that NTDs oblige. The most effective approach for reducing these diseases is still prevention, due to the absence of affordable or effective curative therapies and the deficiency of preventive vaccines. Between such relevant public health issues and many lives directly or indirectly affected by NTDs, there is education that offers a solution to connect NTD prevention to treatment efforts.

Acknowledgements

NPV would like to thank her sister Karina Pacheco Vaz for drawing the scheme in **Figure 2** and for the final art for all the figures available on this chapter.

Author details

Nelissa Pacheco Vaz

Address all correspondence to: nelissavaz@gmail.com

Natural Products Chemistry, Chemistry Department, Federal University of Paraná—UFPR, Curitiba, Paraná, Brazil

References

[1] Faitanin R, Gomes J, Menezes L, Brasileiro B, Jamal C. Phytochemical screening, cytotoxic and thrombolytic activity evaluation of *Myrciaria strigipes* O. Berg, *Ipomoea alba* L. and *Solanum cordifolium* dunal leaves. Pharmacology OnLine. 2015;**3**:131-135.

[2] Leite P, Castilho R, Ribeiro A, Martins M. Consumption of medicinal plants by patients with heart diseases at a pharmacist-managed anticoagulation clinic in Brazil. International Journal of Clinical Pharmacy. 2016;**38**:223-227. DOI 10.1007/s11096-016-0270-0

[3] Vahermo M, Krogerus S, Nasereddin A, Kaiser M, Brun R, Jaffe C, Yli-Kauhaluoma J, Moreira V. Antiprotozoal activity of dehydroabietic acid derivatives against *Leishmania donovani* and *Trypanosoma cruzi*. Medical Chemical Communications. 2016;**7**:457-463. DOI: 10.1039/c5md00498e

[4] Liu Q, Zhou X. Preventing the transmission of American trypanosomiasis and its spread into non-endemic countries. Infectious Diseases of Poverty. 2015;**4**:60-70. DOI: 10.1186/s40249-015-0092-7

[5] Ferreira D S, Esperandim V R, Marçal M G, Neres N B R, Cunha N L, Andrade e Silva M L, Cunha W R. Natural products and Chagas' disease: the action of triterpenes acids isolated from Miconia species. Universitas Scientiarum. 2013;**18**:243-256. DOI: 10.11144/Javeriana.SC18-2.npcd

[6] Mackey T, Liang B, Cuomo R, Hafen R, Brouwer K, Lee D. Emerging and reemerging neglected tropical diseases: a review of key characteristics, risk factors, and the policy and innovation environment. Clinical Microbiology Reviews. 2014;**27**:949-979. DOI: 10.1128/CMR.00045-14

[7] Bonney K. Promoting civic engagement with neglected tropical disease education. Brazilian Journal of Biological Sciences. 2016;**3**:23-26. DOI: 10.21472/bjbs.030502

[8] Abdel-Sattar E, Maes L, Salama M. In vitro activities of plant extracts from Saudi Arabia against malaria, leishmaniasis, sleeping sickness and Chagas disease. Phytotherapy Research. 2010;**24**: 1322-1328. DOI: 10.1002/ptr.3108

[9] Coura J, Dias J. Epidemiology, control and surveillance of Chagas disease—100 years after its discovery. Memórias do Instituto Oswaldo Cruz. 2009;**104**:31-40. DOI: 10.1590/S0074-02762009000900006

[10] Martínez-Díaz R, Ibáñez-Escribano A, Burillo J, Heras L, Prado G, Agulló-Ortuño M, Julio L, González-Coloma A. Trypanocidal, trichomonacidal and cytotoxic components of cultivated Artemisia absinthium Linnaeus (Asteraceae) essential oil. Memórias do Instituto Oswaldo Cruz. 2015;**110**:693-699. DOI: 10.1590/0074-02760140129

[11] Meira C, Guimarães E, Santos J, Moreira D, Nogueira R, Tomassini T, Ribeiro I, Souza C, Santos R, Soares M. In vitro and in vivo antiparasitic activity of *Physalis angulata* L. concentrated ethanolic extract against *Trypanosoma cruzi*. Phytomedicine. 2015;**22**: 969-974. DOI: 10.1016/j.phymed.2015.07.004

[12] Londoño F, Cardona W, Alzate F, Cardona F, Vélez I, Upegui Y, Ospina V, Muñoz J, Robledo S. Antiprotozoal activity and cytotoxicity of extracts from *Solanum arboreum* and *S. ovalifolium* (Solanaceae). Journal of Medicinal Plants Research. 2016;**10**:100-107. DOI: 10.5897/JMPR2015.5923

[13] Pirttimaa M, Nasereddin A, Kopelyanskiy D, Kaiser M, Yli-Kauhaluoma J, Oksman-Caldentey K, Brun R, Jaffe C, Moreira V, Alakurtti S. Abietane-type diterpenoid amides with highly potent and selective activity against *Leishmania donovani* and *Trypanosoma cruzi*. Journal of Natural Products. 2016;**79**:362-368. DOI: 10.1021/acs. jnatprod.5b00990

[14] Coura J, Viñas P, Junqueira A. Ecoepidemiology, short history and control of Chagas disease in the endemic countries and the new challenge for non-endemic countries. Memórias do Instituto Oswaldo Cruz. 2014;**109**:856-862. DOI: 10.1590/0074-0276140236

[15] Lozano E, Barrera P, Spina R, Sosa M. Terpenoid derivatives as potential trypanocidal agents. Medicinal Chemistry (Los Angeles). 2016;**6**:319-321. DOI: 10.4172/2161-0444. 1000363

[16] Calixto Júnior J, Morais S, Gomez C, Molas C, Rolon M, Boligon A, Athayde M, Oliveira C, Tintino S, Coutinho H. Phenolic composition and antiparasitic activity of plants from the Brazilian Northeast "Cerrado". Saudi Journal of Biological Sciences. 2016;**23**:434-440. DOI: 10.1016/j.sjbs.2015.10.009

[17] Nogueira N, Saraiva F, Sultano P, Cunha P, Laranja G, Justo G, Sabino K, Coelho M, Rossini A, Atella G, Paes M. Proliferation and differentiation of *Trypanosoma cruzi* inside its vector have a new trigger: redox status. PLoS One. 2015;**10**:1-16. DOI: 10.1371/journal.pone.0116712

[18] Vaz N, Costa E, Santos E, Mikich S, Marques F, Braga R, Delarmelina C, Duarte M, Ruiz A, Souza V, Carvalho J, Maia B. Caavuranamide, a novel steroidal alkaloid from the ripe fruits of *Solanum caavurana* vell. (Solanaceae). Journal of the Brazilian Chemical Society. 2012;**23**:361-366. DOI: 10.1590/S0103-50532012000200025

[19] Martins G, Moreira R, Planeta C, Almeida A, Bastos J, Salgueiro L, Cavaleiro C, Sousa M. Effects of the extract and glycoalkaloids of *Solanum lycocarpum* St. Hill on Giardia lamblia trophozoites. Pharmacognosy Magazine. 2015;**11**(S1):S161–S165. DOI: 10.4103/0973-1296.157721

[20] Moreira R, Martins G, Magalhães N, Almeida A, Pietro R, Silva F, Cicarelli R. In vitro trypanocidal activity of solamargine and extracts from *Solanum palinacanthum* and *Solanum lycocarpum* of Brazilian cerrado. Anais da Academia Brasileira de Ciências. 2013;**85**:903-907. DOI: 10.1590/S0001-37652013000300006

[21] Jesus J, Lago J, Laurenti M, Yamamoto E, Passero L. Antimicrobial activity of oleanolic and ursolic acids: an update. Evidence-Based Complementary and Alternative Medicine. 2015;1-14. DOI:10.1155/2015/620472

[22] Gonzalez M. Aromatic abietane diterpenoids: their biological activity and synthesis. Natural Products Reports. 2015;**32**:684-704. DOI: 10.1039/c4np00110a

[23] Leite N, Sobral-Souza C, Albuquerque R, Brito D, Lavor A, Alencar L, Tintino S, Ferreira J, Figueredo F, Lima L, Cunha F, Pinho A, Coutinho H. In vitro cytotoxic and antiparasitic activity of caryophyllene and eugenol against *Trypanosoma cruzi* and *Leishmania brasiliensis*. Revista Cubana de Plantas Medicinales. 2013;**18**:522-528.

[24] Grecco S, Reimão J, Tempone A, Sartorelli P, Cunha R, Romoff P, Ferreira M, Fávero O, Lago J. In vitro antileishmanial and antitrypanosomal activities of flavanones from Baccharis retusa DC. (Asteraceae). Experimental Parasitology. 2012;**130**:141-145. DOI: 10.1016/j.exppara.2011.11.002

[25] Dan X, Liu W, Ng T. Development and applications of lectins as biological tools in biomedical research. Medicinal Research Reviews. 2016;**36**:221-247. DOI: 10.1002/med. 21363.

[26] Iordache F, Ionita M, Mitrea L, Fafaneata C, Pop A. Antimicrobial and antiparasitic activity of lectins. Current Pharmaceutical Biotechnology. 2015;**16**:152-161.

[27] Neira L, Stashenko E, Escobar P. Activity of Colombian plant extracts derived from the Euphorbiaceae family. Revista de la Universidad Industrial de Santander (Salud). 2014;**46**:15-22.

[28] Paula J, Desoti V, Sampirona E, Martins S, Ueda-Nakamura T, Ribeiro S, Bianco E, Silva S, Oliveira G, Nakamura C. Trypanocidal activity of organic extracts from the Brazilian and Spanish marine sponges. Revista Brasileira de Farmacognosia. 2015;**25**:651-656. DOI: 10.1016/j.bjp.2015.08.011

[29] Schama R, Pedrini N, Juárez M, Nelson D, Torres A, Valle D, Mesquita R. Rhodnius prolixus supergene families of enzymes potentially associated with insecticide resistance. Insect Biochemistry and Molecular Biology. 2016;**69**:91-104. DOI: 10.1016/j.ibmb.2015.06.005

[30] Sarwar M. Usage of biorational pesticides with novel modes of action, mechanism and application in crop protection. International Journal of Materials Chemistry and Physics. 2015;**1**:156-162.

[31] Dambolena J, Zunino M, Herrera J, Pizzolitto R, Areco V, Zygadlo J. Terpenes: natural products for controlling insects of importance to human health: a structure-activity relationship study. Psyche: A Journal of Entomology. 2016;**2016**:17 pages. DOI: 10.1155/2016/4595823

[32] Nieto-Sanchez C, Baus E, Guerrero D, Grijalva M. Positive deviance study to inform a Chagas disease control program in southern Ecuador. Memórias do Instituto Oswaldo Cruz. 2015;**110**:299-309. DOI: 10.1590/0074-02760140472

Chapter 5

Plant-Derived Compounds as an Alternative Treatment Against Parasites in Fish Farming: A Review

Alison Carlos Wunderlich,
Érica de Oliveira Penha Zica,
Vanessa Farias dos Santos Ayres,
Anderson Cavalcante Guimarães and
Renata Takeara

Additional information is available at the end of the chapter

http://dx.doi.org/10.5772/67668

Abstract

Aquaculture has grown rapidly for food production around the world. However, outbreaks of infectious diseases have also increased in aquaculture, causing serious economic losses. For many years, fish farmers have applied conventional treatments such as anti-parasitics and chemical treatments to control fish parasites. However, previous studies have revealed an accumulation of these chemical residues in fish tissues, and a negative environmental impact from farms to aquatic organisms. As an alternative to conventional methods, many plant-derived compounds such as essential oils (e.g. *Origanum* sp. and *Lippia* spp.) and plant extracts (e.g. *Allium sativum* and *Mentha* spp.) have been used as an efficient treatment to control parasites in freshwater, brackishwater and marine aquaculture systems. Our objective with this review is to highlight the advantages of the use of plant extracts as an alternative treatment against parasites in aquaculture (e.g. protozoans, myxozoans and monogeneans) and to show the possible negative environmental impacts of conventional treatments used in fish farming systems. Finally, we also highlight the potential of discovering new plant-derived bioactive compounds that have been increased in the last year due to the use of new tools such as the application of nanotechnology and microencapsulation to control diseases in fish farming.

Keywords: plant extract, anthelmintic activity, fish parasites, fish farming

1. Introduction

Aquaculture has grown rapidly for food production around the world [1], but infection in aquaculture is an important factor affecting food production [2]. Outbreaks of the infectious diseases have caused significant economic losses in freshwater, brackish water and marine aquaculture systems [2–5]. For instance, although the salmon farming has supplied 53% of the world market [6], their losses due to attack by the salmon louse (*Lepeophtheirus salmonis*) increase farming salmon costs with a global annual cost exceeding $400 million [7].

The increase of the parasites in the farming system led to the development of several chemical treatments [8, 9]. For many years, fish farmers have applied conventional treatments such as anti-parasitics, chemotherapeutics and insecticides to prevent or control parasitic infections in aquaculture [4, 10]. Indeed, the use of traditional parasiticides is well known in the control of helminths [11], such as praziquantel [12], mebendazole [13] and trichlorphon [14]. However, previous studies have revealed side effects of chemical parasiticides, including an accumulation in fish tissues [15], and adverse consequences on the indigenous microflora of the fish [16, 17].

Also, the accumulation of anti-parasitics and chemical residues in water has caused impacts on the environment [18, 19], especially in aquaculture in open waters where drugs are not easily controlled [10]. These chemical residues may have lethal or sub-lethal effects on non-target organisms in the environment [20] (**Figure 1**). For example, when pesticides such as Neguvon and Nuvon were used to control *L. salmonis* in the salmon net-pen farming in Norway, there have been harmful effects on several crustaceans near the farms [21].

During the last years, the search for new and natural treatment to mitigate the side effects of chemicals used in aquaculture included bioactive chemicals from plants [22]. Plants are a rich source of bioactive compounds like alkaloids and glycosides, and they might be an alternative source of natural parasitic control [23]. Medicinal plants have been reported as appetite stimulation, antimicrobial, immunostimulant, anti-inflammatory, biopesticides and anti-parasitic properties and their use in traditional medicine has been known for thousands of years around the world [15, 24–26]. Nowadays, natural products are preferred because of their biodegradability in the environment [23] (**Figure 1**). As an alternative to the conventional methods, different essential oils and plant extracts have been tested and used as an efficient and alternative treatment against parasites in aquaculture [9, 15]. For example, plant-derived compounds have been used either as immunostimulants [17] or as anti-parasitic activity against fish parasites, especially monogeneans and protozoans [15, 27].

The use of the plant-derived compounds has been concentrated in protozoans and especially in monogeneans [27]. Monogeneans (e.g. *Dactylogyrus* spp. and salmon fluke *Gyrodactylus salaris*) and protozoans (e.g. Ich *Ichthyophthirius multifiliis* and *Trichodina* spp.) are very common ectoparasites living on the gills of freshwater and marine fish [28, 29]. Recently, a few studies have used these plant-derived compounds to control myxozoan species such as *Myxobolus* spp. and *Enteromyxum* spp. [30, 31]. For example, essential oil of *Origanum* has been reported to provide varying degrees of protection and therapy in fish infected with myxosporean parasites [30–32].

http://dx.doi.org/10.5772/67668

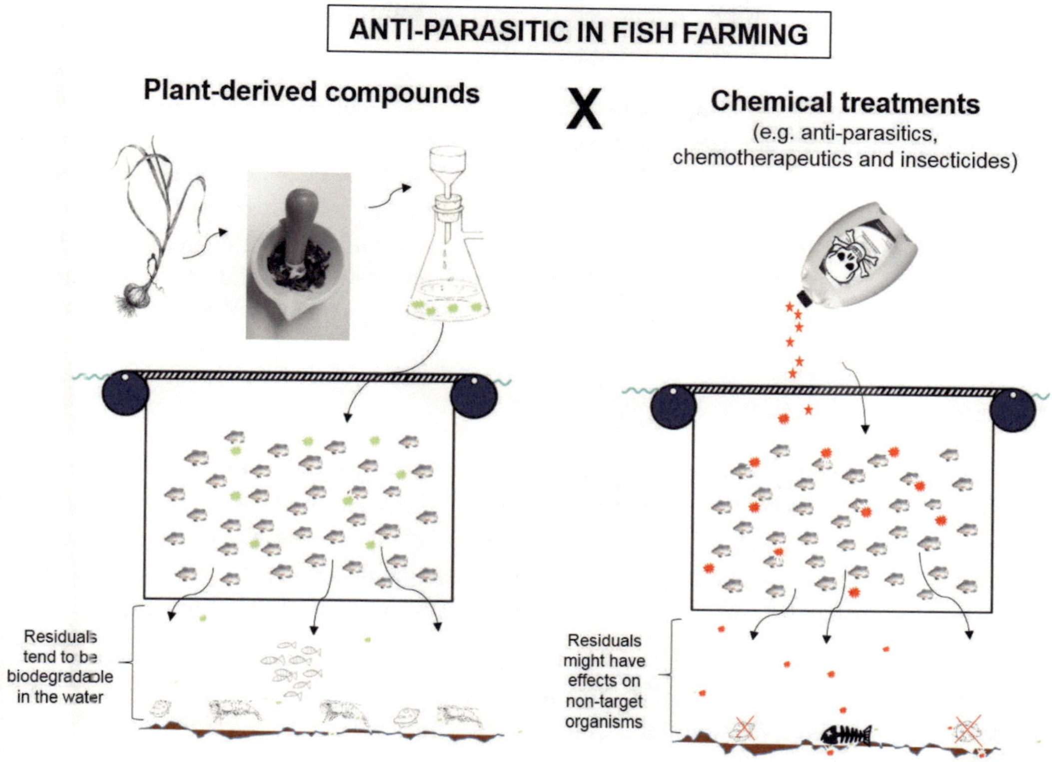

Figure 1. Effects of the residues between plant-derived compounds and conventional anti-parasitic treatments used in fish farming in the environment. Left: Residues from plant-derived compounds treatments tend to be biodegradable in the water. Right: Residues from conventional anti-parasitic treatments might have effects on non-target organisms (e.g. fishes, crustaceans).

In this review, we will begin with an overview of the use of plant-derived compounds as anthelmintic activity in fish aquaculture and identify the advances made by phytotherapy in this research field. We will also describe essential oils, plant extracts and isolated substances that have been used to control parasites in fish farming. Overall, we will illustrate the use of these compounds with several case studies for which information exists on anti-parasitic activity against protozoans, myxozoans and helminths (monogeneans), which are one of the most economically important parasite species in fish farming. Therefore, our main objective in this review is to highlight the advantages of the use of plant extracts as an alternative treatment against parasites in aquaculture and discuss the environmental impacts of conventional treatments used in fish farming systems.

2. Plant-derived compounds as fish anti-parasitics

Historically, plant-derived compounds have long been used in traditional medicine for the treatment of many diseases [33]. Numerous plants have been used to investigate the effects of their compounds to enhance the immune responses and increase the protective abilities against pathogenic agents in fish farming [17, 34].

Many studies have shown that essential oils, extracts and isolated substances from plants might be an important and alternative oral and immersion treatment against parasites in aquaculture (For a review see [27]). In addition, these plant extracts are capable of enhancing immune responses and disease resistance of cultured fish, serving as a great phytotherapeutics against infections in aquaculture [15]. To date, more than 60 plant species have been studied for the use as phytochemicals to control and prevent parasites such as protozoans (**Table 1**), myxozoans (**Table 2**) and monogeneans (**Table 3**) in freshwater and marine aquaculture [9, 15].

2.1. Anti-protozoan activity

Plant-derived compounds to control protozoans have been recently experimented and tested [9, 27]. Research on essential oils for controlling protozoans that inhibit the growth of fingerlings is still scarce. Soares et al. [35] analysed the essential oil of *Lippia alba* (bushy matagrass) leaves at concentrations of 100 and 150 mg/L and obtained efficacies of 40.7 and 50.3% against the *I. multifiliis* protozoan, which is a parasite of *Colossoma macropomum* (tambaqui).

Recent studies of medicinal plants have also shown promising results in the treatment of protozoal diseases in aquaculture [27]. The results revealed that the exposure of methanol extract of *Magnolia officinalis* (2.45 mg/L) and *Sophora alopecuroides* (pea flowered tree) (3.43 mg/L) caused the highest mortality against *I. multifiliis*, a pathogenic ciliate that infects fresh and marine fish farming [36]. These extracts revealed the highest antiprotozoal activity against theronts, which are released from infective stages (i.e. tomites) as swarmers to seek new hosts [36] actively. Extracts of *Eclipta* prostrate (false daisy), *Lycium chinense* (Chinese matrimony vine), *Ophiopogon bodinieri* and *Trichosanthes kirilowii* (Chinese cucumber) showed high antiprotozoal activity against *I. multifiliis* in fish *Carassius auratus*, ranging from 80 to 100% mortality [36]. *Allium sativum* (garlic) and *Matricaria chamomilla* (chamomile) extracts were also active in the control of *I. multifiliis* in *Poecilia latipinna* (sailfin molly) [37]. These results suggest, therefore, that the use of essential oil and medicinal plant extracts is viable and has a significant efficacy for the control of these protozoans in fish farming.

2.2. Anti-myxozoan activity

Recently, a few studies have used the essential oils to control myxosporean species such as *Myxobolus* spp. and *Enteromyxum* spp. [30, 31]. For example, *Origanum* essential oils have exhibited differential degrees of protection against myxosporean infections in gilthead and sharpsnout sea bream tested in land-based experimental facilities [30, 32]. Athanassopoulou et al. [30] tested the essential oil of *Origanum* and found a reduction of the prevalence of *Myxobolus* sp., but with a high level of fish mortality in *Puntazzo puntazzo* (sharpsnout sea bream). This same oil showed a reduction in the prevalence of the myxozoan *Polysporoplasma sparis* in *Sparus aurata* (gilthead sea bream) from 50% to less than 4% [32]. Cojocaru et al. [38] showed a decrease from about 40 to 20% in the prevalence of the infestation of the *Enteromyxum leei* in *S. aurata* after a month of oral and bath treatments using several essential oils. The essential

Plant	Fish	Type of extract	Isolated substances	Type of administration	Protozoan species	References [number]
Allium sativum	*Poecilia latipinna*			Bath	*Ichthyophthirius multifiliis*	Gholipour-Kanani et al. [37]
Allium sativum	*Pterophyllum scalare*	Essential oil	*E,Z*-Ajoene	Oral/Bath	*Spironucleus vortens*	Williams et al. [39]
Eclipta prostrate	*Carassius auratus*	Methanol		Bath	*Ichthyophthirius multifiliis*	Yi et al. [36]
Lippia alba	*Colossoma macropomum*	Essential oil (leaves)		Bath	*Ichthyophthirius multifiliis*	Soares et al. [35]
Lycium chinense	*Colossoma acropomum*	methanol		Bath	*Ichthyophthirius multifiliis*	Yi et al. [36]
Macleaya microcarpa	*Colossoma acropomum*		Dihydrosanguinarine, dihydrochelerythrine	Bath	*Ichthyophthirius multifiliis*	Yao et al. [40]
Magnolia officinalis	*Carassius auratus*	methanol		Bath	*Ichthyophthirius multifiliis*	Yi et al. [36]
Matricaria chamomilla	*Poecilia latipinna*			Bath	*Ichthyophthirius multifiliis*	Gholipour-Kanani et al. [37]
Ophiopogon bodinieri	*Carassius auratus*	methanol		Bath	*Ichthyophthirius multifiliis*	Yi et al. [36]
Psoralea corylifolia	*Carassius auratus*	methanol	Isopsoralen, psoralidin	Bath	*Ichthyophthirius multifiliis*	Song et al. [41]
Sophora alopecuroides	*Carassius auratus*	methanol		Bath	*Ichthyophthirius multifiliis*	Yi et al. [36]
Toddalia asiatica	*Carassius auratus*	Methanolic (leaves)	Chelerythrine and chloroxylonine		*Ichthyophthirius multifiliis*	Xiao-feng et al. [42]
Trichosanthes kirilowii	*Carassius auratus*	methanol		Bath	*Ichthyophthirius multifiliis*	Yi et al. [36]

Table 1. Medicinal plants with activity against protozoan species in fish farming.

Plant	Fish	Type of extract	Type of administration	Myxozoan species	References [number]
Achillea millefolium	*Sparus aurata*	essential oil/ water/ Ethanol	Oral/Bath	*Enteromyxum leei*	Cojocaru et al. [38]
Betula alba					
Calendula officinalis					
Cerasus sativa					
Crategus monogyna					
Equissetum arvensis					
Hypericum perforatum					
Matricaria chamomilla					
Mentha piperita					
Origanum spp.	*Diplodus puntazzo*	essential oil	Oral	Myxobolus sp.	Karagouni et al. [31]
Origanum minutiflorum	*Puntazzo puntazzo*	essential oil	Oral	*Myxobolus* sp.	Athanassopoulou et al. [30]
Origanum spp.	*Sparus aurata*	essential oil	Oral	*Polysporoplasma sparis*	Athanassopoulou et al. [32]
Ocinum basilicum	*Sparus aurata*	essential oil/ water/ethanol	Oral/Bath	*Enteromyxum leei*	Cojocaru et al. [38]
Prunus spinosus					
Rosa canina					
Sambucus nigra					
Thymus serpillum					
Tilia sp.					
Vaccinium myrtilus					
Viola tricolor					

Table 2. Medicinal plants with activity against myxozoan species in fish farming.

oil of *Origanum minutiflorum* (spartan oregano) decreased the prevalence of *Myxobolus* sp. in *P. puntazzo* from 37 to 39% in all oral treatments in comparison to untreated fish [31].

Also, medicinal plant extracts have also shown good results as anti-myxozoan agents. Aqueous and methanol extracts of the species *Achillea millefolium* (milenrama milfoil), *Betula alba* (silver birch), *Calendula officinalis* (marigold), *Cerasus sativa* (sweet chestnuts), *Crategus monogyna*

Plant	Fish	Type of extract	Isolated substances	Type of administration	Anthelmintic activity	References [number]
Allium sativum	*Poecilia reticulata*	Water		Oral/Bath	*G. turnbulli*, *Dactylogyrus* sp.	Fridman et al. [43]
Allium sativum	*Cyprinus carpio*	Hexane		Bath	*Capillaria* sp.,	Peña et al. [44]
Artemisia annua	*Heterobranchus longifilis*	Ethanol (leaves)		Bath	Monogenean	Ekanem and Brisibe [45]
Bixa orellana	*Colossoma macropomum*	Acetone (seeds)	Bixin and geraniol	Bath	*A. spathulatus*	Andrade et al. [46]
Brucea javanica	*Carassius auratus*	Methanolic (fruits)	bruceine A and bruceine D	Bath	*D. intermedius*	Wang et al. [47]
Bupleurum chinense	*Carassius auratus*	PE, CHL, EA, ME, water		Bath	*D. intermedius*	Wu et al. [48]
Caulis spatholobi,	*Carassius auratus*	PE, CHL, EA, ME, water		Bath	*D. intermedius*	Liu et al. [49]
Cimicifuga foetida L.	*Carassius auratus*	PE, CHL, EA, ME, water		Bath	*D. intermedius*	Wu et al. [48]
Cinnamomum cassia	*Carassius auratus*	PE, CHL, EA, ME, water		Bath	*D. intermedius*	Ji et al. [50]
Dioscorea zingiberensis	*Carassius auratus*				*Dactylogyrus* sp.	Jiang et al. [51]
Dryopteris crassirhizoma	*Carassius auratus*	PE, CHL, EA, ME, acetone		Bath	*D. intermedius*	Lu et al. [52]
Dryopteris crassirhizoma	*Carassius auratus*	PE, EA, ME (roots)	Protocatechuic acid, sutchuenoside A, and kaempferitrin	Bath	*D. intermedius*	Jiang et al. [53]
Euphorbia fischeriana	*Carassius uratus,*	PE, EA, ME, n-butanol, water		Bath	*D. vastator*	Zhang et al. [54]
Fructus bruceae	*Carassius auratus*	PE, CHL, EA, ME, water		Bath	*D. intermedius*	Liu et al. [49]
Fructus cnidii	*Carassius auratus*	Ethanol (fruits)	Osthol and isopimpinellin	Bath	*D. intermedius*	Wang et al. [55]

Plant	Fish	Type of extract	Isolated substances	Type of administration	Anthelmintic activity	References [number]
Ginkgo biloba	*Anguilla anguilla*	PE (exopleura)	Ginkgolic acid C13:0 and C15:1	Bath	*Pseudodactylogyrus* sp.	Wang et al. [56]
Ginkgo biloba	*Carassius auratus*				*Dactylogyrus*	Jiang et al. [51]
Kochia scoparia	*Carassius auratus*	PE, CHL, EA, ME, acetone		Bath	*D. intermedius*	Lu et al. [52]
Lippia alba	*Colossoma macropomum*	Essential oil (leaves)		Bath	*A. spathulatus, N. janauachensis, M. boegeri*	Soares et al. [35]
Lindera aggregata	*Carassius auratus*	PE, CHL, EA, ME, water		Bath	*D. intermedius*	Ji et al. [50]
Lippia sidoides	*Oreochromis niloticus*	Essential oil (leaves)		Bath	*C. tilapiae; C. thurstonae; C. halli; S. longicornis*	Hashimoto et al. [57]
Macleaya Microcarpa	*Carassius auratus*	Ethanol (aerial parts)	Sanguinarine, cryptopine, β-allocryptopine, protopine, 6-methoxyl-dihydro-chelerythrine	Bath	*D. intermedius*	Wang et al. [58]
Mentha piperita	*Arapaima gigas*	Essential oil (Leaves and inflorescences)		Bath	*Dawestrema* spp.	Malheiros et al. [59]
Mentha piperita	*Oreochromis niloticus*	Essential oil (leaves)		Bath	*C. tilapiae; C. thurstonae; C. halli; S. longicornis*	Hashimoto et al. [57]
Momordica cochinchinensis Spreng	*Carassius auratus*	PE, CHL, EA, ME, water		Bath	*D. intermedius*	Wu et al. [48]
Ocimum gratissimum	*Colossoma macropomum*	Essential oil (leaves)		Bath	Monogenean	Boijink et al. [60]
Paris polyphylla			polyphyllin D and dioscin		*D. intermedius*	Wang et al. [61]
Peucedanum decursivum (Miq.)	*Carassius auratus*	PE, CHL, EA, ME, water		Bath	*D. intermedius*	Wu et al. [48]

Plant	Fish	Type of extract	Isolated substances	Type of administration	Anthelmintic activity	References [number]
Piper guineense	*Carassius auratus auratus*	Methanolic (seeds)	Piperanine, *N*-isobutyl (E,E)-2,4 decadienamide, $\Delta\alpha$-β-dihydrowasanine	Oral	*G. elegans, D. extensus*	Ekanem et al. [62]
Polygala tenuifolia	*Carassius auratus*	PE, CHL, EA, ME, acetone		Bath	*D. intermedius*	Lu et al. [52]
Prunus amygdalus Batsch	*Carassius auratus*	PE, CHL, EA, ME, water		Bath	*D. intermedius*	Wu et al. [48]
Pseudolarix kaempferi	*Carassius auratus*	PE, CHL, EA, ME, water		Bath	*D. intermedius*	Ji et al. [50]
Radix angelicae pubescentis	*Carassius auratus*	PE, CHL, EA, ME, water		Bath	*D. intermedius*	Liu et al. [49]
Radix angelicae pubescentis	*Carassius auratus)*	Ethanol	Osthol	Bath	*D. intermedius*	Wang et al. [22]
Santalum album	*Carassius auratus*	CHL, EA, ME, water		Bath	*Dactylogyrus* sp., *Gyrodactylus* spp.	Tu et al. [63]
Semen aesculi	*Carassius auratus*	PE, CHL, EA, ME, water		Bath	*D. intermedius*	Liu et al. [49]
Semen pharbitidis	*Carassius auratus*	PE, CHL, EA, ME, water		Bath	*D. intermedius*	Liu et al. [49]

PE, petroleum ether; CHL, chloroform; EA, ethyl acetate; ME, methanol.

Table 3. Medicinal plants with anthelmintic activity in fish farming.

(hawthorn), *Equissetum arvensis* (horsetail), *Hypericum perforatum* (st. johnswort), *M. chamomilla, Mentha piperita*(peppermint), *Ocinum basilicum, Prunus spinosus* (blackthorn), *Rosacanina* (dogrose), *Sambucus nigra* (elder), *Thymus serpillum* (wild thyme), *Tilia* sp., *Vaccinium myrtilus* (bilberry) and *Viola tricolor* (johnny Jump up) were evaluated for 1 month of oral and bath treatments against *Enteromyxum leei* infection in cultured gilthead sea bream, *S. aurata* [38]. They decreased the infection of *E. leei* in *S. aurata*, from approximately 40 to 20% compared with the control [38]. Also, these extracts decreased the spore's level from the water, suggesting that the extract might eliminate some stages that are released into water [38].

2.3. Anthelmintic activity

Essential oils have been used against helminths, especially to control and prevent monogeneans [9]. Studies of essential oils from various plant species have shown the oils to have excellent biological activity when tested against various fish parasites [27]. For instance, essential oils of *Lippia sidoides* (pepper rosemary) and *M. piperita* have shown to be active at a concentration of 40 mg/L when tested in vivo against monogenean species (*Cichlidogyrus tilapiae, C. thurstonae, C. halli* and *Scutogyrus longicornis*). In that case, a therapeutic bath was recommended as an alternative treatment against monogeneans in Nile tilapia *Oreochromis niloticus*, due to a decrease of 70% of the parasite prevalence in Nile tilapia culture [57]. Moreover,in a therapeutic bath with the essential oil of *Ocimum gratissimum* (clove basil), the authors found an anti-parasite efficacy (percentage reduction in parasite count) around of 100% on the gills of juvenile tambaquis C. macropomum in concentrations of 10 and 15 mg/L^{-1} [60]. Soares *et al.* [35] demonstrated an anthelmintic activity against monogeneans species (*Anacanthorus spathulatus, Notozothecium janauachensis* and *Mymarothecium boegeri*) using essential oil of *L. alba* on the gills of *C. macropomum* after 20 minutes of exposure at concentrations of 1280 and 2560 mg/L. Similar results were found by Malheiros et al. [59] using the essential oil of *M. piperita*, yielding an anti-parasitic effect in the in vitro assay against *Dawestrema cycloancistrium* and *D. cycloancistrioides*, while in the in vivo test to evaluate the toxicity, the result was not satisfactory and caused changes in fish gill tissues. Thus, it is necessary to create therapeutic strategies capable of increasing the efficacy of the use of essential oils as phytotherapeutic agents to reduce their toxicity in *Arapaima gigas* (pirarucu).

Furthermore, recent reviews also have shown that plant extracts indicated efficient anthelmintic properties in numerous fish species [9, 15, 27]. Alcoholic or organic solvents have a greater efficiency in the isolation of bioactive substances. For example, the ethanol extract of the leaves of *Artemisia annua* (sweet wormwood), in 1 hour of exposure, at a concentration of 200 mg/L, killed 85% of the parasites without any mortality of juvenile *Heterobranchus longifilis* (vundu) [45]. The aqueous and methanol extract of *Semen aesculi* (buckeye seed) [49]; ethyl acetate, methanol and chloroform extracts of *Radix Bupleuri chinensis* (schisandra fruit) [48]; methanol extract of *Dryopteris crassirhizoma* (thick stemmed wood fern), *Kochia scoparia* (kochia) and *Polygala tenuifolia* (yuan zhi) [52] and methanol extracts of *Cinnamomum cassia* (cinnamon), *Lindera aggregata* (evergreen lindera) and *Pseudolarix kaempferi* [50] proved to be efficient against monogeneans *Dactylogyrus intermedius* in gold fish *C. auratus* (goldfish). Among the ethyl acetate, petroleum ether, n-butanol and water extracts from *Euphorbia fischeriana* (Lang-Du), only the ethyl acetate extract showed a killing effect in the in vitro and in vivo test on *D. vastator*, a monogenean of *C. auratus*. Moreover, the extract showed anthelmintic activity 40% higher than mebendazole or phoxim and had effects similar to those observed for praziquantel and trichlorfon, chemicals often used against *Dactylogyrus* spp. These results suggest that this extract can serve as a potent anti-parasitic agent in the aquaculture industry [54].

Fridman et al. [43] used an aqueous extract of garlic *A. sativum* in an in vivo assay (30 mL/L), and it caused the separation and decreased movement of two species of monogeneans (*Gyrodactylus turnbulli* and *Dactylogyrus* sp.). In the oral (10 and 20%) and bath (7.5 and 12 mL/L) test, the extract showed a significant reduction of parasites when compared to the control group [43]. Previous studies have shown 75% of the anthelmintic activity of the hexane extract of *A. sativum* against *Capillaria* sp., a nematode of *Cyprinus carpio* (common carp) [44]. The extracts of *Ginkgo biloba* (ginkgo) and *Dioscorea zingiberensis* (yellow ginger) showed potent, synergistic, anti-parasitic effects when combined against *Dactylogyrus* spp. in *C. auratus* under in vivo conditions [51].

2.4. Isolated substances from plants with anthelmintic activity

Chemicals of different classes such as alkaloids, flavonoids, saponins, coumarins, quinones, quassinoids, phenolics, lignans and terpenoids have been isolated. Andrade et al. [46] evaluated the efficacy of the extract of *Bixa orellana* (achiote) seeds against monogenean *A.spathulatus*, a parasite of *C. macropomum* in an in vivo test and achieved 100% efficacy. This activity may be related to the bixin and geranylgeraniol terpenoids present in the ketone extract. Studies indicated that the parasiticidal activity is due to the presence of these lipophilic substances since they can cross the surfaces of the membranes, causing a rupture and killing the parasites [64].

Wang et al. [55] isolated the osthol and isopimpinellin coumarins of the *Fructus cnidii* fruit (cnidium), which were 100% effective at concentrations of 1.6 and 9.5 mg/L, respectively, against *D. intermedius*, a parasite of goldfish *C. auratus*. Osthol is an important coumarin with extensive medical activity, including anti-tumour [65, 66], prevention of atherosclerosis [67], anti-aging and anti-proliferative [68]. However, there are few reports of anti-parasitic effects. Osthol was also isolated from *Radix angelicae pubescent* (pubescent angelica root) and exhibited excellent activity against *Dactylogyrus intermedius* achieving 100% mortality at a concentration of 1.6 mg/L and did not show any toxicity to *C. auratus* at a dose of up to 6.2 mg/L [22].

Wang et al. [47] isolated the bruceina A and bruceina D quassinoids from the methanol extract of *Bruceajavanica* fruits (macassar kernels). There was strong anthelmintic activity against *D. intermedius* with EC50 (i.e. defined as the concentration of the sample leading to 50% reduction of *D. intermedius*) values of 0.49 and 0.57 mg/L after 48 hours, respectively. The substances were twice as efficient as mebendazole, which is often used to control *Dactylogyrus* spp. In the toxicity test, these substances proved to be safe for use in goldfish in concentrations of up to 5 mg/L. Bruceina A and D are similar in structure compared to the C-20 type quassinoids. This indicates that the mode of action of these substances may be similar to quassinoids. Several studies discuss the quassinoid action in different parasite species, emphasising that the primary targets of these molecules are the proteins of the cell [69–72]. Fukamiya et al. [71] demonstrated that the C-8-to-C-13 epoxymethano bridge and the hydroxyl group at C-11 and C-12 of the quassinoids are important to inhibit protein synthesis. In a previous study, quassinoids showed anti-malarial activity by inhibiting protein synthesis [72]. Therefore, the anti-parasitic activity of bruceina A and D can be related to the action mechanism that inhibits protein synthesis [47].

Sanguinarine, criptopine, β-allocriptopine, protopine and 6-methoxy-dihydro-chelerythrine alkaloids were isolated from the aerial parts of *Macleaya microcarpa* (kelway's coral plume) and were 100% efficient in monogenean *D. intermedius*, a parasite of *C. auratus* [58]. Ekanem et al. [62] showed that the methanol extract from *Piper guineense* (English West African black pepper) seeds was active against *G. elegans* and *D. extensus* in concentrations of 0.5 to 2.0 mg/L in vitro and in vivo assays. The substances identified in the extracts were piperanine, N- isobutyl (E,E)-2,4-decadienamide and Δα, β-dihydrowasanine.

Wang et al. [61] isolated the steroidal saponins dioscin and polyphyllin D from the crude extract of the rhizome of *Paris polyphylla* (ginseng) and achieved excellent results for the monogenean *D. intermedius*. Wang et al. [56] isolated ginkgolic acid C13:0 (M1) and C15:1 (M2) from *G. biloba* and were 100% effective at concentrations of 2.5 and 6.0 mg/L, with ED50 values of 0.72 and 2.88 mg/L, respectively, for *Pseudodactylogyrus* sp., a parasite of juvenile eels (*Anguilla anguilla*). The flavonoids sutchuenoside A and kaempferitrin, isolated from the rhizome of *D. rhamnosides*, had satisfactory anthelmintic activity in the in vivo test against *D. intermedius* and were safe for the *C. auratus* host [53]. These studies reveal the potential of these isolated substances as anthelmintic activity in fish farming.

2.5. Isolated substances from plants with anti-protozoan activity

Several species of medicinal plants have shown efficiency in the control of protozoans in aquaculture, but there are few reports describing the isolation of bioactive molecules responsible for the anti-protozoan activity. For example, the alkaloids dihydrosanguinarine and dihydrocheleritrine, isolated from *M. microcarpa* were active against the protozoan *I. multifiliis*, a parasite of *C. macropomum* with EC50 values of 5.18 and 9.43 mg/L, respectively, which points to strong anti-parasitic possibilities for fish [40]. Xiao-Feng et al. [42] demonstrated that the alkaloids cheleritrine and chloroxylonine, isolated from the leaves of *Toddalia asiatica* (orange climber) were 100% effective against *I. multifiliis*, a parasite of *C. auratus*, in concentrations of 1.2 and 3.5 mg/L, with average effective concentrations (EC50) of 0.55 and 1.90 mg/L, respectively. In the in vivo test, the fish treated with cheleritrine and chloroxylonine at concentrations of 1.8 and 8.0 mg/L had fewer parasites than the control. The acute toxicity (LC50) was 3.3 mg/L for chelerythrine for goldfish. Direct action in the mitochondria may be involved in the eradication of the parasites since this organelle is responsible for controlling and regulating cell apoptosis, but further studies are still required to detail the action mechanism of these substances [42, 73]. Song et al. [41] isolated isopsoralene and psoralidin, which showed potent anti-protozoan activity. In the in vitro assay with psoralidin, 100% mortality of the protozoan *I. multifiliis* was observed at a concentration of 0.8 mg/L in 4 hours of exposure, which was more active than isopsoralene. Ajoene components (*Allium sativum*) showed inhibition of *Spironucleus vortens*, a protozoan fish parasite of *Pterophyllum scalare* (angelfish) with a minimum inhibitory concentration of

40 ug/mL, while the substance (Z)-ajoene (minimum inhibitory concentration = 16 ug/L) isolated from the essential oils proved to be more active that its isomer (E)-ajoene [39]. When compared with metronidazole (MTZ), the ajoene components were 10-fold greater than that of MTZ (4g/ml), the drug of choice for treatment of *S. vortens* infections [39].

2.6. Environmental impacts of anti-parasitics used in fish farming

The use of anti-parasitics, insecticides, pesticides and antibiotics has been used in several freshwater, brackishwater and marine farming fish systems to control parasites and pathogens [8, 9]. Although the use of these chemical treatments reduces infection rates in fish farming systems, their excessive use might lead to a build-up of drug resistance in the pathogen or parasite [8, 17]. For example, the loss of salmon stock to sea lice infestation (*L. salmonis*) led to the use of two chemical treatments in a marine aquaculture system. One insecticide called dichlorvos and one chemical (i.e. hydrogen peroxide), with the germicidal property. The frequent and widespread use of these chemicals might lead to reduced efficacy caused by the resistance that developed the parasite [8]. Umeda et al. [74] also observed a drug resistance in the use of an organophosphate insecticide (e.g. trichlorfon) and praziquantel in bath treatments for ectoparasites such as monogeneans.

Moreover, the bioaccumulation of the chemicals or the presence of residual antibiotic in the final fish product might have potential consequences on human health [9, 75]. An important issue is the transfer of resistant pathogens from fish farming to humans. As the resistance to antibiotics is transmitted from one bacterium to another, it might have a risk of transference of antibiotic resistance to healthy bacteria in the human gut [20].

Chemical and biocides used in fish farming might also have lethal or sub-lethal effects on non-target organisms in the environment [20]. The encapsulated antibiotics of the uneaten feed accumulated on the seabed beneath fish cages can affect microbial communities in the immediate vicinity, leading to a reduction in their diversity [8]. For example, the release of antibiotics into the environment can negatively affect the biodiversity of planktonic, algae, microcrustaceans and benthic communities [19].

According to Kemper [76], little is known about the effects of anti-parasitics and chemical compounds pollution to either humans or the environment, but the increasing resistance to antibiotics by bacteria and the diminishing effectiveness of therapeutic drugs have been considered a global concern. The anti-parasitics and antibiotics might remain in the water until degraded by natural processes or are accumulated in the sediment. Some chemical treatments used in fish farming may deteriorate most rapidly, but most are persistent [76].

Therefore, the use of the plant-derived compounds as an alternative treatment against parasites in fish farming has been representing few or no adverse impact on the environment because its residuals are usually biodegradable in the water [23]. Differently, of the traditional chemotherapeutics, the administration of the plant-derived compounds in fish has been associated with few or no side effects [15]. Although the persistence of plant-derived compounds in the environment and their side effects to human health have been still little emphasised, more studies are necessary to verify the real impact of these plant-derived compounds into the environment and their effects on human.

3. Conclusions and future perspectives

This review showed that the plant-derived compounds have a great potential to prevent and control parasites in fish farming, especially about protozoans, myxozoans and monogeneans. Many compounds isolated from plant extracts, for example, osthol, geraniol and bruceina A and D may have a useful role for controlling parasites in fish farming, although more studies are necessary to determine the sufficient concentration during the administration, seems that oral administration has been the most suitable for aquaculture [9]. Also, the potential for discovering new essential oils, plant extracts and bioactive compounds is increasing each year due to the use of new tools of analysis and the interest of the researchers in their pharmacological activities to control fish diseases. The use of these plant-derived compounds may become a powerful phytotherapy, although more studies are necessary to prove the efficiency of these plant-derived compounds as a natural parasitic control.

Moreover, novel applications of nanotechnology and microencapsulation are growing rapidly in agriculture, food and aquaculture sector industries [77–79]. The synthesis of the plant-based materials for the production of nanomaterials can be used to enhance the ability of fish to absorb the bioactive from the plants in the control of fish diseases in aquaculture and at the same time its products are safe for the environment [80, 81]. Another application is the microencapsulation that has been used for the incorporation of numerous compounds such as proteins, lipids, carbohydrates, vitamins, minerals, hormones, probiotics and plant extracts necessary for the growth and health of fishes [79]. Both applications might help the growing of aquaculture and enhance the treatment against parasites in fish farming.

Furthermore, there is a need to look for alternative treatments to control and prevent fish parasites in aquaculture, which are at the same time environmentally friendly and highly efficient. Studies of essential oils, crude extracts and chemicals of medicinal plants have shown them to be viable and cheap. Thus, conventional parasiticides might be replaced by the use of phytotherapeutic agents in aquaculture.

Fish health is a challenging task in the search for a sustainable aquaculture, for which the plant-derived compounds offer viable alternatives to deal with the outbreaks of infectious diseases in fish farming. Therefore, plant-derived compounds seem to represent a promising alternative to control fish diseases in aquaculture.

Author details

Alison Carlos Wunderlich[1,2*], Érica de Oliveira Penha Zica[2], Vanessa Farias dos Santos Ayres[3], Anderson Cavalcante Guimarães[3] and Renata Takeara[3]

*Address all correspondence to: awunderlich@gmail.com

1 School of Biological Sciences, Royal Holloway, University of London, Egham, UK

2 São Paulo State University, Department of Parasitology, Botucatu, São Paulo, Brazil

3 Federal University of Amazonas, Institute of Science and Technology, Itacoatiara/AM, Brazil

References

[1] FAO (Food and Agriculture Organization UN). The State of World Fisheries and Aquaculture. Report FAO, Rome; 2012.

[2] Lafferty K.D., Harvell C.D., Conrad J.M., Friedman C.S., Kent M.L., Kuris A.M., Powell E.N., Rondeau D., Saksida S.M. Infectious diseases affect marine fisheries and aquaculture economics. Annual Review of Marine Science. 2015;**7**:471-496. doi:10.1146/annurev-marine-010814-015646.

[3] Murray A.G., Peeler E.J. A framework for understanding the potential for emerging diseases in aquaculture. Preventive Veterinary Medicine. 2005;**67**:223-235.

[4] Woo P.T.K., Buchmann K., editors. Fish Parasites: Pathobiology and Protection, 1st ed. Wallingford, UK: CABI; 2012, 383 p.

[5] Perumal S., Thirunavukkarasu A.R., Pachiappan P., editors. Advances in Marine and Brackish Water Aquaculture, 1st ed. New Delhi, India: Springer; 2015, 262 p. doi:10.1007/978-81-322-2271-2.

[6] FAO (Food and Agriculture Organization UN). The State of World Fisheries and Aquaculture. Report FAO, Rome; 2007.

[7] Costello M.J. The global economic cost of sea lice to the salmonid farming industry. Journal of Fish Diseases. 2009;**32**(1):115-118. doi:10.1111/j.1365-2761.2008.01011.x.

[8] Kaiser M.J., Attrill M.J., Jennings S., Thomas D.N., Barnes D.K.A., editors. Marine Ecology: Processes, Systems, and Impacts, 2nd ed. Oxford, UK: Oxford University Press; 2011, 501 p.

[9] Reverter M., Bontemps N., Lecchini D., Banaigs B., Sasal P. Use of plant extracts in fish aquaculture as an alternative to chemotherapy: current status and future perspectives. Aquaculture. 2014;**433**:50-61. doi:http://dx.doi.org/10.1016/j.aquaculture.2014.05.048.

[10] Noga E.J. Fish Disease: Diagnosis and Treatment, 2nd ed. Iowa: Wiley-Blackwell; 2010, 519 p.

[11] Mehlhorn H., editor. Nature Helps...How Plants and Other Organisms Contribute to Solve Health Problems, 1st ed. Heidelberg: Springer-Verlag; 2011. 372 p. doi:10.1007/978-3-642-19382-8.

[12] Schmahl G., Mehlhorn H. Treatment of fish parasites. I. Praziquantel effective against Monogenea (*Dactylogyrus vastator, Dactylogyrus extensus, Diplozoon paradoxum*). Zeitschrift für Parasitenkunde. 1985;**71**:727-737.

[13] Buchmann K., Slotved H.C., Dana D. Epidemiology of gill parasite infections in *Cyprinus carpio* in Indonesia and possible control methods. Aquaculture.1993;**118**:9-21.

[14] Prost M., Studnicka P. Investigations on the use of organic esters of phosphoric acid in the control of external parasites of farmed fish: II. Control of the invasion of parasites of *Dactylogyrus* and *Gyrodactylus*. Medical Veterinary. 1966;**22**:644-650.

[15] Bulfon C., Volpatti D., Galeotti M. Current research on the use of plant-derived products in farmed fish. Aquaculture Research. 2015;**46**:513-551. doi:doi:10.1111/are.12238.

[16] Sakai M. Current research status of fish immunostimulants. Aqua culture. 1999;**172** (1-2):63-92.

[17] Caipang C.M.A., Lazado C.C. Nutritional impacts on fish mucosa: immunostimulants, pre- and probiotics. In: Beck B.H., Peatman E., editors. Mucosal Health in Aquaculture, 1st ed. London, UK: Academic Press; 2015, pp. 211-272.

[18] Carey D.E., McNamara P.J. The impact of triclosan on the spread of antibiotic resistance in the environment. Frontiers in Microbiology. 2015;**5**(780):1-11. doi:10.3389/fmicb.2014.00780.

[19] Boyd C.E., McNevin A.A. Aquaculture: Resource Use, and the Environment, 1st ed. Hoboken, NJ: John Wiley & Sons; 2015, 337 p.

[20] Pillay T.V.R. Aquaculture and the Environment, 2nd ed. Oxford, UK: Blackwell; 2004, 196 p.

[21] Egidius E., Moster B. Effect of NEGUVON and NUVAN treatment on crab (*Cancer pagurus, C. maenas*), lobster (*Homarus gammarus*) and blue mussel (*Mytilus edulis*). Aquaculture. 1987;**60**:165-168.

[22] Wang K.-Y., Yao L., Du Y.-H., Xie J.-B., Huang J.-L., Yin Z.-Q. Anthelmintic activity of the crude extracts, fractions, and osthole from *Radix angelicae* pubescentis against *Dactylogyrus intermedius* in goldfish (*Carassius auratus*) in vivo. Parasitology Research. 2011;**108**:195-200. doi:10.1007/s00436-010-2058-9.

[23] Rahuman A.A. Efficacies of medicinal plant extracts against blood-sucking parasites. In: Mehlhorn H., editor. Nature Helps...How Plants and Other Organisms Contribute to Solve Health Problems, 1st ed. Heidelberg: Springer-Verlag; 2011, pp. 19-53. doi:10.1007/978-3-642-19382-8_2.

[24] Mehlhorn H., Wu Z., Ye B., editors. Treatment of Human Parasitosis in Traditional Chinese Medicine, 1st ed. Heidelberg: Springer-Verlag; 2014, 274 p.

[25] Khater H.F. Prospects of botanical biopesticides in insect pest. 2012;**3**. Bioactivity of essential oils as green. In: Govil J.N., Bhattacharya S., editors. Recent Progress in Medicinal: Plants, Vol. 37, Essential oils II, 1st ed. Houston: Studium Press LLC; 2013, pp. 153-220

[26] Khater H.F. Prospects of botanical biopesticides in insect pest management. Pharmacologia. 2012;**3**(12):641-656. doi:10.5567/pharmacologia.2012.641.656

[27] Valladão G.M.R., Gallani S.U., Pilarski F. Phytotherapy as an alternative for treating fish disease. Journal of Veterinary Pharmacology and Therapeutics. 2015;**38**:417-428. doi:10.1111/jvp.12202.

[28] Rohde K., editor. Marine Parasitology, 1st ed. Collingwood: CSIRO; 2005, 565 p.

[29] Woo P.T.K., editor. Fish Diseases and Disorders. Volume 1: Protozoan and Metazoan Infections, 2nd ed. Wallingford: CABI; 2006, 791 p.

[30] Athanassopoulou F., Karagouni E., Dotsika E., Ragias V., Tavla J., Christofilloyanis P., Vatsos I. Efficacy and toxicity of orally administrated anti-coccidial drugs for innovative treatments of *Myxobolus* sp. infection in *Puntazzo puntazzo*. Diseases of Aquatic Organisms. 2004;**62**:217-226. doi:10.3354/dao062217

[31] Karagouni E., Athanassopoulou F., Lytra A., Komis C., Dotsika E. Antiparasitic and immunomodulatory effect of innovative treatments against Myxobolus sp. infection in *Diplodus puntazzo*. Veterinary Parasitology. 2005;**134**:215-228. doi:10.1016/j.vetpar.2005.07.020.

[32] Athanassopoulou F., Karagouni E., Dotsika E., Ragias V., Tavla J., Christofilloyanis P. Efficacy and toxicity of orally administered anticoccidial drugs for innovative treatments of *Polysporoplasma sparis* (Sitja-Bobadilla and Alvarez-Pellitero 1985) infection in *Sparus aurata* L. Journal of Applied Ichthyology. 2004; **20**(5): 345-354. doi:10.1111/j.1439-0426.2004.00580.x.

[33] Duke J.A. Handbook of Medicinal Herbs, 5th ed. Boca Raton, FL: CRC Press; 1987, 696 p.

[34] Harikrishnan R., Balasundaram C., Heo M.S. Impact of plant products on innate and adaptive immune system of cultured finfish and shellfish. Aquaculture. 2011;**317**:1-15. doi:10.1016/j.aquaculture.2011.03.039.

[35] Soares B.V., Neves L.R., Oliveira M.S.B., Chaves F.C. M., Dias M.K.R., Chagas E.C. Antiparasitic activity of the essential oil of *Lippia alba* on ectoparasites of *Colossoma macropomum* (tambaqui) and its physiological and histopathological effects. Aquaculture. 2016;**452**:107-114. doi:10.1016/j.aquaculture.2015.10.029.

[36] Yi Y.-L., Lu C., Hu X.-G., Ling F., Wang G.-X. Antiprotozoal activity of medicinal plants against *Ichthyophthirius multifiliis* in goldfish (*Carassius auratus*). Parasitology Research. 2012;**111**:1771-1778. doi:10.1007/s00436-012-3022-7.

[37] Gholipour-Kanani H., Sahandi J., Taheri A. Influence of garlic (*Allium sativum*) and mother worth (*Matricaria chamomilla*) extract on *Ichthyophtirius multifilus* parasite treatment in sail fin molly (*Poecilia latipinna*) ornamental fish. APCBEE Procedia. 2012;**4**:6-11. doi:10.1016/j.apcbee.2012.11.002

[38] Cojocaru C.D. Prevalence, pathogenicity and control of the fish parasites in the Banat region, Romania. In: Mattiucci S., editor. 7th International Symposium on Fish Parasites, 24-28 September; Viterbo; 2007, p. 49(2):370.

[39] Williams C.F., Vacca A.R., Dunham L., Lloyd D., Coogan M.P., Evans G., Graz M., Cable J. The redox-active drug metronidazole and thiol-depleting garlic compounds act synergistically in the protist parasite Spironucleus vortens. Molecular & Biochemical Parasitology. 2016;**206**:20-28. doi:10.1016/j.molbiopara.2016.03.001.

[40] Yao J.-Y., Zhou Z.-M, Li X.-L., Yin W.-L., Ru H.-S., Pan X.-Y., Hao G.-J., Xu Y., Shen J. Antiparasitic efficacy of dihydrosanguinarine and dihydrochelerythrine from *Macleaya microcarpa* against *Ichthyophthirius multifiliis* in richadsin (*Squaliobarbus curriculus*). Veterinary Parasitology. 2011;**183**:8-13. doi:10.1016/j.vetpar.2011.07.021.

[41] Song K., Ling F., Huang A., Dong W., Liu G., Jiang C., Zhang Q., Wang G. In vitro and in vivo assessment of the effect of antiprotozoal compounds isolated from *Psoralea corylifolia* against *Ichthyophthirius multifiliis* in fish. International Journal for Parasitology: Drugs and Drug Resistance.2015;5:58-64. doi:10.1016/j.ijpddr.2015.04.001.

[42] Xiao-feng S., Qing-feng M., Yuan-huan K., Yu B., Yun-hang G., Wei-li W., Ai-dong Q. Isolation of active compounds from methanol extracts of *Toddalia asiatica* against *Ichthyophthirius multifiliis* in goldfish (*Carassius auratus*). Veterinary Parasitology. 2014;**199**:250- 254. doi:10.1016/j.vetpar.2013.10.021.

[43] Fridman S., Sinai T., Zilberg T. Efficacy of garlic based treatments against monogenean parasites infecting the guppy (*Poecilia reticulata* (Peters). Veterinary Parasitology. 2014;**203**:51-58. doi:10.1016/j.vetpar.2014.02.002.

[44] Peña N., Auró A., Sumano H. A comparative trial of garlic, its extract and ammoniumpotassium tartrate as anthelmintics in carp. Journal of Ethnopharmacology. 1988;**24**:199-203. doi:10.1016/0378-8741(88)90152-3.

[45] Ekanem A.P., Brisibe E.A. Effects of ethanol extract of *Artemisia annua* L. against monogenean parasites of *Heterobranchus longifilis*. Parasitology Research. 2010;**106**:1135-1139. doi:10.1007/s00436-010-1787-0.

[46] Andrade J.I.A., Jerônimo G.T., Brasil E.M., Nunes C.V., Gonçalves E.L.T., Ruiz M.L., Martins M.L. Efficacy of seed extract of Bixa orellana against monogenean gill parasites and physiological aspects of *Colossoma macropomum* after bath treatment. Aquaculture. 2016;**462**:40-46. doi:10.1016/j.aquaculture.2016.04.024.

[47] Wang Y., Wu Z.-F., Wang G.-X., Wang F., Liu Y.-T., Li F.-Y., Han J. In vivo anthelmintic activity of bruceine A and bruceine D from *Bruceajavanica* against Dactylogyrus intermedius (Monogenea) in goldfish (*Carassius auratus*). Veterinary Parasitology. 2011;**177**:127-133. doi:10.1016/j.vetpar.2010.11.040.

[48] Wu Z.-F., Zhu B., Wang Y., Lu C., Wang G.-X. In vivo evaluation of anthelmintic potential of medicinal plant extracts against *Dactylogyrus intermedius* (Monogenea) in goldfish (*Carassius auratus*). Parasitology Research. 2011;**108**:1557-1563. doi:10.1007/s00436-010-2211-5.

[49] Liu Y.T., Wang F., Wang G.-X., Han J., Wang Y., Wang Y.-H. In vivo anthelmintic activity of crude extracts of Radix angelicae pubescentis, Fructus bruceae, Caulis spatholobi, Semen aesculi, and Semen pharbitidis against *Dactylogyrus intermedius* (Monogenea) in goldfish (*Carassius auratus*). Parasitology Research. 2010;**106**:1233-1239. doi:10.1007/s00436-010-1799-9.

[50] Ji J., Lu C., Kang Y., Wang G.-X., Chen P. Screening of 42 medicinal plants for in vivo anthelmintic activity against Dactylogyrus intermedius (Monogenea) in goldfish (*Carassius auratus*). Parasitology Research. 2012;**111**:97-104. doi:10.1007/s00436-011-2805-6.

[51] Jiang C., Wu Z.-Q., Liu L., Wang G.-X. Synergy of herbal ingredients combination against Dactylogyrus spp. In an infected goldfish model for monogenean management. Aquaculture. 2014;**33**:115-118. doi:10.1016/j.aquaculture.2014.05.045.

[52] Lu C., Zhang H.-Y., Ji J., Wang G.-X. In vivo anthelmintic activity of *Dryopteris crassirhizoma, Kochia scoparia,* and *Polygala tenuifolia* against Dactylogyrus intermedius (Monogenea) in goldfish (*Carassius auratus*). Parasitology Research. 2012;**110**:1085-1090. doi:10.1007/s00436-011-2592-0.

[53] Jiang B., Chi C., Fu Y.-W., Zhang Q.-Z., Wang, G.-X. In vivo anthelmintic effect of flavonol rhamnosides from *Dryopteris crassirhizoma* against *Dactylogyrus intermedius* in goldfish (*Carassius auratus*). Parasitology Research. 2013;**112**:4097-4104. doi:10.1007/s00436-013-3600-3.

[54] Zhang X.P., Li W.X., Ai T.S., Zou H., Wu S.G., Wang G.T. The efficacy of four common anthelmintic drugs and traditional Chinese medicinal plant extracts to control *Dactylogyrus vastator* (Monogenea). Aquaculture. 2014;**420-421**:302-307. doi:10.1016/j.aquaculture.2013.09.022.

[55] Wang G., Zhou Z., Cheng C., Yao J., Yang Z. Osthol and isopimpinellin from Fructus cnidii for the control of *Dactylogyrus intermedius* in *Carassius auratus*. Veterinary Parasitology. 2008;**158**:144-151. doi:10.1016/j.vetpar.2008.07.034.

[56] Wang G.-X., Jiang D.-X., Zhou Z., Zhao Y.-K., Shen Y.-H. In vivo assessment of anthelmintic efficacy of ginkgolic acids (C13:0, C15:1) on removal of *Pseudodactylogyrus* in European eel. Aquaculture. 2009;**297**:38-43. doi:10.1016/j.aquaculture.2009.09.012.

[57] Hashimoto G.S.O., Neto F.M., Ruiz M.L., Acchile M., Chagas E.C., Chaves F.C.M., Martins M.L. Essential oils of *Lippia sidoides* and *Mentha piperita* against monogenean parasites and their influence on the hematology of *Nile tilapia*. Aquaculture. 2016;**450**:182-186. doi:10.1016/j.aquaculture.2015.07.029.

[58] Wang G.-X., Zhou Z., Jiang D.-X., Han J., Wang J.-F., Zhao L.-W., Li J. In vivo anthelmintic activity of five alkaloids from *Macleaya microcarpa* (Maxim) Fedde against *Dactylogyrus intermedius* in *Carassius auratus*.Veterinary Parasitology. 2010;**171**:305-313. doi:10.1016/j.vetpar.2010.03.032.

[59] Malheiros D.F., Maciel P.O., Videira M.N., Tavares-Dias M. Toxicity of the essential oil of *Mentha piperita* in *Arapaima gigas* (pirarucu) and antiparasitic effects on Dawestrema spp. (Monogenea). Aquaculture. 2016;**455**:81-86. doi:10.1016/j.aquaculture.2016.01.018.

[60] Boijink C.L., Queiroz C.A., Chagas E.C., Chaves F.C.M., Inoue L.A.K.A. Anesthetic and anthelminthic effects of clove basil (*Ocimum gratissimum*) essential oil for tambaqui (*Colossoma macropomum*). Aquaculture. 2016;**457**:24-28. doi:10.1016/j.aquaculture.2016.02.010.

[61] Wang G.-X., Han J., Zhao L.-W., Jiang D.-X., Liu Y.-T., Liu X.-L. Anthelmintic activity of steroidal saponins from Paris polyphylla. Phytomedicine.2010;**17**:1102-1105. doi:10.1016/j.phymed.2010.04.012.

[62] Ekanem A.P., Wang M., Simon J.E., Obiekezie A.I., Morah, F. In vivo and in vitro activities of the seed extract of *Piper guineense* Schum. and Thonn. against skin and gill monogenean parasites of goldfish (*Carassius auratus auratus*). Phytotherapy Research. 2004;**18**:793-797. doi:10.1002/ptr.1550.

[63] Tu X., Ling F., Huang A., Zhang Q., Wang G. Anthelmintic efficacy of *Santalum album* (Santalaceae) against monogenean infections in goldfish. Parasitology Research. 2013;**112**: 2839-2845. doi:10.1007/s00436-013-3455-7.

[64] Wink M. Evolutionary advantage and molecular modes of action of multi-component mixtures used in phytomedicine. Current Drug Metabolism. 2008;9:996-1009. doi:10.2174/138920008786927794.

[65] Xu X., Zhang Y., Qu D., Jiang T., Li S. Osthole induces G2/M arrest and apoptosis in lung cancer A549 cells by modulating PI3K/Akt pathway. Journal of Experimental & Clinical Cancer Research. 2011;30:33-39. doi:10.1186/1756-9966-30-33

[66] Zhang L., Jiang G., Yao F., He Y., Liang G., Zhang Y., Hu B., Wu Y., Li Y., Liu H. Growth inhibition and apoptosis induced by osthole, a natural coumarin, in hepatocellular carcinoma. PLoS One. 2012;**7**:1-9. doi:10.1371/journal.pone.0037865.

[67] Ogawa H., Sasai N., Kamisako T., Baba K. Effects of osthol on blood pressure and lipid metabolism in stroke-prone spontaneously hypertensive rats. Journal of Ethnopharmacology. 2007;**112**:26-31. doi:10.1016/j.jep.2007.01.028.

[68] Hsieh M.T., Hsieh C.L., Wang W.H., Chen C.S., Lin C.J., Wu C.R. Osthole improves aspects of spatial performance in ovariectomized rats. The American Journal of Chinese Medicine. 2004;**32**:11-20. doi:10.1142/S0192415X04001758.

[69] Liao L.-L., Kupchan M., Horwitz S.B. Mode of action of the antitumor compound bruceantin, an inhibitior of protein synthesis. Molecular Pharmacology. 1976;**12**:167-176.

[70] Kirby G.C., O'Neill M.J., Phillipson J.D., Warhurst D.C. In vitro studies on the mode of action of quassinoids with activity against chloroquine-resistant *Plasmodium falciparum*. Biochemical Pharmacology. 1989;**8**:4367-4374. doi:10.1016/0006-2952(89)90644-8.

[71] Fukamya N., Lee K.-H., Muhammad I., Murakami C., Okano M., Harvey I., Pelletier J. Structure-activity relationships of quassinoids for eukaryotic protein synthesis. Cancer Letters. 2005;**220**:37-48. doi:10.1016/j.canlet.2004.04.023.

[72] Guo Z., Vangapandu S., Sindelar R.W., Walker L.A., Sindelar R.D. Biologically active quassinoids and their chemistry: potential leads for drug design.Current Medicinal Chemistry. 2005;**12**:173-190. doi:10.2174/0929867053363351.

[73] Kemény-Beke A., Aradi J., Damjanovich J., Beck Z., Facskó A., Berta A., Bodnár A. Apoptotic response of uveal melanoma cells upon treatment with chelidonine, sanguinarine and chelerythrine. Cancer Letters. 2006;**237**:67-75. doi:10.1016/j.canlet.2005.05.037.

[74] Umeda N., Nibe H., Hara T., Hirazawa N. Effects of various treatments on hatching of eggs and viability of oncomiracidia of the monogenean *Pseudodactylogyrus anguillae* and *Pseudodactylogyrus bini*. Aquaculture. 2006;**253**:148-153. doi:10.1016/j.aquaculture.2005.08.009.

[75] Cabello F.C. Heavy use of prophylactic antibiotics in aquaculture: a growing problem for human and animal health and for the environment. Environmental Microbiology. 2006;**8**:1137-1144. doi:10.1111/j.1462-2920.2006.01054.x.

[76] Kemper N. Veterinary antibiotics in the aquatic and terrestrial environment. Ecological Indicators. 2008;**8**:1-13. doi:10.1016/j.ecolind.2007.06.002.

[77] Selvaraj B., Subramanian K., Gopal S., Renuga P.S. Nanotechnology as a novel tool for aquaculture industry: a review. World Journal of Pharmaceutical Sciences. 2014;**2**(9): 1089-1096.

[78] Husen A., Siddiqi K.S. Phytosynthesis of nanoparticles: concept, controversy and application. Nanoscale Research Letters. 2014;**9**(229):1-24.

[79] Stoica M., Alexe P., Valsame M. Microencapsulation of biological compounds for cultured fish diet. A brief review. Journal of Agroalimentary Processes and Technologies. 2016;**22**(1):1-6.

[80] Mohanpuria P., Rana N.K., Yadav S.K. Biosynthesis of nanoparticles: technological concepts and future applications. Journal of Nanoparticle Research. 2008;**10**:507-517.

[81] Mahanty A., Mishra S., Bosu S., Maurya U.K., Netam S.P., Sarkar B. Phytoextracts-synthesized silver nanoparticles inhibit bacterial fish pathogen *Aeromonas hydrophila*. Indian Journal of Microbiology. 2013;**53**(4):438-446.

Section 4

Miscellaneous Biorationals

Chapter 6

Involvement of Gap Junction Proteins in Infectious Diseases Caused by Parasites

José Luis Vega, Iván Barría, Juan Güiza,
Jorge González and Juan C. Sáez

Additional information is available at the end of the chapter

http://dx.doi.org/10.5772/67187

Abstract

Parasitic diseases affect low-income nations with health consequences that affect the economy of these countries. Research aimed at understanding their biology and identification of potential targets for drug development is of the highest priority. Inhibitors of channels formed by proteins of the gap junction family such as suramin and probenecid are currently used for treatment of parasitic diseases caused by pathogenic protozoan. Gap junction proteins are present in both vertebrates and invertebrates permitting direct and indirect cellular communication. These cellular specializations are formed by two protein families corresponding to connexins (vertebrates) and innexins (invertebrates). In addition, a third protein family composed by proteins denominated pannexins is present in vertebrates and shows primary sequence homology to innexins. Channels formed by these proteins are essential in many biological processes. Recent evidences suggest that gap junction proteins play a critical role in bacterial and viral infections. Nonetheless, little is known about the role of these channels in parasitic infections. In this chapter, we summarized the current knowledge about the role of gap junction family proteins and channels in parasitic infections.

Keywords: connexins, pannexins, innexins, cellular communication, parasites

1. Introduction

The gap junction protein families include connexin, pannexin, and innexin proteins [1]. Connexin and innexin proteins form gap junction channels, which connect the cytoplasm of neighbouring cells, or connexin, pannexin and innexin proteins form channels (a half of gap junction channel) that connect the intra- and extracellular milieu [1]. In humans, connexins and pannexins are encoded by 21 and 3 genes, respectively [1]. Moreover, it has been identified 25 and 8 innexin genes in *Caenorhabditis elegans* and *Drosophila melanogaster*, respectively [2, 3]. It is known that Panx1 channels participate in response to bacterial and viral infections; however, little is known about the role of Panx1 channels and gap junction channels in infections caused by parasites [4–7] (**Table 1**). For example, *Shigella flexneri*, which is a causative agent of bacillary dysentery, causes opening of hemichannels formed by connexin 26 [4], which favours its spread and invasion [4]. Also, blockade of Panx1 channels has been shown to inhibit HIV replication in CD4(+) T lymphocytes [6]. In this chapter, we summarized the current knowledge about how the parasite infections modulate channels formed by gap junction proteins in host cells and the cellular pathways involved in this phenomenon. We also comment on channel blockers currently used in medicine for treatment of parasitic diseases caused by pathogenic protozoan (**Table 2**).

Gap junction proteins	Parasite	Cell type	Effects	References
Cx43	*Trypanosoma cruzi*	Cardiomyocytes	Downregulated	[43]
		Astrocytes	Downregulated	[44]
		Leptomeningeal cells	Downregulated	[44]
		Cardiomyocytes	Downregulated	[48]
		Cardiomyocytes	Downregulated	[51]
		Cardiomyocytes and heart human biopsies	Downregulated	[50]
	Toxoplasma gondii	Astrocytes	Downregulated	[44]
		Leptomeningeal cells	Downregulated	[44]
Cx26	*Toxoplasma gondii*	Astrocytes	Downregulated	[44]
Cx37	*Trypanosoma cruzi*	Heart from chagasic mouse	Upregulated	[52]
Cx40	*Trypanosoma cruzi*	Heart from chagasic mouse	Not change	[52]
Cx45	*Trypanosoma cruzi*	Heart from chagasic mouse	Not change	[52]
	Trypanosoma cruzi	Cardiomyocytes	Upregulated	[51]
Panx1	*Plasmodium falciparum*	Human erythrocytes	Increased ATP release	[54]
	Entamoeba histolytica	Human monocytic cells	Increased ATP release	[60]
AGAP001476	*Plasmodium falciparum*	Midgut tissues from *Anopheles gambiae*	Upregulated	[61]
	Plasmodium berghei	Midgut tissues from *Anopheles gambiae*	Upregulated	[61]

Table 1. Summary of published works on the effect of parasite infections on the gap junction proteins.

Drug	Commercial name	Presentation and quantity	Company	Country production
Probenecid	Probalan	Tablets 500 mg	Lannett	USA
Probenecid	Probenecid & Colchicine	Tablets 500 mg	Watson	INDIA
Probenecid	Probenecid	Tablets 500 mg	Mylan	USA
Probenecid	Probenecid & Colchicine	Tablets 500 mg	Ingenus	USA
Suramin	Germanin	Vial 1 g	Bayer	Germany

Table 2. Commercial drugs.

2. The family of gap junction proteins

Gap junction proteins are present in both vertebrates and invertebrates from mesozoa to mammals [8]. In chordate animals, gap junction channels are encoded by a family of genes called connexins (Cxs) [9] (**Table 3**). In addition, gap junction communication of invertebrate is mediated via another family of proteins called innexins (Inxs) [8]. Inx homologues have been identified in vertebrates and were termed pannexins (Panxs) [10]. Members of the same protein family oligomerize in hexamers forming channels, which are inserted into the plasma membrane connecting the intra- and extracellular milieu [8]. Whereas, docking of two channels forms intercellular channels (gap junction channels) that connect the cytoplasm of two cells [8]. It has been proposed that Panx-based channels do not form gap junction channels due to their post-translational glycosylation [11]. However, this theoretical prediction might be proved wrong because in exogenous cells systems forms functional gap junctions. In support to this possibility is the fact that Panx1 expressed in exogenous cell systems forms functional gap junctions [12, 13].

2.1. Genes

The first Cx gene was cloned in 1986, and there are at least 21 Cx isoforms in the human genome [8, 14]. Most Cx genes have a first exon containing only 5′-untranslated region (UTR) sequences and a large second exon containing the complete coding region sequence (CDS) as well as all remaining untranslated sequences [8]. Exceptions to this gene structure are the Cx32, Cx36, and Cx45 genes [8]. Panx are termed as Panx1, Panx2, and Panx3 and are present both in invertebrate and chordate genomes [15, 16]. The human and mouse genome contain three Panx-encoding genes [10]. The genomic sequence revealed that human Panx1 contains five exons with four introns [10]. Moreover, Panx2 and Panx3 contain four exons [10]. The first Inx gene was identified in 1998 as a result of genome sequencing of nematode *C. elegans* [17]. Actually, 25 and 8 Inx genes in *C. elegans* and *D. melanogaster* have been identified, respectively [2, 3]. Usually, Inx genes are encoded on multiple exons and have the potential to produce more than one protein by differential splicing [18]. Recently, viral homologs of Panxs/Inxs were identified in *Polydnaviruses* and denominated vinnexins (Vinx) [19].

Abbreviations	Definitions
ATP	Adenosine triphosphate
cAMP	Cyclic adenosine monophosphate
CDS	Coding region sequence
Cx	Connexin
DCSF	Divalent cation solution free
HC	Hemichannel
Inx	Innexin
Panx	Pannexin
P.Falciparum	*Plasmodium falciparum*
PMA	Phorbol 12-myristate 13-acetate
T. cruzi	*Trypanosoma cruzi*
UTR	Untranslated region
Vinx	Vinnexin

Table 3. Abbreviations.

2.2. Secondary structure

Cx, Inx, and Panx proteins share the same membrane topology, characterized by four transmembrane domains connected by two extracellular loops and a single cytoplasmic loop [20]. These extracellular loops contain 2 (for Panxs and Inxs) or 3 (for Cxs) highly conserved cysteine residues [21]. Moreover, the intracellular loop is highly variable [21]. The four transmembrane domains are well-conserved among members of the same family of proteins and form alpha-helical sheets that contribute to the wall of the HC and line its central hydrophilic space [21]. All members of the 3 families have their NH_2- and COOH-terminal region within the cytoplasm [21]. The COOH-terminal region differs in length and sequence in all gap junction proteins [21]. Inx proteins have a highly conserved pentapeptide YYQWV close to, or at, the beginning of the second transmembrane domain [22].

2.3. Gap junctional channels

Gap junctions are specialized cell-to-cell junctions that mediate direct intercellular communication between cells [8]. Depending on whether the two interacting channels are made of the same or different Cxs, gap junction plaques are formed by homo- and heterotypic channels, respectively, with distinct biophysical characteristics [21]. These intercellular channels are essential in several Physiologic tissue functions such as electrical conduction between cardiomyocytes [23], development and regeneration of skeletal muscle [24], endocrine gland secretion [25], and ovarian folliculogenesis [26]. They are also implicated in pathophysiological conditions including hereditary deafness [27], cataract [28], ectodermal dysplasias [29], tumorigenesis [30], and neuroinflammatory responses [31].

http://dx.doi.org/10.5772/67187

2.4. Hemichannels (HCs)

Several studies have shown that HCs allow the bidirectional passage of ions and cytosolic signaling molecules, such adenosine triphosphate (ATP), nicotinamide adenine dinucleotide (NAD^+), glutamate, glutathione, and prostaglandins [32]. Under physiological conditions, HCs are involved in the regulation of cell volume [33], vascular tone [34], hemostasis [35], and neuroglia paracrine interactions [36], among others. However, HCs have been the focus of interest because of their relevance in pathological conditions, including metabolic inhibition [37], stroke [38], myocardial infarction [39, 40], ischemic neuronal death [41], spinal cord injury [42], diarrhoea during infectious enteric disease [5], and keratitis-ichthyosis-deafness syndrome [43].

The presence and functional HCs in the plasma membrane have been determined through several techniques such as electrophysiology, uptake of fluorescent dyes, and release of adenosine triphosphate (ATP) [44]. Due to the existence of non-selective channels in the plasma membrane, there are significant considerations for studying HCs [45]. These criteria are as follows: (i) cell expression of at least one Cx/Panx isoform at the plasma membrane, (ii) the ability of the cells to incorporate or release molecules, (iii) to mediate membrane currents with conductance associated to Cx/Panx HCs, (iv) the abolishment of HC function using a pharmacologic approach (e.g. La^{3+}, probenecid, or carbenoxolone) or mimetic peptide blockers (Gap19, Gap26, Gap27 for specific Cx HCs or ^{10}Panx1 for Panx1 HCs), and (v) to demonstrate that blockade of HCs affect physiological responses [44, 45].

3. Gap junction proteins in parasitic infections

3.1. Connexins (Cxs)

3.1.1. Functional studies

Pioneering studies in the 1990s by de Carvalho et al., 1992 showed that *Trypanosoma cruzi* induces a gap junction alteration in cardiac myocytes [46] (**Table 1**). They showed that *T. cruzi* infection reduces the junctional conductance and Lucifer yellow transfer in cardiomyocytes, revealing that this parasite infection reduces the channel function of host cells [46]. The same researchers also showed that infection caused by *Toxoplasma gondii* reduces intercellular communication in astrocytes and leptomeningeal cells [47]. Recently, we demonstrated that *T. cruzi* increases dye uptake via HCs in non-confluent Cx43-HeLa cells [7]. Suramin, an anti-protozoa drug, inhibits the activity of HCs [48]. Suramin causes a concentration-dependent inhibition of a divalent cation-free solution (DCSF)-induced dye uptake in a rat kidney epithelial cell line [48]. Also, suramin blocks the DCSF-induced ATP release in a rat kidney epithelial cell line [48]. Interestingly, the suppressive effect of suramin on the influx of dye and efflux of ATP was not reproduced by PPADS, a broad-spectrum antagonist of P2 receptors, suggesting that the action of suramin on HCs is independent of its action on P2 purine receptors [48]. Also, suramin (300 μM for 12 h) did not affect the total Cx43 level [48]. Moreover, prolonged incubation of *T. cruzi*-infected LLC-MK2 cells in the presence of suramin (500 μM) causes morphological changes on trypomastigote forms characterized by an accentuated decrease on parasite motility [49]. In trypomastigotes, suramin causes a decrease in ~5% in cell length and an increase in ~43% in cell width [49]. Also, it was observed that 95% of trypomastigotes exposed to suramin present a partial or even total detachment of the flagellum from the cell body [49].

3.1.2. Protein expression alterations

At the protein level, *T. cruzi* reduces Cx43 levels at junctional membrane regions in neonatal rat cardiomyocytes [46, 47]. Other studies in mouse cardiomyocytes showed that *T. cruzi* reduces Cx43 levels at 24-h post-infections [50]. Interestingly, cardiomyocytes with pronounced decrease in Cx43 protein levels showed an increased number of intracellular amastigotes, suggesting a direct relationship between host cell parasitism and Cx43 downregulation in *vitro* [50]. Also, it has been described that infection with *T. cruzi* or *T. gondii* reduces the levels of Cx43 and Cx26 protein in astrocytes or leptomeningeal cells [47]. *In vivo* model of *T. cruzi* infection showed a significant reduction in myocardial Cx43 protein levels [50]. *Swiss Webster* mice infected with *T. cruzi* showed a reduction in Cx43 levels in atrium and ventricles at 11- or 30-day post-infection, respectively [50]. Moreover, brain slices prepared from mice infected with *T. gondii* showed complete absence of Cx43 immunoreactivity within the cysts and marked reduction in the surroundin tissue [47]. The same study described a reduction of Cx43 protein levels in whole brains of *T. cruzi*-infected mice [47]. In monkeys, *T. cruzi* infection causes significant Cx43 loss in the cardiac tissue [51]. Clinical studies described that samples from chagasic patients showed alterations of cardiac Cx levels [52]. Immunohistochemical analysis of left ventricle biopsies from subjects with chronic chagasic disease showed reduction in both mean number (<20%) and size (<2.2 fold) of Cx43 plaques [52].

3.1.3. Gene expression regulation

Gene profiling of *T. cruzi*-infected cardiomyocytes revealed downregulation at 48 h after infection of *GJA1* and *GJC1* genes, which encode for Cx43 and Cx45, respectively [53]. Upregulation of *GJA4* gene encoding Cx37, a major endothelial cell Cx, was also described [54].

3.1.4. Cx knock-out mice and parasitic infections

Hepatic granulomas induced by *Schistosoma mansoni* infection in Cx43 deficient mice showed a higher degree of fibrosis and a reduced index of cell proliferation at 8 and 12 weeks after infection [55]. However, no differences in the average area of granulomas or number of cells per granuloma were observed [55]. The authors of the above mention work suggested that deletion of one allele of Cx43 gene could be the cause of reduced gap junction channels that modifies the interactions between granuloma cells, thereby modifying the characteristics of granuloma [55].

3.2. Pannexins (Panxs)

It has been demonstrated that *Plasmodium falciparum* infection induces ATP release via Panx1 channels in human erythrocytes [56]. A mixture of isoproterenol (β-adrenergic agonist),

http://dx.doi.org/10.5772/67187

forskolin (adenylate kinase activator), and papaverine (phosphodiesterase inhibitor) induce cyclic adenosine monophosphate (cAMP)-dependent ATP release in human erythrocytes, and this effect was 3.8-fold higher in trophozoite-infected erythrocytes compared to uninfected erythrocytes [56]. Interestingly, this effect was reduced by 100 μM carbenoxolone or 100 nM mefloquine, two Panx1 channel blockers [54]. These authors suggest that the increased ATP release from infected red cells could be mediated by by Panx1 channels [56]. Several studies have shown that probenecid has a marked antimalarial effect [57–59]. The incubation of *P. falciparum* with probenecid shows antimalarial activity at concentrations >150 μM at day 2 of treatment [57]. However, probenecid at concentration <150 μM increases the *P. falciparum* sensitivity to antifolate drugs [57]. For example, in the presence of 50 μM probenecid, the IC_{50} (nM) was reduced from 1.42 ± 0.52 to 0.52 ± 0.36, from 215 ± 150 to 36.50 ± 26.80 and from 33.53 ± 12.30 to 1.77 ± 2.70 for pyrimethamine, sulfadoxine, and dapsone, respectively [57]. Probenecid also reverses the chloroquine resistance of *P. falciparum* and increases piperaquine activity *in vitro* [57]. Also, probenecid chemosensitize a multidrug-resistant strain V1S of *P. falciparum* to piperaquine [59]. Moreover, antimalarial drugs such as artemisinin and artesunate also inhibit Panx1 channel [60]. For example, artesunate causes a concentration-dependent inhibition of membrane current mediated by Panx1 channels with an IC_{50} of 450 μM, while 200 μM artemisinin causes a membrane current reduction of about 20% in *Xenopus* oocytes [60]. Moreover, artemisinin also inhibits dye uptake with an IC_{50} of 0.14 μM in frog erythrocytes [60]. Moreover, 100 nM mefloquine significantly reduces voltage-activated Panx1 channel currents in astrocytes from Cx43-null mice [61]. Also, mefloquine blocks dye uptake induced by ATP in astrocytes from Cx43-null mice [61]. In addition, it has been described that *Entamoeba histolytica* induces ATP release into the extracellular space through opening of Panx1 channels in macrophages [62]. Incubation with 500 μM ^{10}Panx1, a mimetic blocking peptide of Panx1 channels, abolished ATP release in response to *E. histolytica* in phorbol 12-myristate 13-acetate (PMA)-differentiated THP-1 human monocytic cells [62]. The same results were observed with 100 μM carbenoxolone or 250 μM probenecid [62].

3.3. Innexins (Inxs)

It has been demonstrated that Inx proteins have a critical role for mediating anti-*Plasmodium* responses in *Anopheles gambiae* [63]. It has been shown that AGAP001476 mRNA levels were induced during *Plasmodium* infection in *Anopheles* midguts [63]. The carbenoxolone-treated mosquitoes showed an increase in both *Plasmodium* oocyst number and infection rate [63].

4. Possible role of gap junction proteins in parasite infections

Although the role of gap junction proteins in parasitic infections has not been fully elucidated, they could participate in responses that include changes in plasma membrane permeability, signalling, and inflammasome activation.

4.1. Alteration of the host cell membrane permeability

A common condition and often necessary for infection is the alteration of the host cell membrane permeability [64, 65], and hemichannel activity can considerably affect the permeability of the cell membrane in mammalian cells [66]. For example, *T. cruzi* alters the plasma membrane permeability in host cells during different stages of the disease [65, 67–69]. Another parasite that alters the plasma membrane permeability is *P. falciparum*. This parasite invades and replicates asexually within human erythrocytes and enhances plasma membrane permeability in different stages of the disease [70, 71]. The apicomplexan *Babesia divergens* also increases the membrane permeability of erythrocyte [64]. The mechanism for such erythrocyte permeabilization is different in transport rates, solutes selectivity, and temperature dependence compared with the alteration induced by *P. falciparum* [64].

4.2. Intracellular Ca^{2+} mobilization

Gap junction proteins participate in Ca^{2+} signalling, and they constitute one pathway for intercellular Ca^{2+} wave propagation in cardiomyocytes, astrocytes, and osteocytes, among other cell types [72]. In addition, Cx26, Cx32 and Cx43 HCs are permeable to Ca^{2+} [73–76] and might be involved in initiation of intracellular rise in Ca^{2+} signals. In protozoan infections, a key process in early stages of invasion is the rise in cytosolic Ca^{2+} concentration [77]. For example, when *T. cruzi* comes into contact with the host cell, triggers a transient increase in cytosolic Ca^{2+} concentration that induces lysosome exocytosis in host cells [65, 77]. This process is required for cell invasion, because chelating the intracellular Ca^{2+} transients in host cells reduces the entry of the parasite into the cell [78]. **Figure 1** shows a model of the possible participation of pannexin channel in intracellular Ca^{2+} mobilization during the invasion by *T. cruzi*.

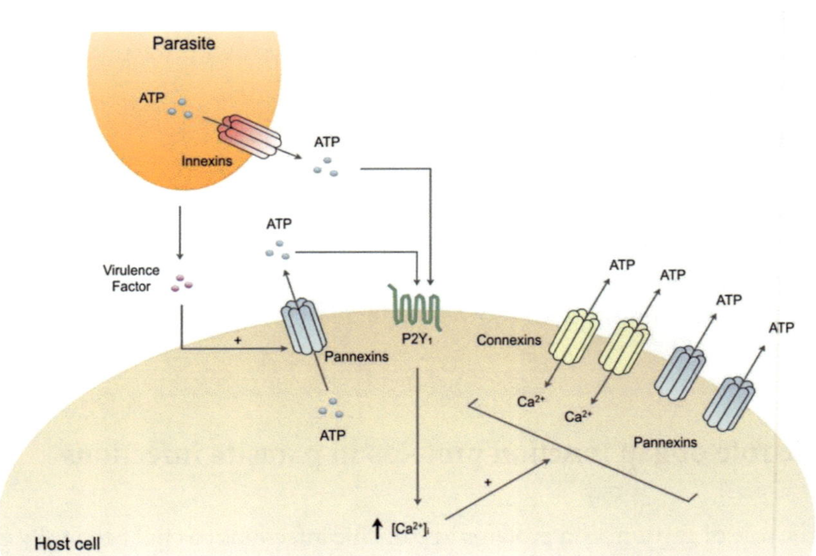

Figure 1. Model of the possible participation of gap junction proteins in the invasion of host cells by *Trypanosoma cruzi*. Parasites release a virulence factor, which opens Pannexin 1 channels allowing the release of ATP to the extracellular milieu. The ATP activates $P2Y_1$ receptors and promotes Ca^{2+} release from intracellular stores generating intracellular Ca^{2+} transients, which induces the opening of new hemichannels formed by connexin or pannexins. These effects promote the *Trypanosoma cruzi* invasion.

4.3. Activation of the inflammasome

The inflammasome activation triggers innate immune defence by inducing the processing of pro inflammatory cytokines, such as IL-1, in a caspase 1-dependent manner [79]. Panx1 channels play a key role in inflammasome activation [79]. It has been proposed that small pathogen-associated molecule patterns (PAMPs) can gain cytosolic access via the $P2X_7$ receptor/Panx1 ($P2X_7R$/Panx1) complex and activate the inflammasome [79].

5. Conclusions

Parasitic infections affect predominantly underprivileged areas of the world and represent serious life-threatening conditions in high-risk groups such as young children, elderly, and immune deficient subjects. Also, therapeutic options include a wide variety of compounds with considerable toxic and undesirable side effects. The introduction of knockout animals and specific inhibitors has increased our understanding about the role of Cx, Panx, and Inx proteins in the pathophysiology of many infectious conditions. However, their participation in infections caused by parasites is not completely elucidated. A variety of methods have been used to evaluate changes in gap junction protein expression during parasite infections. These methods include Western blot, immunofluorescence, or functional studies such dye uptake, dye coupling, or current measurements with electrophysiological techniques. In summary, the available data suggest that the parasite infections modulate gap junction proteins in host cells. In this context, characterization of gap junction proteins and their functions in protozoan parasites might facilitate the design of effective new therapies to fight protozoan infections such as malaria and Chagas disease.

Acknowledgements

This work was partially supported by FONDECYT grants 11130013 (to JLV) and 1131007 (to JG) and ICM-Economía grant P09-022-F (to JCS).

Author details

José Luis Vega[1]*, Iván Barría[1], Juan Güiza[1], Jorge González[2] and Juan C. Sáez[3,4]

*Address all correspondence to: josevega.ua@gmail.com

1 Experimental Physiology Laboratory (EP*hy*L), Antofagasta Institute, Universidad de Antofagasta, Antofagasta, Chile

2 Molecular Parasitology Unit, Medical Technology Department, Faculty of Health Sciences, Universidad de Antofagasta, Antofagasta, Chile

3 Departamento de Fisiología, Pontificia Universidad Católica de Chile, Santiago, Chile

4 Instituto Milenio, Centro Interdisciplinario de Neurociencias de Valparaíso, Universidad de Valparaíso, Valparaíso, Chile

References

[1] Sáez JC, Berthoud VM, Branes MC, Martinez AD, Beyer EC. Plasma membrane channels formed by connexins: their regulation and functions. Physiol Rev. 2003;83:1359-1400. doi:10.1152/physrev.00007.2003

[2] Starich T, Sheehan M, Jadrich J, Shaw J. Innexins in *C. elegans*. Cell Commun Adhes. 2001;8:311-314. doi:10.3109/15419060109080744

[3] Stebbings LA, Todman MG, Phillips R, Greer CE, Tam J, Phelan P, Jacobs K, Bacon JP, Davies JA. Gap junctions in Drosophila: developmental expression of the entire innexin gene family. Mech Dev. 2002;13:197-205. doi:10.1016/S0925-4773(02)00025-4

[4] Tran Van Nhieu G, Clair C, Bruzzone R, Mesnil M, Sansonetti P, Combettes L. Connexin-dependent inter-cellular communication increases invasion and dissemination of Shigella in epithelial cells. Nat Cell Biol. 2003;8:720-6. doi:10.1038/ncb1021

[5] Guttman JA, Lin AE-J, Li Y, Bechberger J, Naus CC, Vogl AW, Finlay BB. Gap junction hemichannels contribute to the generation of diarrhoea during infectious enteric disease. Gut. 2010;59:218-226. doi:10.1136/gut.2008.170464

[6] Orellana JA, Velasquez S, Williams DW, Sáez JC, Berman JW, Eugenin EA. Pannexin1 hemichannels are critical for HIV infection of human primary CD4+ T lymphocytes. J Leukoc Biol. 2013;94:399-407. doi:10.1189/jlb.0512249

[7] Vega JL, Subiabre M, Figueroa F, Schalper KA, Osorio L, González J, Sáez JC. Role of gap junctions and hemichannels in parasitic infections. Biomed Res Int. 2013;2013:589130. doi:10.1155/2013/589130

[8] Meşe G, Richard G, White TW. Gap junctions: basic structure and function. J Invest Dermatol. 2007;127:2516-2524. doi:10.1038/sj.jid.5700770

[9] Goodenough DA. Bulk isolation of mouse hepatocyte gap junctions. Characterization of the principal protein, connexin. J Cell Biol. 1974;61:557-563. doi:10.1083/jcb.61.2.557

[10] Panchin YV. Evolution of gap junction proteins—the pannexin alternative. J Exp Biol. 2005;208:1415-1419. doi:10.1242/jeb.01547

[11] Sosinsky GE, Boassa D, Dermietzel R, Duffy HS, Laird DW, MacVicar B, Naus CC, Penuela S, Scemes E, Spray DC, Thompson RJ, Zhao HB, Dahl G. Pannexin channels are not gap junction hemichannels. Channels (Austin). 2011;5:193-197. doi:10.4161/chan.5.3.15765

[12] Bruzzone R, Hormuzdi SG, Barbe MT, Herb A, Monyer H. Pannexins, a family of gap junction proteins expressed in brain. Proc Natl Acad Sci U S A. 2003;100:13644-13649. doi:10.1073/pnas.2233464100

[13] Lai CP, Bechberger JF, Thompson RJ, MacVicar BA, Bruzzone R, Naus CC. Tumor-suppressive effects of pannexin 1 in C6 glioma cells. Cancer Res. 2007;67:1545-1554. doi:10.1158/0008-5472.CAN-06-1396

[14] Paul DL. Molecular cloning of cDNA for rat liver gap junction protein. J Cell Biol. 1986;103:123-134. doi:10.1083/jcb.103.1.123

[15] Phelan P, Bacon JP, Davies JA, Stebbings LA, Todman MG, Avery L, Baines RA, Barnes TM, Ford C, Hekimi S, Lee R, Shaw JE, Starich TA, Curtin KD, Sun YA, Wyman RJ. Innexins: a family of invertebrate gap-junction proteins. Trends Genet. 1998;14:348-349. doi:10.1016/S0168-9525(98)01547-9

[16] Baranova A, Ivanov D, Petrash N, Pestova A, Skoblov M, Kelmanson I, Shagin D, Nazarenko S, Geraymovych E, Litvin O, Tiunova A, Born TL, Usman N, Staroverov D, Lukyanov S, Panchin Y. The mammalian pannexin family is homologous to the invertebrate innexin gap junction proteins. Genomics. 2004;83:706-716. doi:10.1016/j.ygeno.2003.09.025

[17] C. elegans Sequencing Consortium. Genome sequence of the nematode C. elegans: a platform for investigating biology. Science. 1998 Dec 11;282(5396):2012-8. doi:10.1126/science.282.5396.2012

[18] Crompton D, Todman M, Wilkin M, Ji S, Davies J. Essential and neural transcripts from the Drosophila shaking-B locus are differentially expressed in the embryonic mesoderm and pupal nervous system. Dev Biol. 1995;170:142-158. doi:10.1006/dbio.1995.1203

[19] Kroemer JA, Webb BA. Polydnavirus genes and genomes: emerging gene families and new insights into polydnavirus replication. Annu Rev Entomol. 2004;49:431-56. doi:10.1146/annurev.ento.49.072103.120132

[20] Barbe MT, Monyer H, Bruzzone R. Cell-cell communication beyond connexins: the pannexin channels. Physiology (Bethesda). 2006 Apr;21:103-14. doi:10.1152/physiol.00048.2005

[21] Bosco D, Haefliger JA, Meda P. Connexins: key mediators of endocrine function. Physiol Rev. 2011 Oct;91(4):1393-445. doi:10.1152/physrev.00027.2010

[22] Phelan P. Innexins: members of an evolutionarily conserved family of gap-junction proteins. Biochim Biophys Acta. 2005;1711:225-245. doi:10.1016/j.bbamem.2004.10.004

[23] Kanno S, Saffitz JE. The role of myocardial gap junctions in electrical conduction and arrhythmogenesis. Cardiovasc Pathol. 2001;10:169-177. doi:10.1016/S1054-8807(01)00078-3

[24] Araya R, Eckardt D, Maxeiner S, Krüger O, Theis M, Willecke K, Sáez JC. Expression of connexins during differentiation and regeneration of skeletal muscle: functional relevance of connexin43. J Cell Sci. 2005:118:27-37. doi:10.1242/jcs.01553

[25] Murray SA, Davis K, Gay V. ACTH and adrenocortical gap junctions. Microsc Res Tech. 2003;61:240-246. doi:10.1002/jemt.10332

[26] Gershon E, Plaks V, Dekel N. Gap junctions in the ovary: expression, localization and function. Mol Cell Endocrinol. 2008;282:18-25. doi:10.1016/j.mce.2007.11.001

[27] Kelsell DP, Dunlop J, Stevens HP, Lench NJ, Liang JN, Parry G, Mueller RF, Leigh IM. Connexin 26 mutations in hereditary non-syndromic sensorineural deafness. Nature. 1997;387:80-83. doi:10.1038/387080a0

[28] Xia CH, Chang B, Derosa AM, Cheng C, White TW, Gong X. Cataracts and microphthalmia caused by a Gja8 mutation in extracellular loop 2. PLoS One. 2012;7:e52894. doi:10.1371/journal.pone.0052894

[29] Scott CA, Tattersall D, O'Toole EA, and Kelsell DP. Connexins in epidermal homeostasis and skin disease. Biochimica et Biophysica Acta. 2012;1818:1952-1961. doi:10.1016/j.bbamem.2011.09.004

[30] Naus CC, Laird DW. Implications and challenges of connexin connections to cancer. Nat Rev Cancer. 2010;10:435-441. doi:10.1038/nrc2841

[31] Bennett MVL. Garré JM, Orellana JA, Bukauskas FF, Nedergaard M, Sáez JC. Connexin and pannexin hemichannels in inflammatory responses of glia and neurons. Brain Res. 2012;1487:3-15. doi:10.1016/j.brainres.2012.08.042

[32] Kar R, Batra N, Riquelme MA, Jiang JX. Biological role of connexin intercellular channels and hemichannels. Arch Biochem Biophys. 2012;524:2-15. doi:10.1016/j.abb.2012.03.008

[33] Quist AP, Rhee SK, Lin H, Lal R. Physiological role of gap-junctional hemichannels. Extracellular calcium-dependent isosmotic volume regulation. J Cell Biol. 2000;148:1063-1074. doi:10.1083/jcb.148.5.1063

[34] Billaud M, Sandilos JK, Isakson BE. Pannexin 1 in the regulation of vascular tone. Trends Cardiovasc Med. 2012;22:68-72. doi:10.1016/j.tcm.2012.06.014

[35] Vaiyapuri S, Jones CI, Sasikumar P, Moraes LA, Munger SJ, Wright JR, Ali MS, Sage T, Kaiser WJ, Tucker KL, Stain CJ, Bye AP, Jones S, Oviedo-Orta E, Simon AM, Mahaut-Smith MP, Gibbins JM. Gap junctions and connexin hemichannels underpin hemostasis and thrombosis. Circulation. 2012;125:2479-2491.

[36] Orellana JA, Froger N, Ezan P, Jiang JX, Bennett MVL, Naus CC, Giaume C, Sáez JC. ATP and glutamate released via astroglial connexin 43 hemichannels mediate neuronal death through activation of pannexin 1 hemichannels. J Neurochem. 2011;118:826-840. doi:10.1111/j.1471-4159.2011.07210.x

[37] Contreras JE, Sánchez HA, Eugenin EA, Speidel D, Theis M, Willecke K, Bukauskas FF, Bennett MVL, Sáez JC. Metabolic inhibition induces opening of unapposed connexin 43 gap junction hemichannels and reduces gap junctional communication in cortical astrocytes in culture. Proc Natl Acad Sci U.S.A. 2002;99:495-500. doi:10.1073/pnas.012589799

[38] Thompson RJ, Zhou N, MacVicar BA. Ischemia opens neuronal gap junction hemichannels. Science. 2006;312:924-927. doi:10.1126/science.1126241

[39] Hawat G, Benderdour M, Rousseau G, Baroudi G. Connexin 43 mimetic peptide Gap26 confers protection to intact heart against myocardial ischemia injury. Pflugers Arch. 2010;460:583-592.

[40] Wang N, De Bock M, Antoons G, Gadicherla AK, Bol M, Decrock E, Evans WH, Sipido KR, Bukauskas FF, Leybaert L. Connexin mimetic peptides inhibit Cx43 hemichannel opening triggered by voltage and intracellular Ca^{2+} elevation. Basic Res Cardiol. 2012;107:304. doi:10.1007/s00395-012-0304-2

[41] Orellana JA, Figueroa XF, Sánchez HA, Contreras-Duarte S, Velarde V, Sáez JC. Hemichannels in the neurovascular unit and white matter under normal and inflamed conditions. CNS Neurol Disord Drug Targets. 2011;10:404-414. doi:10.2174/187152711794653869

[42] Chen MJ, Kress B, Han X, Moll K, Peng W, Ji R-R, Nedergaard M. Astrocytic CX43 hemichannels and gap junctions play a crucial role in development of chronic neuropathic pain following spinal cord injury. Glia. 2012;60:1660-1670. doi:10.1002/glia.22384

[43] Levit NA, Mese G, Basaly MGR, White TW. Pathological hemichannels associated with human Cx26 mutations causing Keratitis-Ichthyosis-Deafness syndrome. Biochim Biophys Acta. 2012;1818: 2014-2019. doi:10.1016/j.bbamem.2011.09.003

[44] Retamal MA, Reyes EP, García IE, Pinto B, Martínez AD, González C. Diseases associated with leaky hemichannels. Front Cell Neurosci. 2015;9:267. doi:10.3389/fncel.2015.00267

[45] Sáez JC, Leybaert L. Hunting for connexin hemichannels. FEBS Lett. 2014;588:1205-1211. doi:10.1016/j.febslet.2014.03.004

[46] de Carvalho AC, Tanowitz HB, Wittner M, Dermietzel R, Roy C, Hertzberg EL, Spray DC. Gap junction distribution is altered between cardiac myocytes infected with Trypanosoma cruzi. Circ Res. 1992;70:733-742. doi:10.1161/01.RES.70.4.733

[47] Campos de Carvalho AC, Roy C, Hertzberg EL, Tanowitz HB, Kessler JA, Weiss LM, Wittner M, Dermietzel R, Gao Y, Spray DC. Gap junction disappearance in astrocytes and leptomeningeal cells as a consequence of protozoan infection. Brain Res. 1998;790:304-314. doi:10.1016/S0006-8993(97)01523-0

[48] Chi Y, Gao K, Zhang H, Takeda M, Yao J. Suppression of cell membrane permeability by suramin: involvement of its inhibitory actions on connexin 43 hemichannels. Br J Pharmacol. 2014;171:3448-3462. doi:10.1111/bph.12693

[49] Bisaggio DF, Campanati L, Pinto RC, Souto-Padrón T. Effect of suramin on trypomastigote forms of Trypanosoma cruzi: changes on cell motility and on the ultrastructure of the flagellum-cell body attachment region. Acta Trop. 2006;98:162-175. doi:10.1016/j.actatropica.2006.04.003

[50] Adesse D, Garzoni LR, Huang H, Tanowitz HB, de Nazareth Meirelles M, Spray DC. Trypanosoma cruzi induces changes in cardiac connexin43 expression. Microbes Infect. 2008;10:21-28. doi:10.1016/j.micinf.2007.09.017

[51] Carvalho CM, Silverio JC, da Silva AA, Pereira IR, Coelho JM, Britto CC, Moreira OC, Marchevsky RS, Xavier SS, Gazzinelli RT, da Glória Bonecini-Almeida M, Lannes-Vieira J. Inducible nitric oxide synthase in heart tissue and nitric oxide in serum of Trypanosoma cruzi-infected rhesus monkeys: association with heart injury. PLoS Negl Trop Dis. 2012;6:e1644. doi:10.1371/journal.pntd.0001644

[52] Waghabi MC, Coutinho-Silva R, Feige JJ, Higuchi Mde L, Becker D, Burnstock G, Araújo-Jorge TC. Gap junction reduction in cardiomyocytes following transforming growth factor-beta treatment and Trypanosoma cruzi infection. Mem Inst Oswaldo Cruz. 2009;104:1083-1090. doi:10.1590/S0074-02762009000800004

[53] Goldenberg RC, Iacobas DA, Iacobas S, Rocha LL, da Silva de Azevedo Fortes F, Vairo L, Nagajyothi F, Campos de Carvalho AC, Tanowitz HB, Spray DC. Transcriptomic alterations in *Trypanosoma cruzi*-infected cardiac myocytes. Microbes Infect. 2009;11:1140-1149. doi:10.1016/j.micinf.2009.08.009

[54] Adesse D, Goldenberg RC, Fortes FS, Jasmin, Iacobas DA, Iacobas S, Campos de Carvalho AC, de Narareth Meirelles M, Huang H, Soares MB, Tanowitz HB, Garzoni LR, Spray DC. Gap junctions and chagas disease. Adv Parasitol. 2011;76:63-81. doi:10.1016/B978-0-12-385895-5.00003-7

[55] Oloris SC, Mesnil M, Reis VN, Sakai M, Matsuzaki P, Fonseca Ede S, da Silva TC, Avanzo JL, Sinhorini IL, Guerra JL, Costa-Pinto FA, Maiorka PC, Dagli ML. Hepatic granulomas induced by *Schistosoma mansoni* in mice deficient for connexin 43 present lower cell proliferation and higher collagen content. Life Sci. 2007;80:1228-1235. doi:10.1016/j.lfs.2006.12.030

[56] Alvarez CL, Schachter J, de Sá Pinheiro AA, Silva Lde S, Verstraeten SV, Persechini PM, Schwarzbaum PJ. Regulation of extracellular ATP in human erythrocytes infected with *Plasmodium falciparum*. PLoS One. 2014;9:e96216. doi:10.1371/journal.pone.0096216

[57] Nzila A, Mberu E, Bray P, Kokwaro G, Winstanley P, Marsh K, Ward S. Chemosensitization of *Plasmodium falciparum* by probenecid in vitro. Antimicrob Agents Chemother. 2003;47:2108-2112.

[58] Sowunmi A, Fehintola FA, Adedeji AA, Gbotosho GO, Falade CO, Tambo E, Fateye BA, Happi TC, Oduola AM. Open randomized study of pyrimethamine-sulphadoxine vs. pyrimethamine-sulphadoxine plus probenecid for the treatment of uncomplicated *Plasmodium falciparum* malaria in children. Trop Med Int Health. 2004;9:606-614. doi:10.1128/AAC.47.7.2108-2112.2003

[59] Masseno V, Muriithi S, Nzila A. In vitro chemosensitization of *Plasmodium falciparum* to antimalarials by verapamil and probenecid. Antimicrob Agents Chemother. 2009;53:3131-3134.

[60] Dahl G, Qiu F, Wang J. The bizarre pharmacology of the ATP release channel pannexin1. Neuropharmacology. 2013;75:583-593. doi:10.1016/j.neuropharm.2013.02.019

[61] Iglesias R, Dahl G, Qiu F, Spray DC, Scemes E. Pannexin 1: the molecular substrate of astrocyte "hemichannels". J Neurosci. 2009;29:7092-7097. doi:10.1523/JNEUROSCI.6062-08.2009

[62] Mortimer L, Moreau F, Cornick S, Chadee K. The NLRP3 Inflammasome is a pathogen sensor for invasive *Entamoeba histolytica* via activation of $\alpha 5\beta 1$ integrin at the macrophage-amebae intercellular junction. PLoS Pathog. 2015;11:e1004887. doi:10.1371/journal.ppat.1004887

[63] Li MW, Wang J, Zhao YO, Fikrig E. Innexin AGAP001476 is critical for mediating anti-Plasmodium responses in Anopheles mosquitoes. J Biol Chem. 2014;289:24885-24897. doi:10.1074/jbc.M114.554519

[64] Alkhalil A, Hill DA, Desai SA. Babesia and plasmodia increase host erythrocyte permeability through distinct mechanisms. Cell Microbiol. 2007;9:851-860. doi:10.1111/j.1462-5822.2006.00834.x

[65] Fernandes MC, Cortez M, Flannery AR, Tam C, Mortara RA, Andrews NW. *Trypanosoma cruzi* subverts the sphingomyelinase-mediated plasma membrane repair pathway for cell invasion. J Exp Med. 2011;208:909-921. doi:10.1084/jem.20102518

[66] Schalper KA, Orellana JA, Berthoud VM, Sáez JC. Dysfunctions of the diffusional membrane pathways mediated hemichannels in inherited and acquired diseases. Curr Vasc Pharmacol. 2009;7:486-505. doi:10.2174/157016109789043937

[67] Costales J, Rowland EC. A role for protease activity and host-cell permeability during the process of Trypanosoma cruzi egress from infected cells. J Parasitol. 2007;93:1350-1359. doi:10.1645/GE-1074.1

[68] Osuna A, Rodríguez-Cabezas MN, Castanys S, Mesa-Valle MC, Mascaro MC. A protein secreted by *Trypanosoma cruzi* capable of inducing the entry of inert particles into HeLa cells. Int J Parasitol. 1995;25:1213-1225.

[69] Rossi MA, Silva JS. Permeability alteration of the sarcolemmal membrane, particularly at the site of macrophage contact, in experimental chronic *Trypanosoma cruzi* myocarditis in mice. Int J Exp Pathol. 1990;71:545-555.

[70] Cabantchik ZI. Altered membrane transport of malaria-infected erythrocytes: a possible pharmacologic target. Blood. 1989;74:1464-1471.

[71] Ginsberg H. Alterations caused by the intraerythrocytic malaria parasite in the permeability of its host cell membrane. Comp Biochem Physiol. 1990;95:31-39.

[72] Orellana JA, Schalper KA, Figueroa V, Sanchez H, Sáez JC. Regulation of intercellular calcium signaling through calcium interactions with connexin-based channels. Adv Exp Med Biol. 2012;740:777-794. doi:10.1007/978-94-007-2888-2_34

[73] Sanchez HA, Orellana JA, Verselis VK, Sáez JC. Metabolic inhibition increases activity of connexin-32 hemichannels permeable to Ca^{2+} in transfected HeLa cells. Am J Physiol Cell Physiol. 2009;297:C665-C678. doi:10.1152/ajpcell.00200.2009

[74] Sanchez HA, Mese G, Srinivas M, White TW, Verselis VK. Differentially altered Ca^{2+} regulation and Ca^{2+} permeability in C x 26 hemichannels formed by the A40V and G45E mutations that cause keratitis ichthyosis deafness syndrome. J Gen Physiol. 2010;136:47-62. doi:10.1085/jgp.201010433

[75] Schalper KA, Sanchez HA, Lee SC, Altenberg GA, Nathanson MH, Saez JC. Connexin 43 hemichannels mediate the Ca^{2+} influx induced by extracellular alkalinization. Am J Physiol Cell Physiol. 2010;299:C1504-C1515. doi:10.1152/ajpcell.00015.2010

[76] Fiori MC, Figueroa V, Zoghbi ME, Saez JC, Reuss L. Permeation of calcium through purifed Connexin 26 hemichannels. J Biol Chem. 2012;287:40826-40834. doi:10.1074/jbc.M112.383281

[77] Moreno SN, Silva J, Vercesi AE, Docampo R. Cytosolic-free calcium elevation in *Trypanosoma cruzi* is required for cell invasion. J Exp Med. 1994;180:1535-1540. doi:10.1084/jem.180.4.1535

[78] Tardieux I, Nathanson MH, Andrews NW. Role in host cell invasion of *Trypanosoma cruzi*-induced cytosolic-free Ca^{2+} transients. J Exp Med. 1994;179:1017-1022. doi:10.1084/jem.179.3.1017

[79] Davis BK, Wen H, Ting JP. The inflammasome NLRs in immunity, in ammation, and associated diseases. Annu Rev Immunol. 2011;29:707-735. doi:10.1146/annurev-immunol-031210-101405

Chapter 7

Lactoferrin in the Battle against Intestinal Parasites: A Review

Nidia León-Sicairos, Cynthia Ordaz-Pichardo,
Julio César Carrero and Mireya de la Garza

Additional information is available at the end of the chapter

http://dx.doi.org/10.5772/66819

Abstract

Lactoferrin is an iron-binding glycoprotein of the innate immune system, which is present in some mammalian fluids and secreted into the mucosae; it is also produced by the secondary granules of the polymorphonuclear neutrophils and secreted at infection sites. Lactoferricins (Lfcins) are peptides derived from the N-terminus of Lf. Lf avoids the iron availability to parasites in the body fluids due to its high avidity for iron, maintaining together with transferrin the free-iron concentration in about 10^{-18} M, which is too low to support the pathogenic invader survival. Intestinal parasitic diseases affect people worldwide, mainly in developing countries with poor hygienic conditions; for example, parasites such as *Entamoeba histolytica, Giardia intestinalis,* and *Cryptosporidium parvum* infect the human intestine when are orally ingested as cysts. Human and bovine Lf have been found parasiticidal in experiments *in vitro* and in animal models. Interestingly, Lf synergizes with metronidazole, the main drug used against *E. histolytica* and *G. intestinalis*. The aim of this chapter is to show the benefits of using Lf and Lfcins against intestinal parasitic diseases.

Keywords: antimicrobial, intestinal mucosa, iron, lactoferrin, parasiticide

1. Introduction

Lactoferrin (Lf) is an iron-binding nonheme glycoprotein that possesses an exceptional high iron-binding affinity and retains iron at acidic pH. Lf is mainly devoted to chelate iron in fluids and secretions; in addition, Lf is immunomodulatory. Based on its iron content, Lf can exist in two forms: iron-loaded (holoLf, with one or two ferric ions) and iron-free (apoLf). Lf is a constituent of the mammalian innate-immune defense system. In mucosae, Lf displays antimicrobial activity against a wide range of pathogens [1–5]. Lf is synthesized by the mammary gland and secreted into colostrum and milk, participating in the primary immune response in newborns [5–8]. In humans, Lf concentration ranges from 7 to 15 mg/ml in colostrum and 1.2 mg/ml in mature milk. Lf is also present in tears, saliva, and exocrine secretions of mucosal surfaces located in the respiratory, reproductive, and intestinal tracts [9–12]. Lf has been found in tissues of the stomach, lung, liver, bone marrow, cartilage, and bones [13–16]. In the gastrointestinal tract, Lf concentration varies from 0.75 μg/ml in duodenal juice, 0.71–1.07 μg/ml in whole gut lavage fluid, or 0.3–0.7 μg/g in feces [17].

Lf is also synthesized during the transition from promyelocytes to myelocytes of white cells; thus it is a major component of the secondary granules of polymorphonuclear (PMN) neutrophils present in blood [18]. These cells store Lf (3 μg Lf/10^6 neutrophils) and they release it at the sites of microbial invasion which are of low pH due to the pathogens activity [2, 7, 11, 19]. Lf concentration in plasma is relatively low (0.0004–0.002 mg/ml) and derives from neutrophils; however, in patients with sepsis neutrophils are activated and degranulated, secreting into the bloodstream significant levels of apoLf (~0.2 mg/ml) [9]. Lf in feces is also due to the neutrophils action and its concentration noticeably increases in bowel inflammatory diseases (BID) due to pathogenic bacteria, such as ulcerative colitis and Crohn's disease. Thus, Lf is used in a test as an inflammatory marker in intestine, test that discriminates between people suffering BID from those that only have irritable bowel syndrome (IBS), who show normal values of Lf [20]. A test of latex agglutination using anti-Lf antibodies demonstrated that cases with either shigellosis or bacterial urinary infections revealed a high Lf titer which was positively correlated with the number of PMN. In contrast, cases with parasitic infections such as *Entamoeba histolytica* or *Schistosoma haematobium* were characterized by a relatively lower inflammatory process as expressed by mild Lf titer which was also correlated with the PMN count [21]. Ascites Lf can also offer a promising biomarker for bacterial peritonitis, and Lf in pancreatic juice and stone could provide pathophysiological information [22].

2. Structure and biological properties of lactoferrin

Lf was initially identified from bovine milk [23], and simultaneously isolated from bovine [24] and human [25] milk more than 55 years ago. Both glycoproteins (hLf and bLf) share 70% in amino acid sequence [26] and are monomeric, with an approximated molecular weight of 80 kDa; both are highly cationic with a basic isoelectric point (8.5–9). Tertiary structure of Lf consists in two main N and C lobes that are in turn organized in domains N1, N2, and C1 and C2. Both lobes are linked at N1 and C1 domains by a three-turn alpha chain [27, 28] and are able to bind one ferric ion ($Kd = 10^{-23}$ M); this ion derives from the diet or from iron-charged transferrin (holoTf) [29]; Tf is a similar glycoprotein present in plasma and lymph but it has lower affinity for iron than Lf. HoloLf structure is conformationally more rigid and stable compared with apoLf [30–32].

In the N1 terminus of Lf, there is a region lacking iron-chelating activity, known as a lactoferricin (Lfcin) domain, characterized by its strong cationic charge. Lfcin can be obtained from Lf by enzymatic proteolysis with stomach pepsin; the antibacterial properties of Lf are due to this Lfcin domain [33–35]. Several Lfcins have been employed against pathogens, and they are termed according to the residues number they contain. Moreover, antimicrobial peptides have been synthesized and can be used in combination with drugs [36]. Synthetic Lfcin17-30 and lactoferrampin (Lfampin265-284), and a fusion peptide of both, Lfchimera, have been assayed against multiresistant bacteria, and also those that form biofilms [37–39]. Lfchimera also has been tested against parasitic protozoa [40–42].

Microbes that colonize mucosal surfaces in the different body tracts will likely be exposed to different concentrations of Lf, to different complexes of Lf with other proteins, and to different levels of Lf derivatives [43]. As a plus of the beneficial effects of Lf in the intestinal tissues, many studies report its property as growth-promoting on bifidobacteria [44]. All these findings suggest that Lf and Lfcins can be of potential use as adjuncts to conventional antibiotics and drugs in the pharmacological use against pathogens.

3. Importance of iron in infections and the role of lactoferrin

Due to the iron toxicity, all organisms need to regulate its concentration and maintain iron homeostasis [45, 46]. This transition element is mainly linked to proteins, like the heme group in hemoglobin, as cofactor of enzymes, bound to other proteins like iron-chelating proteins, or stored in ferritin [9, 45, 47, 48].

To multiply and cause disease, parasites must acquire iron within their vertebrate hosts. However, mammals have evolved a universal strategy against microbial invaders, consisting in the expression of iron-sequestering systems for dropping the free iron concentration that pathogens need to survive inside a host. The iron-chelating property of Lf and Tf in fluids leads to a concentration of 10^{-18} M, a quantity too low to sustain the microbial life [9, 49, 50]. In addition, infections are often associated with a reduction in the circulating iron in fluids, a host response known as hypoferremia of infection [10]. So, pathogens must have systems needed to gain the iron retained in human proteins such as Lf; if not, they succumb by the iron restriction. This is the reason by which Lf is microbiostatic.

Furthermore, Lf can damage the functional integrity of the microbial surface and being bactericide [1]; diverse authors have shown that bLf and hLf display activity against Gram-positive and Gram-negative bacteria, including antibiotic multiresistant bacteria [35, 51–53]. Lf is also able to affect and kill certain unicellular parasites, such as *Toxoplasma*, *Entamoeba*, and *Giardia*. In consequence, Lf can be parasiticide [54–56].

On the other hand, Lf is considered a modulatory molecule of both the innate and adaptive immune systems. Lf is able to modify the production of humoral mediators and the activity of cell components involved in specific immune responses, such as the increase of T-cell proliferation and maturation [57–60]. Lf is capable of modulating the response of macrophages to induce a Th1 response essential to combat intracellular pathogens [61–64]. Effects of Lf on inflammation correlate with a decrease of the proinflammatory mediator tumor necrosis factor (TNF), interleukin (IL)-6, and IL-1 and, in some cases, with an increase of anti-inflammatory interleukins, IL-4 and IL-10 [65–68]. Lf from neutrophils decreases the TNF release and modulates the recruitment and activation of phagocytes to sites of inflammation. Also the peptide Lfcin has shown anti-inflammatory effect [69]. In addition, several researchers have proven that orally administrated bLf prevents cancer progression, which could be due to an improvement of immunity against the tumor cells, or a direct interaction with these cells, or to both effects [16, 70].

4. Lactoferrin against intestinal infections caused by parasites

The identification of natural compounds with antiparasitic activity has always been a pivotal aim of parasitology research. Alternative therapies against parasites have been explored mainly in chronic infections, or when drugs cause adverse effects, or when microbes are resistant to all treatments. As a consequence to be part of the mammalian natural defense, Lf has been searched as an antimicrobial in assays *in vitro,* and a minimal inhibitory concentration (MIC) has been established for each microorganism tested. Experimental infections have also been performed *in vivo* in animal models in which different doses of Lf and administration via have been employed, and the reduction of lesions is evidenced. In a wide range of bacteria and in less number of fungi and parasites, Lf has been tested as microbicide, in some cases with promissory results. It has been shown that Lf inhibits the growth of protozoan parasites, such as *Toxoplasma gondii* [55], *Plasmodium falciparum* [71], *Trypanosoma cruzi* [72], and *E. histolytica* [73, 74]. *T. cruzi* is an emerging parasite responsible for frequent outbreaks of acute cases of Chagas disease contracted orally and causing high mortality [75]. In this chapter, the interactions of some intestinal protozoa with the innate immune-system protein Lf are discussed, as examples of the Lf parasiticidal action. **Table 1** shows the cases of parasites affected by Lf and its natural or synthetic derived peptides.

4.1. Entamoeba histolytica and amoebiasis

Amoebiasis is a parasitic disease caused by the protozoan *E. histolytica* and a major medical problem in developing countries. This infection is responsible for 50 million cases of tissue invasion and 60,000 deaths per year [76]. Amoebiasis is primarily spread in food and water contaminated by human feces [77, 78]. Only about 10% people show invasive symptoms and the rest of them can remain asymptomatic due to the host defense. In addition, *Entamoeba dispar,* a morphologically indistinguishable noninvasive amoeba, is involved in many asymptomatic cases. Distinguishing *E. histolytica* from *E. dispar* requires molecular or enzymatic characterization [79].

Furthermore, the pattern of amoebic infection, the presence of antibodies, manifestations of disease, an approach to investigations, and strategies for management remain complex [80]. *E. histolytica* trophozoites (amoebae) can damage the large intestine causing ulcers and sometimes they move to the liver, forming abscesses that could be fatal if not treated. *E. histolytica* can also affect nonhuman primates in captivity or wild life [81, 82]. The *in vitro* studies of amoebic pathogenesis have demonstrated three essential processes in the interaction of *E. histolytica* with target cells: (1) adherence of amoebae to cells, which is mediated in virulent strains by a GalNAc-inhibitable amoebic adhesin; (2) contact-dependent target cell lysis, and (3) amoebic phagocytosis of target cells [83, 84]. Many factors have been involved in promoting the invasiveness, pathogenicity, and virulence of *E. histolytica* [85].

Noteworthy, incidence of amoebiasis remains high nowadays when compared to the last century, in spite of the high efficacy of metronidazole treatment. However, this drug causes nausea, vomiting, and other side effects, in addition to be found mutagenic in bacterial cultures, and carcinogenic to experimental animal models [86, 87]. These findings, and the obtaining of resistant strains to metronidazole *in vitro*, encourage us to the development and/

Parasite	Protein and/or peptides	Experiments performed	References
Amoebozoa *Entamoeba histolytica*	**hLf bLF Lfcin4-14 LFcin17-30 LFampin265-284 LFchimera**	***In vitro* assays** Viability assays; *E. histolytica* trophozoites were incubated with the Lfs or peptides.Viability was established.Also, synergy of Lf with metronidazole was assayed.	[40, 73, 74]
	bLF	***In vivo***Murine intestinal amoebiasis model;Mice were intracecal inoculated with *E. histolytica* trophozoites, and then intestinal amoebiasis was developed. bLF was orally administered. Viability and infection of mice was determined.	[99]
	bLF	***In vivo***Amoebic liver abscess; mice were intraportal inoculated with *E. histolytica* trophozoites until liver abscess development, and then hepatic amoebiasis was developed. hLF was orally administered.Viability and infection of mice was determined.	[108]
Metamonada *Giardia intestinalis*	**hLf bLf Lfcin4-14**	***In vitro* assays** Viability assays; *G. intestinalis* cultures were incubated with hLf, bLF, and natural Lfcins. Viability was assessed.	[54]
	bLF LFcin17-30 LFampin265-284 LFchimera	***In vitro* assays** Viability assays, clinical isolates of *G. intestinalis* were incubated with bLF and the synthetic bLF derived peptides.Viability of cultures was determined.	[42]
	bLf	**Clinical trials** bLF versus placebo were administered to children for the prevention of diarrhea by *G. intestinalis.*	[103]
Apicomplexa *Cryptosporidium parvum*	**hLf bLf hLfcin bLfcin**	**Infectivity assay on host cell cultures** Preincubation of sporozoites with Lf or peptides and then, infection of Caco-2 cells.	[135]
Microsporidia *Encephalitozoon intestinalis*	**hLf bLfcin4-14**	**Spore germination assay on host cell cultures** Intestinal epithelial cells were infected with clinical isolates of *E. intestinalis* and then, were treated with hLf or bLFcin4-14.	[143]
Fungi *Candida albicans*	**pLf**	***In vivo* assay** Oral administration with porcine Lf-rich milk in mice pups infected with *C. albicans*	[147]
Apicomplexa *Toxoplasma gondii*	**bLF Lfcin**	***In vitro* assays** Viability assays; *T. gondii* was incubated with the Lfs or peptides. Viability and infectivity established. ***In vivo* assays** Infection of mice and pretreated or treated with bLF administered orally. Infectivity, parasitemia, and survival of mice were determined.	[148, 149] [150, 151]
Helminths *Haemonchus contortus*	**cLf**	***In vitro* assays** Effect of cLf on egg hatching and worm motility inhibition	[152]

Table 1. Parasites affected by lactoferrin and its natural or synthetic derived peptides.

or identification of new antiamoebic drugs that could replace metronidazole or synergize with it allowing a diminution in the dose of drug necessary for an effective treatment [88–90]. Up to date, there is no direct evidence of a protective role of Lf in human intestinal and hepatic amoebiasis. However, results from studies *in vitro* and in experimental animal models allow us to consider the use of Lf for both types of amoebiasis.

4.1.1. Studies in vitro *of use of lactoferrin against* E. histolytica *trophozoite growth*

Our group of research fractionated human milk and tested each fraction against amoebae in an axenic culture to search an effect of Lf, lysozyme, and secretory immunoglobulin A (sIgA); we also sought any combined effect among these molecules, and tested human, bovine, and swine milk against the parasite. For that, trophozoites of the strain HM-1:IMSS were treated with 5–20% of each milk, with 10% of human milk fractions, or with 1 mg/ml of isolated human milk Lf or sIgA, or chicken egg white lysozyme. From milks, only human and bovine milk were amoebicidal showing a concentration-dependent effect, which increased in the absence of iron. Human milk protein fractions (Lf, lysozyme, and sIgA) were amoebicidal, and Lf showed the major effect [74]. Regarding the mechanism of action, Lf bound to the amoebic membrane causing cell rounding, lipid disruption, and damage.

In another work, the microbicidal action of hLf, bLf, and Lfcin4-14 was established on the viability of *E. histolytica* trophozoites. Both Lfs and Lfcin were able to kill amoebae in a concentration-dependent manner. The effect was modulated according to the culture age, pH, and temperature and prevented by Fe^{2+} and Fe^{3+}. Mg^{2+} and Ca^{2+} prevented the killing effect of Lf but not of Lfcin. Parasites obtained from the stationary phase were more susceptible to Lf than those from the exponential phase. A synergistic effect was observed with metronidazole, decreasing about fivefold the concentration necessary to kill most amoebae [73, 74]. This observation is important, since as we mentioned before, metronidazole has been found toxic and mutagenic at the used concentrations. These data suggest that both Lfs and bLfcin might be used in amoebiasis if they are administered with low doses of metronidazole to have less toxicity of this drug. After that, we used the synthetic peptides Lfcin17-30, Lfampin256-284, and Lfchimera to search for an effect against *E. histolytica*. At 50 μM of each peptide, Lfcin and Lfampin showed a moderate amoebicidal effect, with 45–50% of amoeba viable at 24 h culture. However, at 50 μM Lfchimera, about 75% of amoebae were killed, whereas at 100 μM all parasites died. These data indicate that N-terminal Lf-peptides, mainly Lfchimera, have amoebicidal activity in a time- and concentration-dependent manner [40].

4.1.2. Effect of lactoferrin on a murine intestinal-amoebiasis model

Infection with *E. histolytica* may be confined to the intestinal lumen, or can result in invasion of the colonic mucosa (intestinal amoebiasis, IA). Pathologic changes of this mucosa initially are nonspecific but are followed by ulceration [77]. In a study with 3000 patients, it was found that the clinic-pathologic forms of the disease were: ulcerative rectocolitis (95%), typhloappendicitis (3%), amoeboma (1.5%), and fulminating colitis with toxic megacolon (0.5%) [91].

In addition to the studies *in vitro*, human breast milk and saliva secretions have been well documented to possess antiamoebic activity and, in addition to the sIgA antibodies, Lf could be one of the active molecules in IA [92–95]. Around 35 years ago, it was suggested that Lf present in milk could be involved in protecting against IA in some population groups. Prospective studies carried out on Turkana and Maasai African nomads that consume milk as the major item in their diet showed amoeba seronegativity or freedom from intestinal infection with *E. histolytica*, respectively, in contrast to similar nomads having a mixed diet. In both studies, the milk-drinker group showed iron deficiency, probably due to the poor supply of iron in the milk, and it was proposed that the low intestinal content of iron affected the growth of *E. histolytica*. Noteworthy, it was also proposed that Lf and Tf present in the milk may actively compete with amoeba for intestinal iron [92, 96]. Likewise, newborns are protected against infectious agents including amoeba while they are being breastfed. In a study carried out with 322 Egyptian infants of 2–6 months old, the group who had been breastfed since birth showed significantly lower incidence of parasitic infections than the other group who only received formula (38.5% versus 75.2%, respectively). Reduction in infections by *Cryptosporidium* spp., *E. histolytica/E. dispar, G. lamblia,* and *Blastocystis* spp., as well as mixed parasite infections, was observed. These studies suggested that cattle and breast milk contain components that can combat intestinal infections in humans [97].

In contrast to the well-documented antiamoebic potential of Lf *in vitro*, almost nothing is known about its effect on an intestinal model of infection. The only study of this type has been addressed by our group in a murine model of cecal amoebiasis with high success [98]. The model uses mice of the C3H/HeJ strain, which has a spontaneous mutation in the toll-like receptor 4 gene, Tlr4Lps-d, making these mice more resistant to endotoxin. Intracecal inoculation with virulent *E. histolytica* cultured trophozoites results in an inflammatory and ulcerative disease highly reminiscent of human IA, starting with tiny erosions of the surface epithelium at 5 days, which evolve to deeper and extensive destructive lesions of the cecal wall at 21 days, including flask-shaped ulcers, intestinal perforations, and intramural abscesses formation, without evidence of tissue invasion by amoebae. In this model, we found that a simple oral dose of bLf to mice controls the infection already established in the cecum [99]. Details of this experiment are included below paragraphs.

Germ-free mice of the C3H/HeJ strain were intracecally infected by 10^6 virulent amoebae (strain HM1:IMSS). Fourteen days post challenge, by which time amoeba-induced lesions are expected [98], a group of mice was orally treated with bLf (20 mg/kg), daily for 7 days. At 21 days, all mice were sacrificed and the ceca exscinded, fixed, and embedded in paraffin (**Figure 1**, upper cartoon). Finally, tissue sections were stained with hematoxylin-eosin for histological analysis. The results showed that infected mice receiving bLf cured IA in 63.14% as neither trophozoites nor tissue damage were found in sections of the ceca (**Figure 1A**). The rest of treated mice showed partial resolve of the infection, evidenced by reduction in the number of amoebae and tissue damage, compared with the untreated mice, which had inflamed and vascularized ceca with abundant mucus, amoebae, and microhemorrhages (**Figure 1B**). Intriguingly, a similar protocol of treatment with 200 mg/kg did not resolve the infection, which could be due to the formation of immune complexes between bLf and sIgA antibodies present in the intestinal lumen, and/or formation of anionic aggregates that occur

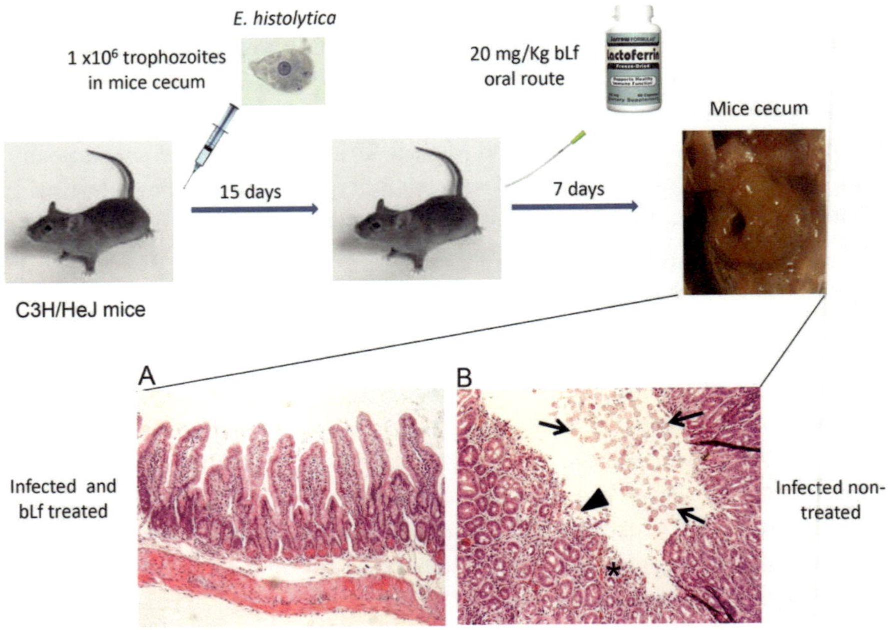

Figure 1. Treatment protocol with bLf against intestinal amoebiasis in a murine model. Above: Mice strain C3H/HeJ was intracecally infected with virulent E. histolytica trophozoites. Two weeks post-infection, mice were treated daily by oral route with 20 mg/kg bLf for 1 week. Upon completion of treatment, the mice were sacrificed and the ceca processed for histological analysis. Below: The treated mice showed absence of infection (left tissue section) compared to the ceca of infected but untreated mice (right tissue section), which showed many trophozoites in the lumen (arrows) and extensive damage of the intestinal epithelium, with loss of epithelial integrity (arrow head) and micro-hemorrhages (asterisk).

when high amounts of Lf are prepared in high salt concentrations [100]. It is worthy of noting that resolution of the IA by bLf correlated both with an increased production of total sIgA and an anti-inflammatory response, determined in cecum tissue extracts or tissue sections, respectively. The average of total sIgA levels in cured mice was twofold higher than that observed in the infected ones, and also higher in completely cured mice when compared to sIgA levels in mice with partial resolution of the infection. Also, whereas high expression of proinflammatory INFγ and TNFα as well as of regulatory IL-10 and TGFβ cytokines were observed in the ceca of infected mice, only high expression of IL-4 was observed in the bLf treated and cured mice. The immune-regulatory activity of Lf has been well documented, mainly downregulating the inflammatory response and reestablishing intestinal homeostasis, but also upregulating the humoral response [101, 102].

In conclusion, Lf might exert a protective effect against IA, through multiple mechanisms because of its multifaceted properties. Directly, Lf may perform amoebicidal activity disrupting the parasite membrane as suggested from the *in vitro* studies. Indirectly, Lf may boost the intestinal secretory immune response increasing the production of both, unspecific and specific antiamoeba IgA antibodies that could block the adherence of amoebae to the gut epithelium, or inhibit the growth of parasites by competing for local iron. Based on our studies aforementioned, and that the therapeutic use of Lf for treating infections causing diarrhea in humans is highly safe [103, 104], we suggest that oral daily treatment with a relatively low dose of bLf for 1 week, either alone or in combination with metronidazole, could represent a new therapeutic strategy for curing the human intestinal infection caused by *E. histolytica*.

4.1.3. *Effect of lactoferrin on the amoebic liver abscess*

Intestinal amoebiasis may complicate by spreading of amoebae via the portal venous to the liver, or perforation of the intestinal wall, resulting in peritonitis or fistulas. Amoebic liver abscesses (ALA) may perforate into the peritoneal, pleural, or pericardial cavities. Hematogenous spreading of amoebae can also result in abscess formation in more distant sites, such as the brain [105]. ALA is the most important for no intestinal infection, due to its high frequency of occurrence and serious clinical concerns, since ALA occurs in up to 95% of fatal cases of amoebiasis. The abscess is composed of a thin capsular wall whose inner surface has "shaggy" appearance; microscopically, the abscess fluid is granular with eosinophilic debris and few or no cells. Smaller abscesses have been felt by some authors to form larger abscesses by coalescence; portal fibrosis and bile duct proliferation have been noted as part of a healing process [106].

ALA can be induced in animal models by intraportal inoculation of amoebae, and it presents a PMN infiltrate within the first 12 hours. As the neutrophils and hepatocytes lyse, the amoebae remain in debris of basophilic material. Later in the progression of abscess formation, these form a more organized capsule with collagen fibers and fibroblasts surrounded by macrophages and epithelioid cells. Experimental amoebiasis has been conducted to evaluate therapeutic regimens, immunology, or pathology of invasive amoebiasis [106, 107]. In this sense, we evaluated the therapeutic effect of bLf in a model of ALA in hamsters. Interestingly, hamsters treated intragastrically with Lf (2.5 mg/100 g body weight) over a period of 8 days, showed no clinical signs of disease and ALA was effectively decreased with only 0.63% detectable lesion, compared with 63% in untreated animals. Furthermore, liver function and blood cells approached normal levels in hamsters receiving bLf treatment [108]. These results suggest that bLf may aid in the therapy of amoebiasis, most likely without producing side effects in patients.

4.2. Giardia intestinalis

Giardia intestinalis (also known as *Giardia lamblia* or *Giardia duodenalis*) is a flagellated unicellular binucleated parasite that causes giardiasis, a diarrheal disease spread throughout the world [109]. Giardiasis is the most common cause of waterborne outbreaks of diarrhea. The prevalence of this parasitic disease commonly ranges from 20 to 30% of the population in developing countries or 3 to 7% in developed ones. Giardiasis is reported more frequently in young children (between 6 months and 5 years of age), and in chronically infected and immune-suppressed people, and also in susceptible travelers [109, 110].

Giardia species have two major stages in their lifecycle. First, infection with *G. intestinalis* initiates when the cysts are ingested in contaminated water or, less commonly, foods. The cyst is relatively inert, allowing prolonged survival in a variety of environmental conditions. Cysts excyst into trophozoites in the proximal small intestine, and then they attach to the lining of the small intestine and reproduce, interfering with the absorption of fats and carbohydrates from digested foods, causing diarrhea and malabsorption [111]. After exposure to biliary fluid, some trophozoites form cysts in the jejunum and pass to the feces, allowing for completion the transmission cycle by infecting a new host [112, 113]. When the clinical signs of infection are present, they may include diarrhea, nausea, weight loss, and abdominal pain. Giardiasis is an established cause of failure to thrive in children; it also causes diminished cognitive functions and chronic fatigue. In adults, giardiasis may lead to postinfectious gastrointestinal disorders such as IBS and dyspepsia. In addition to diarrhea, *G. intestinalis* causes iron deficiency anemia, micronutrient deficiencies, protein-energy malnutrition, growth and cognitive retardation, and malabsorption. A few cases of *Giardia* associated with tumor masses have also been reported, but cause-to-effect relationship between giardiasis and cancer has yet to be established [114].

When giardiasis develops symptoms, a standard treatment mainly consists of metronidazole therapy. However, in addition to this drug causes side effects in patients, it has been associated with significant failure rates in clearing parasites from the gut [109]. Also, an increasing incidence of nitroimidazole-refractory giardiasis has been reported in travelers from India [115]. A correct fluid and electrolyte management is critical, mainly [22] in patients with large-volume diarrheal losses, and children with acute or chronic diarrhea in whom Giardia organisms have been identified [116–118]. In some patients, giardiasis resolves within a few days, whereas in others the symptoms last for years, even in the presence of circulating antigiardia antibodies in serum, or sIgA antibodies at mucosal sites and the cell-mediated immunity. Because of its biological features, it is likely that nonimmune factors play a role in the susceptibility or duration and severity of the disease. Both humoral and cell-mediated immune responses play a role in giardiasis, but the mechanisms involved are poorly known [119]. For example, human milk kills *G. duodenalis* trophozoites independently of specific sIgA antibodies [120]. The giardicidal factors present in milk are conjugated bile salts and unsaturated and free fatty acids [121–124]. Also, human neutrophil defensins and indolicidin were giardicides when they were added to the culture medium [111, 125].

It has been tested the effect of hLf, bLf, hLfcin, and bLfcin against *G. intestinalis, in vitro* [54]. On a molar basis, bLfcin had the most potent giardicidal activity, followed by hLfcin, bLf, and hLf; this effect was concentration-dependent and the activity estimated during 2 h of incubation. In addition, trophozoites from early stationary phase cultures were more susceptible to the parasiticidal effect. Intestinal factors and physiologic conditions present in the intestine did not have effect on the activity exhibited by Lfs and Lfcins. On the other hand, $MgCl_2$, $CaCl_2$, and $CoCl_2$ protected against the activity of hLf and bLf, but not of Lfcins against *G. intestinalis*. In the presence of ferric iron, neither Lfs nor Lfcins presented parasiticidal activity, indicating that iron has protective effects [54]. This finding is interesting, since Lfcins did not have any site for iron binding. Under electron microscopy, it was detected that giardias treated with Lfs and Lfcins showed striking and complex morphologic changes in plasmalemma, endomembrane, and cytoskeleton, and increased the electron density of lysosome-like peripheral vacuoles. Also, it was observed by confocal microscopy that Lfs and Lfcins are able to be bound by *G. intestinalis* membranes [126].

Recently, the effect of synthetic bovine Lfcins on the growth of *G. intestinalis* culture was studied. The peptides Lfcin17-30 and Lfampin265-284 and the fusion of both Lfchimera

http://dx.doi.org/10.5772/66819

showed microbicidal activity against *G. intestinalis* trophozoites. Apparently, the best effect was exerted by Lfchimera, since the first hour of incubation. Additionally, low concentrations of this peptide combined with low concentrations of metronidazole or albendazole had a better effect on the inhibition of *G. intestinalis* cultures than the drugs or peptides used alone. When the mechanism of action was explored by transmission and scanning electron microscopy, trophozoites treated with the synthetic Lfcins showed damage on membrane and internal structures [42].

The effect of bovine Lf has been also tested in patients. A randomized, double-blind, placebo-controlled trial was conducted, in a supplementation with bLf (0.5 g twice daily for 9 months), for the prevention of diarrhea in 26 children of 12–36 months of age, in Peru. In the comparison of results, the overall diarrhea incidence and prevalence rates were similar between the two groups (the Lf group versus the placebo group). However, there was a lower prevalence of colonization with *Giardia* species and better growth among children in the Lf group [103]. In conclusion, data from experiments *in vitro* and those from patients support the idea that Lf and Lfcins can be used in the defense against giardiasis.

4.3. Cryptosporidium parvum

Cryptosporidium parvum is an apicomplexan parasite of human and veterinary importance that causes diarrhea and gastroenteritis. Infection is common in children of developing countries with poor hygiene practices and no potable water supplies, where it has high seroprevalence rates and specific IgG seropositivity after 1 year of age, with recurrent infections and relapsing diarrhea [127–129]. The main risk factors are the ingestion of contaminated water, contact with infected persons or animals, and travel to endemic areas of the disease. The *Cryptosporidium* life cycle is divided into six major developmental phases; the infective sporozoites are produced after excystation of oocysts [130] that attach to the cell apical surfaces and become internalized within an intracellular but extra-cytoplasmic compartment, which is separated from the cytoplasm by an electron-dense layer that appears to be predominantly of host origin. In this compartment, parasite is protected from the hostile gut environment and supplied with energy and nutrients by the host cell through a feeder organelle, which is unique among apicomplexan parasites [131]. It has also been reported that *C. parvum* may have extracellular gregarine-like life stages [132].

In immunocompetent patients, diarrhea due to *C. parvum* is self-limited; however, cryptosporidiosis is recognized as an important disease in immunosuppressed people such as AIDS patients. By immunological and molecular techniques, researchers have identified over 25 putative virulence factors, which are proposed to be involved in aspects of host-pathogen interactions from adhesion and locomotion to invasion and proliferation [131, 133]. It has been investigated the increase of Lf in feces as an indicator of inflammation in healthy adult volunteers experimentally infected with oocysts, and in children with diarrhea that have naturally acquired *C. parvum*. Of the 21 specimens taken post challenge, only one of 14 *Cryptosporidium*-seropositive patients had Lf titer >1:50. In contrast, 12 of 17 specimens from children with only *Cryptosporidium* infection had mild to moderate elevation of fecal Lf. These results suggest that there may be a mild subclinical inflammatory component in cryptosporidiosis in children with diarrhea. Also, that Lf increase is a good tool to detect inflammation in cryptosporidiosis [134].

Currently, there are no consistently effective parasite-specific pharmaceuticals or immunotherapies for control of cryptosporidiosis. Thus, several alternative therapies have been studied to combat this disease, among them, some natural compounds from the innate immune system. Some *in vitro* assays have been performed to demonstrate whether bLf, bLfcin, and a bLf pepsin hydrolysate (bLfh) have some effect against *C. parvum*. For that, freshly excysted sporozoites were incubated for 15 min in MEM containing 10 μg/ml of Lf or its derivative peptides; further, an infection to Caco-2 cells was done. The authors found that only the bLfh and bLfcin were highly parasiticidal decreasing sporozoite viability by 45–69% when compared to the control. In addition, these compounds strongly reduced sporozoite infectivity to the cells. The viability percentage was similar when the bLfh and bLfcin were used [135]. From these experiments, we can deduce that it would be remarkable the use of bLf derivatives to prevent or cure the infection by *C. parvum*.

4.4. Fungi

4.4.1. Microsporidia

Microsporidia are unicellular, obligate intracellular fungal parasites that affect a variety of vertebrate and invertebrate hosts. The phylum Microsporidia comprises 150 genera with more than 1200 species, from which only seven genera infect humans [136]. These parasites have been found in water sources and in wild, domestic, laboratory, and food-producing farm animals; thus, microsporidia can also cause zoonotic diseases. In addition, microsporidiosis is an emergent infection because the parasites are opportunistic agents in patients with HIV, or in those immunosuppressed by organ transplant, or in children and old people, affecting the gastrointestinal tract, nasopharynx, lungs, eyes, and skin [136, 137]. In the gastrointestinal tract, infection of differentiated mucosal epithelial cells most likely results from impalement via spores containing a unique coiled tube used to impale target cells and inject the infectious sporoplasm [138]. Spores germinate in the lumen in close proximity to the target cells [136, 139, 140]. In addition to the unique way in which microsporidia infect cells, *Encephalitozoon cuniculi* spores enter nonprofessional phagocytes by phagocytosis and traffic into a late endosomal-lysosomal compartment; after being phagocytosed, spores germinate within the cell [141, 142]. The pathogenesis of intestinal disease is related to excess death of enterocytes as a result of cellular infection. Clinically, microsporidiosis most often presents with diarrhea and weight loss as a result of small intestinal injury and malabsorption [140]. *Enterocytozoon bieneusi* is the most common microsporidial cause of human intestinal disease. A second species, *Encephalitozoon intestinalis* (originally named *Septata intestinalis*) is associated with disseminated as well as intestinal disease, and the second most common cause of intestinal microsporidiosis. Therapeutic options are few; *E. intestinalis* responds well to albendazole, whereas no antiparasitic therapy has documented efficacy in *E. bieneusi* infections [140].

Leitch and Ceballos [143] [E-CE3] studied clinical isolates of *E. intestinalis*. A spore germination assay and a cultured intestinal epithelial cell-infection assay were used to determine if hLf and bLfcin, in addition to lysozyme and defensins, could inhibit the infection. In this assay, cells were cultured on collagen-coated chamber slides, and at 7 days post confluence, monolayers were infected with 4 × 10^5 spores per well. After 24 hours p.i., the excess of spores was removed with Opti-MEM containing 1 mg/ml chondroitin sulfate and the wells refilled with medium. At 3 days p.i., cells were fixed and stained to visualize parasite sporogonial stages [144] and detect host cell and parasite nuclei. The *Encephalitozoon* species were unaffected in germination by Lf up to a concentration of 2 mg/ml, or by bLfcin. However, bLf was able to significantly diminish the infection to enterocytes.

4.4.2. *Candida albicans*

Besides microsporidia, numerous *in vitro* and *in vivo* studies have been conducted demonstrating the potent capacity of Lf and derived peptides to inhibit the growth and infectivity of other fungal pathogens that can affect mucous membrane of the upper digestive tract, mouth, and pharynx, such as *Candida albicans.* Candida organisms commonly colonize the human gastrointestinal tract as a component of the resident microbiota. Their presence is generally benign. However, high-level colonization by *Candida* could delay healing of inflammatory lesions and that inflammation promotes colonization. Both BID and gastrointestinal *Candida* colonization are associated with elevated levels of the proinflammatory cytokine IL-17. Because *Candida* is a frequent colonizer, these effects have the potential to impact many people [145]; in addition, *C. albicans* gut colonization in mice aggravates inflammation in allergic and autoimmune diseases, not only in the gut but also in the extra-gut tissues and underscores the necessity of investigating the pathogenic role of *C. albicans* gut colonization in immune diseases in humans [146]. Since research about the effect of Lf has been ample in *Candida,* it could be interesting to perform experiments to demonstrate that Lf can help against both the gut inflammation and the pathogen. Despite not being an intestinal pathogen, there is a work that reports the benefit of lactation of mice pups with porcine Lf-rich milk against an oral infection with *C. albicans* [147]. Thus, treated CD1 mice showed lower bacterial counts when compared with normal fed controls as well as a healthier architecture in the small intestine [148], suggesting that porcine Lf can be used as a selective decontamination of the digestive tract regimen.

4.5. *Toxoplasma gondii*

Toxoplasma gondii is an obligatory deadly intracellular parasitic protozoan transmitted by ingestion of uncooked infected meat; this parasite resides in every nucleated cell causing severe complications in immunocompromised hosts. Tanaka et al. [149] examined the effect of bovine Lfcin (LFcin-B), a peptide composed of 25 amino acid residues, on the viability and infectivity of *T. gondii* parasites, both *in vitro* and *in vivo.* After treatment of *T. gondii* with Lfcin at 100 μg/ml for 1 h, 65% of the parasites became oval in shape and had lost the ability to exclude the trypan blue dye, a vital staining. Interestingly, approximately 96% of the parasites treated with Lfcin at 1000 μg/ml for 0.5 h lost the dye exclusion ability. In contrast, more than 80% of the parasites incubated with bLf or a C-terminal peptide at 1000 μg/ml for 4 h retained the dye exclusion ability. On the other hand, the loss of infectivity of the parasites and/or cystozoites in cyst was confirmed by inoculation of mice. Five mice inoculated with 10^2 untreated parasites died within 9 days post challenge. Similarly, parasites pretreated with bLf at 1000 μg/ml caused 100% mortality of inoculated mice within 9 days post challenge. In contrast, four of five mice inoculated with the same dose of parasites pretreated with Lfcin at 1000 μg/ml survived for more than 30 days post challenge. In the case of parasites pretreated with Lfcin at 100 μg/ml, one of five mice survived up to 30 days post challenge. In conclusion, this Lfcin peptide derived from bLf could be used against human toxoplasmosis. To study the effector pathway of *Toxoplasma* growth inhibitory activity induced by bLf in murine macrophage, the role of reactive oxygen intermediates (O^{2-}) and inorganic nitric oxide (NO) was examined by Tanaka et al. [150]. Production of O^{2-} was diminished in cultures of macrophages supplemented with bLf and the effect was dose and time dependent. Production of NO was enhanced in cultures of peritoneal macrophages supplemented with interferon-gamma, but not with bLf. Their findings suggested that this *Toxoplasma* growth-inhibitory activity induced by bLf in macrophages is not mediated by O^{2-} or NO molecules; it may be mediated by an L-arginine-dependent effector pathway that does not involve NO production. The same group of work [151] administered orally or intraperitoneally bLfcin (5 and 0.1 mg/mouse, respectively). Afterward, the researchers challenged mice with cysts of *T. gondii* at a dose of LD90. Although only a small number of mice were used, both administration routes of Lfcin prevented the death in the 100% mice.

Lf also has shown antimicrobial properties in its nanoformulation using alginate chitosan calcium phosphate bLf nanocapsules (AEC-CCo-CP-bLf-NCs). Anand et al. [152] analyzed and compared the effect of bLf in its native as well as nanoformulation AEC-CCo-CP-bLf-NC against coccidian parasite *T. gondii*. The J7741 macrophage cell line culture model showed a significant increase in NO production and low parasitemia. In their *in vivo* BALB/c mice model, after treatment with NCs substantially increased the bioavailability of the protein and showed comparatively increased levels of reactive oxygen species, NO production, and Th1 cytokine which helped in parasite clearance. Regarding to the mechanism of action of NCs, immunoreactivity analysis showed accumulation of Lf in macrophages of various visceral organs, which are the site of parasite multiplication.

4.6. Helminths

Antipathogenic properties of camel milk have been investigated to substitute for drugs hence overcome drug resistance. Recently, Alimi et al. [153] investigated the antihelminthic activity of the chemical compounds of camel milk. *In vitro,* the antihelminthic effects of camel milk against *Haemonchus contortus* (nematode) from sheep were ascertained by egg hatching and worm motility inhibition, in comparison to milks from cow, ewe, and goat, and to the reference drug albendazole. Chemical compounds revealed that camel milk has higher contents of protective protein Lf and vitamin C than other species' milk; for example, the camel milk contains sevenfold more Lf than the cow milk. Camel milk showed ovicidal activity at all tested concentrations and completely inhibited egg hatching at concentrations close to 100 mg/ml (IC50 = 42.39 mg/ml). Also, camel milk revealed *in vitro* activity against adult parasites in terms of the paralysis and/or death of the worms at different hours post-treatment. After 8 h of exposure, camel milk induced 100% mortality at the highest tested concentration. In contrast, there was 82.3% immobility of worms in albendazole at 8 h postexposition. Bioactive compounds such as Lf and vitamin C may be involved in such an effect.

5. High-scale production of lactoferrin

Lf is considered as a nutraceutical protein by certain countries. Because of its versatile properties on health and the null toxicity to humans, Lf can be added to different foods and nutritional supplements, in addition to be used in medicine as an immune modulator, antimicrobial, antiviral, and anticarcinogenic, among other properties, some of them unknown so far. Since the finding of the regulatory property of Lf, much research has been published about this molecule; nowadays we can found almost 7500 references in Pubmed for this glycoprotein.

Currently, Lf is one of the most studied proteins in order to have it commercially available and with full biological activity. Concerning this, Lf from different origins, mainly from human and bovine, but also from camel, buffalo, and other animals, has been obtained from milk and colostrum. To have a better quality and production of Lf, since 25 years ago Lf has been cloned in different vectors and expressed overall in eukaryotic systems which can glycosylate it, such as yeasts and fungi [154–156]. From these organisms, Lf has been highly purified as a recombinant protein and its biological role, mainly antibacterial, has been confirmed. In addition, human Lf has been cloned in transgenic cows and plants [156–159]. Interestingly, recombinant hLf expressed in cows enhanced systematic and intestinal immune responses in piglets, used as a model of infants [160]. In addition, when researchers analyzed the composition of meat from the offspring of hLF transgenic cows, which can express hLf protein in their mammary gland, they did not found any abnormality on the meat nutrient composition of hLF bulls [161]. Therefore, the ample use of Lf in the human health care is promissory.

Commercially available Lf is now offered by several companies for using in research, as a food supplement, as antibacterial or to increase immunity to improving health. Mainly skim milk and cheese whey that have not undergone rigorous heating can be sources of bLF. Because Lf has a cationic nature, it has been purified by cation exchange chromatography in bLF-supplying companies [162–164]. The Japanese Morinaga Milk Co. was the pioneer in research and development of bLf and in the addition of this protein to milk formula and other products are also in the use of Lf in clinical trials. Nowadays, there are numerous patents of Lf from companies that produce Lf of high quality. As examples, those of Nestle for infant memory and learning and promotion of brain maturation in children or another one to be used as antidiarrhea; Fonterra and Tatua, from New Zealand; Pharming Group from The Netherlands; Abial Biotech from Spain; Tatura-Bio from Australia, and NRL-Pharma from Japan, which produces enteric-coating Lf for use in adults in who the whole Lf molecule can rise the intestine. Highly purified Lf without LPS is produced by Taradon Laboratory. On the other hand, recombinant hLF for use in animal and human clinical studies has been produced in the fungus *Aspergillus niger* var. *awamori* by Agennix Inc., for the potential treatment of cancers, asthma, and chronic wounds; in transgenic cows by Pharming Technologies N.V. as a nutraceutical; and in rice by Ventria Bioscience for diarrhea and iron deficiency [164].

6. Conclusion and perspectives

Lf and its derived peptides Lfcins could be an option in the treatment of intestinal parasitic diseases, based mainly on results *in vitro* and in animal models. Research in this glycoprotein has generally been leaded with success, although it is necessary to deep in the understanding of the mechanisms of action of Lf against parasites. In general, drugs used in the therapy antiparasites cause toxic side effects, and/or the parasites can become resistant to them. Lf is an innocuous protein that could be used as adjunct with drugs, with the considerable advantage of using low doses of drugs due to the synergic effect of Lf. It would be required more studies in animal models and carry out strict clinical trials with methodologic accuracy and a large number of patients, in order to extend the use of Lf as a parasiticide.

Acknowledgements

We thank to Consejo Nacional de Ciencia y Tecnologia (CONACYT) for the grants obtained to support our research: No. CB-2012-179251 (Mireya de la Garza), No. CB-2011-167788 (Julio César Carrero), and No. CB-2014-236546 (Nidia León-Sicairos). JCC also thanks to Programa de Apoyo a Proyectos de Investigación e Innovación Tecnológica (PAPIIT-UNAM) for grant No. IN206316. We also thank Dr. Luisa Samaniego and Mr. Carlos Villasana for their technical assistance.

Abbreviations

ALA	Amoebic liver abscess
apoLf	Apolactoferrin
bLf	Bovine Lf
BID	Bowel inflammatory disease
INFγ	Gamma interferon
holoLf	Hololactoferrin
HIV	Human immune deficiency virus
hLf	Human Lf
IL	Interleukin
IA	Intestinal amoebiasis
IBS	Irritable bowel syndrome
Lf	Lactoferrin
Lfcin	Lactoferricin
MEM	Minimal essential medium
MIC	Minimal inhibitory concentration

PMN	Polymorphonuclear
p.i.	Post-infection
sIgA	Secretory immunoglobulin A
Tf	Transferrin
TGF?	Tumor growth factor beta
TNF?	Tumor necrosis factor alpha

Author details

Nidia León-Sicairos[1], Cynthia Ordaz-Pichardo[2], Julio César Carrero[3] and Mireya de la Garza[4*]

*Address all correspondence to: mireya@cell.cinvestav.mx

1 Investigation Department, Pediatric Hospital of Sinaloa, Mexico. Investigation Unity, CIASaP, Faculty of Medicine, Autonomous University of Sinaloa, Mexico

2 Laboratory of Cell Biology and Natural Products, National School of Medicine and Homeopathy, National Polytechnic Institute, Mexico

3 Immunology Department, Institute of Biomedical Investigations, Autonomous National University of Mexico, Mexico

4 Cell Biology Department, Center for Research and Advanced Studies of the National Polytechnic Institute, San Pedro Zacatenco, Mexico City, Mexico

References

[1] Jenssen H, Hancock REW. Antimicrobial properties of lactoferrin. Biochimie 2009;91:19–29. doi:10.1016/j.biochi.2008.05.015.

[2] Weinberg ED. The therapeutic potential of lactoferrin. Expert Opin Investig Drugs 2003;12:841–51. doi:10.1517/13543784.12.5.841.

[3] Sánchez L, Calvo M, Brock JH. Biological role of lactoferrin. Arch Dis Child 1992;67:657–61.

[4] Brock JH. The physiology of lactoferrin. Biochem Cell Biol 2002;80:1–6.

[5] Masson PL, Heremans JF. Lactoferrin in milk from different species. Comp Biochem Physiol B 1971;39:119–29.

[6] Masson PL, Heremans JF, Dive CH. An iron-binding protein common to many external secretions. Clin Chim Acta 1966;14:735–9. doi:10.1016/0009-8981(66)90004-0.

[7] Legrand D, Elass E, Pierce A, Mazurier J. Lactoferrin and host defence: an overview of its immuno-modulating and anti-inflammatory properties. BioMetals 2004;17:225–9.

[8] Vorland LH. Lactoferrin: a multifunctional glycoprotein. APMIS 1999;107:971–81.

[9] Bullen JJ. The significance of iron in infection. Rev Infect Dis 1981;3:1127–38.

[10] Van Snick JL, Masson PL, Heremans JF. The involvement of lactoferrin in the hyposideremia of acute inflammation. J Exp Med 1974;140:1068–84.

[11] Levay PF, Viljoen M. Lactoferrin: a general review. Haematologica 1995;80:252–67.

[12] Hirai Y, Kawakata N, Satoh K, Ikeda Y, Hisayasu S, Orimo H, et al. Concentrations of lactoferrin and iron in human milk at different stages of lactation. J Nutr Sci Vitaminol (Tokyo) 1990;36:531–44.

[13] Mason DY, Taylor CR. Distribution of transferrin, ferritin, and lactoferrin in human tissues. J Clin Pathol 1978;31:316–27.

[14] Tuccari G, Giuffrè G, Scarf R, Simone A, Todaro P, Barresi G. Immunolocalization of lactoferrin in surgically resected pigmented skin lesions. Eur J Histochem 2005;49:33–8.

[15] Ieni A, Barresi V, Grosso M, Speciale G, Rosa MA, Tuccari G. Does lactoferrin behave as an immunohistochemical oncofetal marker in bone and cartilage human neoplasms? Pathol Oncol Res 2011;17:287–93. doi:10.1007/s12253-010-9311-5.

[16] Tuccari G, Barresi G. Lactoferrin in human tumours: immunohistochemical investigations during more than 25 years. BioMetals 2011;24:775–84. doi:10.1007/s10534-011-9450-5.

[17] Uchida K, Matsuse R, Tomita S, Sugi K, Saitoh O, Ohshiba S. Immunochemical detection of human lactoferrin in feces as a new marker for inflammatory gastrointestinal disorders and colon cancer. Clin Biochem 1994;27:259–64.

[18] Rado TA, Bollekens J, St Laurent G, Parker L, Benz EJ. Lactoferrin biosynthesis during granulocytopoiesis. Blood 1984;64:1103–9.

[19] Masson PL, Heremans JF, Schonne E. Lactoferrin, an iron-binding protein in neutrophilic leukocytes. J Exp Med 1969;130:643–58.

[20] Kane S V, Sandborn WJ, Rufo PA, Zholudev A, Boone J, Lyerly D, et al. Fecal lactoferrin is a sensitive and specific marker in identifying intestinal inflammation. Am J Gastroenterol 2003;98:1309–14. doi:10.1111/j.1572-0241.2003.07458.x.

[21] Aly SM, El-Zawawy LA, Said DE, Fathy FM, Mohamed ON. The utility of lactoferrin in differentiating parasitic from bacterial infections. J Egypt Soc Parasitol 2005;35:1149–62.

[22] Hayakawa T, Jin CX, Ko SBH, Kitagawa M, Ishiguro H. Lactoferrin in gastrointestinal disease. Intern Med 2009;48:1251–4. doi: 10.2169/internalmedicine.48.2199.

[23] Sorensen M, Sorensen SPL. The proteins in whey. CR Trav Lab 1939;23:55–9.

[24] Groves ML. The isolation of a red protein from milk 2. J Am Chem Soc 1960;82:3345–50. doi:10.1021/ja01498a029.

[25] Montreuil J, Tonnelat J, Mullet S. [Preparation and properties of lactosiderophilin (lactotransferrin) of human milk]. Biochim Biophys Acta 1960;45:413–21.

[26] Lambert LA. Molecular evolution of the transferrin family and associated receptors. Biochim Biophys Acta 2012;1820:244–55. doi:10.1016/j.bbagen.2011.06.002.

[27] Baker EN, Baker HM. A structural framework for understanding the multifunctional character of lactoferrin. Biochimie 2009;91:3–10. doi:10.1016/j.biochi.2008.05.006.

[28] Moguilevsky N, Retegui LA, Masson PL. Comparison of human lactoferrins from milk and neutrophilic leucocytes. Relative molecular mass, isoelectric point, iron-binding properties and uptake by the liver. Biochem J 1985;229:353–9.

[29] Testa U. Proteins of iron metabolism. Boca Raton, Florida: CRC Press; 2002.[A4]

[30] Anderson BF, Baker HM, Dodson EJ, Norris GE, Rumball SV, Waters JM, et al. Structure of human lactoferrin at 3.2-A resolution. Proc Natl Acad Sci (U S A) 1987;84:1769–73.

[31] Moore SA, Anderson BF, Groom CR, Haridas M, Baker EN. Three-dimensional structure of diferric bovine lactoferrin at 2.8 A resolution. J Mol Biol 1997;274:222–36. doi:10.1006/jmbi.1997.1386.

[32] Coddeville B, Strecker G, Wieruszeski JM, Vliegenthart JF, van Halbeek H, Peter-Katalinić J, et al. Heterogeneity of bovine lactotransferrin glycans. Characterization of alpha-D-Galp-(1–>3)-beta-D-Gal and alpha-NeuAc-(2–>6)-beta-D-GalpNAc-(1–>4)-beta-D-GlcNAc-substituted N-linked glycans. Carbohydr Res 1992;236:145–64.

[33] Gifford JL, Hunter HN, Vogel HJ. Lactoferricin: a lactoferrin-derived peptide with antimicrobial, antiviral, antitumor and immunological properties. Cell Mol Life Sci 2005;62:2588–98. doi:10.1007/s00018-005-5373-z.

[34] Tomita M, Wakabayashi H, Shin K, Yamauchi K, Yaeshima T, Iwatsuki K. Twenty-five years of research on bovine lactoferrin applications. Biochimie 2009;91:52–7. doi:10.1016/j.biochi.2008.05.021.

[35] Samaniego[E-CE5]-Barron L, Luna-Castro S, Piña-Vázquez C, Suárez-Güemes F. Two outer membrane proteins are bovine lactoferrin-binding proteins in Mannheimia haemolytica A1. Vet Res 2016;47:93. doi: 10.1186/s13567-016-0378-1.

[36] Brouwer CPJM, Rahman M, Welling MM. Discovery and development of a synthetic peptide derived from lactoferrin for clinical use. Peptides 2011;32:1953–63. doi:10.1016/j.peptides.2011.07.017.

[37] Bolscher JGM, Adão R, Nazmi K, van den Keybus PAM, van 't Hof W, Nieuw Amerongen AV, et al. Bactericidal activity of LFchimera is stronger and less sensitive to ionic strength than its constituent lactoferricin and lactoferrampin peptides. Biochimie 2009;91:123–32. doi:10.1016/j.biochi.2008.05.019.

[38] Xu G, Xiong W, Hu Q, Zuo P, Shao B, Lan F, et al. Lactoferrin-derived peptides and lactoferricin chimera inhibit virulence factor production and biofilm formation in Pseudomonas aeruginosa. J Appl Microbiol 2010;109:1311–8. doi: 10.1111/j.1365-2672.2010.04751.x

[39] Flores-Villaseñor H, Canizalez-Román A, Reyes-Lopez M, Nazmi K, de la Garza M, Zazueta-Beltrán J, et al. Bactericidal effect of bovine lactoferrin, LFcin, LFampin and LFchimera on antibiotic-resistant Staphylococcus aureus and Escherichia coli. BioMetals 2010;23:569–78. doi:10.1007/s10534-010-9306-4.

[40] López-Soto F, León-Sicairos N, Nazmi K, Bolscher JG, de La Garza M. Microbicidal effect of the lactoferrin peptides lactoferricin 17–30, lactoferrampin 265–284, and lactoferrin chimera on the parasite Entamoeba histolytica. BioMetals 2010;23:563–8. doi:10.1007/s10534-010-9295-3.

[41] Omata Y, Satake M, Maeda R, Saito a, Shimazaki K, Yamauchi K, et al. Reduction of the infectivity of Toxoplasma gondii and Eimeria stiedai sporozoites by treatment with bovine lactoferricin. J Vet Med Sci 2001;63:187–90. doi:10.1292/jvms.63.187.

[42] Aguilar-Díaz H, Canizalez-Roman A, Nepomuceno-Mejia T, Gallardo-Vera F, Hornelas-Orozco Y, Nazmi K, et al. Parasiticidal effect of synthetic bovine lactoferrin peptides on the enteric parasite Giardia intestinalis. Biochem Cell Biol 2016; In revision.

[43] Ling JML, Schryvers AB. Perspectives on interactions between lactoferrin and bacteria. Biochem Cell Biol 2006;84:275–81. doi:10.1139/o06-044.

[44] Oda H, Wakabayashi H, Yamauchi K, Abe F. Lactoferrin and bifidobacteria. BioMetals 2014;27:915–22. doi:10.1007/s10534-014-9741-8.

[45] Dunn LL, Suryo Rahmanto Y, Richardson DR. Iron uptake and metabolism in the new millennium. Trends Cell Biol 2007;17:93–100. doi:10.1016/j.tcb.2006.12.003.

[46] Zhang AS, Enns CA. Molecular mechanisms of normal iron homeostasis. Hematology Am Soc Hematol Educ Program 2009;207–14. doi: 10.1182/asheducation-2009.1.207

[47] Griffiths E. Iron in biological systems. In: Bullen JJ, Griffith E, editors. Iron and infection: molecular, physiological and clinical aspects, Chichester, UK: John Wiley … Sons,; 1987, pp. 1–25.

[48] Ong ST, Ho JZS, Ho B, Ding JL. Iron-withholding strategy in innate immunity. Immunobiology 2006;211:295–314. doi:10.1016/j.imbio.2006.02.004.

[49] Nairz M, Schroll A, Sonnweber T, Weiss G. The struggle for iron - a metal at the host-pathogen interface. Cell Microbiol 2010;12:1691–702. doi:10.1111/j.1462-5822.2010.01529.x.

[50] Weinberg ED. Iron availability and infection. Biochim Biophys Acta 2009;1790:600–5. doi:10.1016/j.bbagen.2008.07.002.

[51] Arnold RR, Brewer M, Gauthier JJ. Bactericidal activity of human lactoferrin: sensitivity of a variety of microorganisms. Infect Immun 1980;28:893–8.

[52] Nibbering PH, Ravensbergen E, Welling MM, van Berkel LA, van Berkel PH, Pauwels EK, et al. Human lactoferrin and peptides derived from its N terminus are highly effective against infections with antibiotic-resistant bacteria. Infect Immun 2001;69: 1469–76. doi:10.1128/IAI.69.3.1469-1476.2001.

[53] Luna-Castro S, Aguilar-Romero F, Samaniego-Barrón L, Godínez-Vargas D, de la Garza M. Effect of bovine apo-lactoferrin on the growth and virulence of Actinobacillus pleuropneumoniae. BioMetals 2014;27:891–903. doi:10.1007/s10534-014-9752-5.

[54] Turchany JM, Aley SB, Gillin FD. Giardicidal activity of lactoferrin and N-terminal peptides. Infect Immun 1995;63:4550–2.

[55] Tanaka T, Omata Y, Saito A, Shimazaki K, Igarashi I, Suzuki N. Growth inhibitory effects of bovine lactoferrin to Toxoplasma gondii parasites in murine somatic cells. J Vet Med Sci 1996;58:61–5.

[56] Ordaz-Pichardo C, Leon-Sicairos N, Canizales-Román A, Cornejo-Cortés M, Ortiz-Estrada G, de la Garza M. Lactoferrin: a protein of the innate immune system capable of killing parasitic protozoa. In: Erzinger, GS Editor. Parasites: Ecology, Diseases and Management, Hauppauge, NY, Nova Science Publishers, Inc.; 2013, pp.177-213

[57] Actor J, Hwang S-A, Kruzel M. Lactoferrin as a natural immune modulator. Curr Pharm Des 2009;15:1956–73.

[58] Zimecki M, Mazurier J, Spik G, Kapp JA. Human lactoferrin induces phenotypic and functional changes in murine splenic B cells. Immunology 1995;86:122–7.

[59] Bi BY, Lefebvre AM, Duś D, Spik G, Mazurier J. Effect of lactoferrin on proliferation and differentiation of the Jurkat human lymphoblastic T cell line. Arch Immunol Ther Exp (Warsz) 1997;45:315–20.

[60] Dhennin-Duthille I, Masson M, Damiens E, Fillebeen C, Spik G, Mazurier J. Lactoferrin upregulates the expression of CD4 antigen through the stimulation of the mitogen-activated protein kinase in the human lymphoblastic T Jurkat cell line. J Cell Biochem 2000;79:583–93.

[61] de la Rosa G, Yang D, Tewary P, Varadhachary A, Oppenheim JJ. Lactoferrin acts as an alarmin to promote the recruitment and activation of APCs and antigen-specific immune responses. J Immunol 2008;180:6868–76.

[62] Spadaro M, Caorsi C, Ceruti P, Varadhachary A, Forni G, Pericle F, et al. Lactoferrin, a major defense protein of innate immunity, is a novel maturation factor for human dendritic cells. FASEB J 2008;22:2747–57. doi:10.1096/fj.07-098038.

[63] Sorimachi K, Akimoto K, Hattori Y, Ieiri T, Niwa A. Activation of macrophages by lactoferrin: secretion of TNF-alpha, IL-8 and NO. Biochem Mol Biol Int 1997;43:79–87.

[64] Wilk KM, Hwang S-A, Actor JK. Lactoferrin modulation of antigen-presenting-cell response to BCG infection. Postępy Hig I Med Doświadczalnej 2007;61:277–82.

[65] Håversen LA, Baltzer L, Dolphin G, Hanson LA, Mattsby-Baltzer I. Anti-inflammatory activities of human lactoferrin in acute dextran sulphate-induced colitis in mice. Scand J Immunol 2003;57:2–10.

[66] Håversen LA, Engberg I, Baltzer L, Dolphin G, Hanson LA, Mattsby-Baltzer I. Human lactoferrin and peptides derived from a surface-exposed helical region reduce experimental Escherichia coli urinary tract infection in mice. Infect Immun 2000;68:5816–23.

[67] Togawa J-I, Nagase H, Tanaka K, Inamori M, Nakajima A, Ueno N, et al. Oral administration of lactoferrin reduces colitis in rats via modulation of the immune system and correction of cytokine imbalance. J Gastroenterol Hepatol 2002;17:1291–8.

[68] Zimecki M, Miedzybrodzki R, Szymaniec S. Oral treatment of rats with bovine lactoferrin inhibits carrageenan-induced inflammation; correlation with decreased cytokine production. Arch Immunol Ther Exp (Warsz) 1998;46:361–5.

[69] Oo TZ, Cole N, Garthwaite L, Willcox MDP, Zhu H. Evaluation of synergistic activity of bovine lactoferricin with antibiotics in corneal infection. J Antimicrob Chemother 2010;65:1243–51. doi:10.1093/jac/dkq106.

[70] Fujita K, Ohnishi T, Sekine K, Iigo M, Tsuda H. Down-regulation of 2-amino-3, 8-dimethylimidazo[4,5-f]quinoxaline (MeIQx)-induced CYP1A2 expression is associated with bovine lactoferrin inhibition of MeIQx-induced liver and colon carcinogenesis in rats. Japan J Cancer Res 2002;93:616–25.

[71] Fritsch G, Sawatzki G, Treumer J, Jung A, Spira DT. Plasmodium falciparum: inhibition in vitro with lactoferrin, desferriferrithiocin, and desferricrocin. Exp Parasitol 1987;63: 1–9.

[72] Lima MF, Kierszenbaum F. Lactoferrin effects on phagocytic cell function. I. Increased uptake and killing of an intracellular parasite by murine macrophages and human monocytes. J Immunol 1985;134:4176–83.

[73] Leon-Sicairos N, Reyes-López M, Ordaz-Pichardo C, de la Garza M. Microbicidal action of lactoferrin and lactoferricin and their synergistic effect with metronidazole in Entamoeba histolytica. Biochem Cell Biol 2006;84:327–36. doi: 10.1139/o06-060

[74] León-Sicairos N, López-Soto F, Reyes-López M, Godínez-Vargas D, Ordaz-Pichardo C, de la Garza M. Amoebicidal activity of milk, apo-lactoferrin, sIgA and lysozyme. Clin Med Res 2006;4:106–13.

[75] Yoshida N, Tyler KM, Llewellyn MS. Invasion mechanisms among emerging food-borne protozoan parasites. Trends Parasitol 2011;27:459–66. doi: 10.1016/j.pt.2011.06.006

[76] Stanley SL. Amoebiasis. Lancet (London, England) 2003;361:1025–34. doi:10.1016/S0140-6736(03)12830-9.

[77] Espinosa-Cantellano M, Martínez-Palomo A. Recent developments in amoebiasis research. Curr Opin Infect Dis 2000;13:451–6.

[78] Bercu TE, Petri WA, Behm JW. Amebic colitis: new insights into pathogenesis and treatment. Curr Gastroenterol Rep 2007;9:429–33.

[79] Rivera WL, Tachibana H, Silva-Tahat MR, Uemura H, Kanbara H. Differentiation of Entamoeba histolytica and E. dispar DNA from cysts present in stool specimens by

polymerase chain reaction: its field application in the Philippines. Parasitol Res 1996;82:585–9.

[80] Choudhuri G, Rangan M. Amebic infection in humans. Indian J Gastroenterol 2012;31:153–62. doi:10.1007/s12664-012-0192-2.

[81] Legesse M, Erko B. Zoonotic intestinal parasites in Papio anubis (baboon) and Cercopithecus aethiops (vervet) from four localities in Ethiopia. Acta Trop 2004;90:231–6. doi:10.1016/j.actatropica.2003.12.003.

[82] Regan CS, Yon L, Hossain M, Elsheikha HM. Prevalence of Entamoeba species in captive primates in zoological gardens in the UK. Peer J 2014;2:e492. doi:10.7717/peerj.492.

[83] Petri W, [E-CE7] Ravdin JI. In vitro models of amebic pathogenesis. Amebiasis, Human Infection by Entamoeba histolytica, Wiley Medical Publication; Chichester, UK 1988, pp. 191–204.

[84] Abou-el-Magd I, Soong CJ, El-Hawey AM, Ravdin JI. Humoral and mucosal IgA antibody response to a recombinant 52-kDa cysteine-rich portion of the Entamoeba histolytica galactose-inhibitable lectin correlates with detection of native 170-kDa lectin antigen in serum of patients with amebic colitis. J Infect Dis 1996;174:157–62.

[85] Meerovitch E, Chadee K, Ravdin JI. In vivo models for pathogenicity in Amebiasis. Amebiasis, Human Infection by Entamoeba histolytica, Wiley Medical Publication; Chichester, UK 1988, pp. 177–90.

[86] Goldman P. Metronidazole: proven benefits and potential risks. Johns Hopkins Med J 1980;147:1–9.

[87] Roe FJ. Toxicologic evaluation of metronidazole with particular reference to carcinogenic, mutagenic, and teratogenic potential. Surgery 1983;93:158–64.

[88] Stranz MH, Bradley WE. Metronidazole (Flagyl IV, Searle). Drug Intell Clin Pharm 1981;15:838–46.

[89] Kapoor K, Chandra M, Nag D, Paliwal JK, Gupta RC, Saxena RC. Evaluation of metronidazole toxicity: a prospective study. Int J Clin Pharmacol Res 1999;19:83–8.

[90] Espinosa A, Clark D, Stanley SL. Entamoeba histolytica alcohol dehydrogenase 2 (EhADH2) as a target for anti-amoebic agents. J Antimicrob Chemother 2004;54:56–9. doi:10.1093/jac/dkh280.

[91] Cardoso JM, Kimura K, Stoopen M, Cervantes LF, Flizondo L, Churchill R, et al. Radiology of invasive amebiasis of the colon. AJR Am J Roentgenol 1977;128:935–41. doi:10.2214/ajr.128.6.935.

[92] Murray MJ, Murray A, Murray CJ. The salutary effect of milk on amoebiasis and its reversal by iron. Br Med J 1980;280:1351–2.

[93] Akisu C. Effect of human milk and colostrum on Entamoeba histolytica. World J Gastroenterol 2004;10:741. doi:10.3748/wjg.v10.i5.741.

[94] Carrero JC, Díaz MY, Viveros M, Espinoza B, Acosta E, Ortiz-Ortiz L. Human secretory immunoglobulin A anti-Entamoeba histolytica antibodies inhibit adherence of amebae to MDCK cells. Infect Immun 1994;62:764–7.

[95] Carrero JC, Cervantes-Rebolledo C, Aguilar-Díaz H, Díaz-Gallardo MY, Laclette JP, Morales-Montor J. The role of the secretory immune response in the infection by Entamoeba histolytica. Parasite Immunol 2007;29:331–8. doi:10.1111/j.1365-3024.2007.00955.x.

[96] Murray MJ, Murray AB, Murray CJ. An ecological interdependence of diet and disease? A study of infection in one tribe consuming two different diets. Am J Clin Nutr 1980;33:697–701.

[97] Abdel-Hafeez EH, Belal US, Abdellatif MZM, Naoi K, Norose K. Breast-feeding protects infantile diarrhea caused by intestinal protozoan infections. Korean J Parasitol 2013;51:519–24. doi:10.3347/kjp.2013.51.5.519.

[98] Ghosh PK, Mancilla R, Ortiz-Ortiz L. Intestinal amebiasis: histopathologic features in experimentally infected mice. Arch Med Res 1994;25:297–302.

[99] León-Sicairos N, Martínez-Pardo L, Sánchez-Hernández B, de la Garza M, Carrero JC. Oral lactoferrin treatment resolves amoebic intracecal infection in C3H/HeJ mice. Biochem Cell Biol 2012;90:435–41. doi:10.1139/o2012-008.

[100] Mela I, Aumaitre E, Williamson A-M, Yakubov GE. Charge reversal by salt-induced aggregation in aqueous lactoferrin solutions. Colloids Surf B Biointerfaces 2010;78:53–60. doi:10.1016/j.colsurfb.2010.02.011.

[101] Hartog A, Leenders I, van der Kraan PM, Garssen J. Anti-inflammatory effects of orally ingested lactoferrin and glycine in different zymosan-induced inflammation models: evidence for synergistic activity. Int Immunopharmacol 2007;7:1784–92. doi:10.1016/j.intimp.2007.09.019.

[102] González-Chávez SA, Arévalo-Gallegos S, Rascón-Cruz Q. Lactoferrin: structure, function and applications. Int J Antimicrob Agents 2009;33:301.e1–8. doi:10.1016/j.ijantimicag.2008.07.020.

[103] Ochoa TJ, Chea-Woo E, Campos M, Pecho I, Prada A, McMahon RJ, et al. Impact of lactoferrin supplementation on growth and prevalence of Giardia colonization in children. Clin Infect Dis 2008;46:1881–3. doi:10.1086/588476.

[104] Ochoa TJ, Chea-Woo E, Baiocchi N, Pecho I, Campos M, Prada A, et al. Randomized double-blind controlled trial of bovine lactoferrin for prevention of diarrhea in children. J Pediatr 2013;162:349–56. doi:10.1016/j.jpeds.2012.07.043.

[105] Pérez-Tamayo R, Montfort I, García AO, Ramos E, Ostria CB. Pathogenesis of acute experimental liver amebiasis. Arch Med Res 2006;37:203–9. doi:10.1016/j.arcmed.2005.10.007.

[106] Tsutsumi V, Ravdin JI. Pathology of experimental amebiasis. Amebiasis, Human Infection by Entamoeba histolytica, Wiley Medical Publication; 1988, Chichester, UK pp. 147–65.

[107] Tsutsumi V, Shibayama M. Experimental amebiasis: a selected review of some in vivo models. Arch Med Res 2006;37:210–20. doi:10.1016/j.arcmed.2005.09.011.

[108] Ordaz-Pichardo C, Leon-Sicairos N, Hernández-Ramírez V, Talamás-Rohana P, de la Garza M. Effect of bovine lactoferrin in a therapeutic hamster model of hepatic amoebiasis. Biochem Cell Biol 2012;90:425–34. doi:10.1139/o11-084.

[109] Watkins RR, Eckmann L. Treatment of giardiasis: current status and future directions. Curr Infect Dis Rep 2014;16:396. doi:10.1007/s11908-014-0396-y.

[110] Painter JE, Gargano JW, Collier SA, Yoder JS. Centers for Disease Control and Prevention. Giardiasis surveillance – United States, 2011–2012. MMWR Suppl 2015;64:15–25.

[111] Eckmann L. Mucosal defences against Giardia. Parasite Immunol 2003;25:259–70.

[112] Adam RD. Biology of Giardia lamblia. Clin Microbiol Rev 2001;14:447–75. doi:10.1128/CMR.14.3.447-475.2001.

[113] Carranza PG, Lujan HD. New insights regarding the biology of Giardia lamblia. Microbes Infect 2010;12:71–80. doi:10.1016/j.micinf.2009.09.008.

[114] Halliez MCM, Buret AG. Extra-intestinal and long term consequences of Giardia duodenalis infections. World J Gastroenterol 2013;19:8974–85. doi:10.3748/wjg.v19.i47.8974.

[115] Nabarro LEB, Lever RA, Armstrong M, Chiodini PL. Increased incidence of nitroimidazole-refractory giardiasis at the Hospital for Tropical Diseases, London: 2008–2013. Clin Microbiol Infect 2015;21:791–6. doi:10.1016/j.cmi.2015.04.019.

[116] Domínguez-López ME, González-molero I, Ramírez-Plaza CP, Soriguer F, Olveira G. [Chonic diarrhea and malabsorption due to common variable immunodeficiency, gastrectomy and giardiasis infection: a difficult nutritional management]. Nutr Hosp 2011;26:922–5. doi:10.1590/S0212-16112011000400037.

[117] Hill DR. Giardiasis. Issues in diagnosis and management. Infect Dis Clin North Am 1993;7:503–25.

[118] Vesy CJ, Peterson WL. Review article: the management of Giardiasis. Aliment Pharmacol Ther 1999;13:843–50.

[119] Faubert G. Immune response to Giardia duodenalis. Clin Microbiol Rev 2000;13:35–54, table of contents.

[120] Gillin FD, Reiner DS, Wang CS. Human milk kills parasitic intestinal protozoa. Science 1983;221:1290–2.

[121] Gillin FD. Giardia lamblia: the role of conjugated and unconjugated bile salts in killing by human milk. Exp Parasitol 1987;63:74–83.

[122] Hernell O, Ward H, Bläckberg L, Pereira ME. Killing of Giardia lamblia by human milk lipases: an effect mediated by lipolysis of milk lipids. J Infect Dis 1986;153:715–20.

[123] Reiner DS, Wang CS, Gillin FD. Human milk kills Giardia lamblia by generating toxic lipolytic products. J Infect Dis 1986;154:825–32.

[124] Rohrer L, Winterhalter KH, Eckert J, Köhler P. Killing of Giardia lamblia by human milk is mediated by unsaturated fatty acids. Antimicrob Agents Chemother 1986;30:254–7.

[125] Aley SB, Zimmerman M, Hetsko M, Selsted ME, Gillin FD. Killing of Giardia lamblia by cryptdins and cationic neutrophil peptides. Infect Immun 1994;62:5397–403.

[126] Turchany JM, McCaffery JM, Aley SB, Gillin FD. Ultrastructural effects of lactoferrin binding on Giardia lamblia trophozoites. J Eukaryot Microbiol 1997;44:68–72.

[127] Zu SX, Li JF, Barrett LJ, Fayer R, Shu SY, McAuliffe JF, et al. Seroepidemiologic study of Cryptosporidium infection in children from rural communities of Anhui, China and Fortaleza, Brazil. Am J Trop Med Hyg 1994;51:1–10.

[128] Ungar BL, Gilman RH, Lanata CF, Perez-Schael I. Seroepidemiology of Cryptosporidium infection in two Latin American populations. J Infect Dis 1988;157:551–6.

[129] Newman RD, Sears CL, Moore SR, Nataro JP, Wuhib T, Agnew DA, et al. Longitudinal study of Cryptosporidium infection in children in northeastern Brazil. J Infect Dis 1999;180:167–75. doi:10.1086/314820.

[130] Current WL, Garcia LS. Cryptosporidiosis. Clin Microbiol Rev 1991;4:325–58.

[131] Bouzid M, Hunter PR, Chalmers RM, Tyler KM. Cryptosporidium pathogenicity and virulence. Clin Microbiol Rev 2013;26:115–34. doi:10.1128/CMR.00076-12.

[132] Rosales MJ, Cordón GP, Moreno MS, Sánchez CM, Mascaró C. Extracellular like-gregarine stages of Cryptosporidium parvum. Acta Trop 2005;95:74–8. doi:10.1016/j.actatropica.2005.03.009.

[133] Shimelis T, Tassachew Y, Lambiyo T. Cryptosporidium and other intestinal parasitic infections among HIV patients in southern Ethiopia: significance of improved HIV-related care. Parasit Vectors 2016;9:270. doi:10.1186/s13071-016-1554-x.

[134] Alcantara CS, Yang C-H, Steiner TS, Barrett LJ, Lima AAM, Chappell CL, et al. Interleukin-8, tumor necrosis factor-alpha, and lactoferrin in immunocompetent hosts with experimental and Brazilian children with acquired cryptosporidiosis. Am J Trop Med Hyg 2003;68:325–8.

[135] Carryn S, Schaefer D a, Imboden M, Homan EJ, Bremel RD, Riggs MW. Phospholipases and cationic peptides inhibit Cryptosporidium parvum sporozoite infectivity by parasiticidal and non-parasiticidal mechanisms. J Parasitol 2012;98:199–204. doi:10.1645/GE-2822.1.

[136] Didier ES, Weiss LM. Microsporidiosis: current status. Curr Opin Infect Dis 2006;19:485–92. doi:10.1097/01.qco.0000244055.46382.23.

[137] Mathis A, Weber R, Deplazes P. Zoonotic potential of the microsporidia. Clin Microbiol Rev 2005;18:423–45. doi:10.1128/CMR.18.3.423-445.2005.

[138] Keohane EM, Orr GA, Takvorian PM, Cali A, Tanowitz HB, Wittner M, et al. Polar tube proteins of microsporidia of the family encephalitozoonidae. J Eukaryot Microbiol 1999;46:1–5.

[139] Leitch GJ, Ward TL, Shaw AP, Newman G. Apical spore phagocytosis is not a significant route of infection of differentiated enterocytes by Encephalitozoon intestinalis. Infect Immun 2005;73:7697–704. doi:10.1128/IAI.73.11.7697-7704.2005.

[140] Kotler DP, Orenstein JM. Clinical syndromes associated with microsporidiosis. Adv Parasitol 1998;40:321–49.

[141] Couzinet S, Cejas E, Schittny J, Deplazes P, Weber R, Zimmerli S. Phagocytic uptake of Encephalitozoon cuniculi by nonprofessional phagocytes. Infect Immun 2000;68: 6939–45.

[142] Franzen C. Microsporidia: how can they invade other cells? Trends Parasitol 2004;20:275–9. doi:10.1016/j.pt.2004.04.009.

[143] Leitch GJ, Ceballos C. A role for antimicrobial peptides in intestinal microsporidiosis. Parasitology 2009;136:175–81. doi: 10.1017/S0031182008005313.

[144] Didier ES, Orenstein JM, Aldras A, Bertucci D, Rogers LB, Janney FA. Comparison of three staining methods for detecting microsporidia in fluids. J Clin Microbiol 1995;33:3138–45.

[145] Kumamoto CA. Inflammation and gastrointestinal Candida colonization. Curr Opin Microbiol 2011;14:386–91. doi:10.1016/j.mib.2011.07.015.

[146] Sonoyama K, Miki A, Sugita R, Goto H, Nakata M, Yamaguchi N. Gut colonization by Candida albicans aggravates inflammation in the gut and extra-gut tissues in mice. Med Mycol 2011;49:237–47. doi:10.3109/13693786.2010.511284.

[147] Chen H-L, Yen C-C, Lu C-Y, Yu C-H, Chen C-M. Synthetic porcine lactoferricin with a 20-residue peptide exhibits antimicrobial activity against Escherichia coli, Staphylococcus aureus, and Candida albicans. J Agric Food Chem 2006;54:3277–82. doi:10.1021/jf053031s.

[148] Yen C-C, Lin C-Y, Chong K-Y, Tsai T-C, Shen C-J, Lin M-F, et al. Lactoferrin as a natural regimen for selective decontamination of the digestive tract: recombinant porcine lactoferrin expressed in the milk of transgenic mice protects neonates from pathogenic challenge in the gastrointestinal tract. J Infect Dis 2009;199:590–8. doi:10.1086/596212.

[149] Tanaka T, Omata Y, Saito A, Shimazaki K, Yamauchi K, Takase M, et al. Toxoplasma gondii: parasiticidal effects of bovine lactoferricin against parasites. Exp Parasitol 1995;81:614–7. pii: S0014489485711575.

[150] Tanaka T, Omata Y, Narisawa M, Saito A, Shimazaki K, Igarashi I, et al. Growth inhibitory effect of bovine lactoferrin on Toxoplasma gondii tachyzoites in murine macrophages: role of radical oxygen and inorganic nitrogen oxide in Toxoplasma growth-inhibitory activity. Vet Parasitol 1997;68:27–33.

[151] Isamida T, Tanaka T, Omata Y, Yamauchi K, Shimazaki K, Saito a. Protective effect of lactoferricin against Toxoplasma gondii infection in mice. J Vet Med Sci 1998;60:241–4.

[152] Anand N, Sehgal R, Kanwar RK, Dubey ML, Vasishta RK, Kanwar JR. Oral administration of encapsulated bovine lactoferrin protein nanocapsules against intracellular parasite Toxoplasma gondii. Int J Nanomedicine 2015;10:6355–69. doi:10.2147/IJN.S85286.

[153] Alimi D, Hajaji S, Rekik M, Abidi A, Gharbi M, Akkari H. First report of the in vitro nematicidal effects of camel milk. Vet Parasitol 2016;228:153–9. doi:10.1016/j.vetpar.2016.09.003.

[154] Stowell KM, Rado TA, Funk WD, Tweedie JW. Expression of cloned human lactoferrin in baby-hamster kidney cells. Biochem J 1991:349–55.

[155] Xiaonan P, Xiao H, Xuan W, Xiwen C, Jia L, Defu C. Research progress in physicochemical characteristics of lactoferrin and its recombinant expression systems. Yi Chuan 2015;37:873–84. doi:10.16288/j.yczz.15-146.

[156] Iglesias-Figueroa B, Valdiviezo-Godina N, Siqueiros-Cendón T, Sinagawa-García S, Arévalo-Gallegos S, Rascón-Cruz Q. High-Level Expression of Recombinant bovine lactoferrin in Pichia pastoris with antimicrobial activity. Int J Mol Sci 2016;17. doi:10.3390/ijms17060902.

[157] Suzuki YA, Kelleher SL, Yalda D, Wu L, Huang J, Huang N, et al. Expression, characterization, and biologic activity of recombinant human lactoferrin in rice. J Pediatr Gastroenterol Nutr 2003;36:190–9.

[158] Lönnerdal B. Recombinant human milk proteins. Nestlé Nutr Work Ser Paediatr Program 2006;58:207–217. doi:10.1159/000095064.

[159] Yemets AI, Tanasienko I V, Krasylenko YA, Blume YB. Plant-based biopharming of recombinant human lactoferrin. Cell Biol Int 2014;38:989–1002. doi:10.1002/cbin.10304.

[160] Li Q, Hu W, Zhao J, Wang J, Dai Y, Zhao Y, et al. Supplementation transgenic cow's milk containing recombinant human lactoferrin enhances systematic and intestinal immune responses in piglets. Mol Biol Rep 2014;41:2119–28. doi:10.1007/s11033-014-3061-5.

[161] Zhao J, Xu J, Wang J, Li N. Nutritional composition analysis of meat from human lactoferrin transgenic bulls. Anim Biotechnol 2013;24:44–52. doi:10.1080/10495398.2012.739979.

[162] Law BA, Reiter B. The isolation and bacteriostatic properties of lactoferrin from bovine milk whey. J Dairy Res 1977;44:595–9.

[163] Yoshida S, Wei Z, Shinmura Y, Fukunaga N. Separation of lactoferrin-a and -b from bovine colostrum. J Dairy Sci 2000;83:2211–5. doi:10.3168/jds.S0022-0302(00)75104-6.

[164] Wakabayashi H, Yamauchi K, Takase M. Lactoferrin research, technology and applications. Int Dairy J 2006;16:1241–51. doi:10.1016/j.idairyj.2006.06.013.

Chapter 8

Plasmepsin: Function, Characterization and Targeted Antimalarial Drug Development

Peng Liu

Additional information is available at the end of the chapter

http://dx.doi.org/10.5772/66716

Abstract

The devastating malaria, caused by parasites of the genus *Plasmodium*, afflicts nearly half of the world's population and imposes a heavy socio-economic burden particularly to the disease-endemic Sub-Saharan Africa. Sustained efforts in malaria control have been made from the perspectives of medicine- and vaccine-based prevention and treatment of malaria and malaria transmission blockage for the past 15 years, resulting in a decreased mortality rate by 60% and a decreased malaria incidence rate by 37% globally. Nonetheless, due to the emergence and rapid spread of drug-resistant parasite strains, novel antimalarial drugs are urgently required to combat this deadly disease. Plasmepsins are deemed potential targets for novel antimalarial drug design. Plasmepsins represent an aspartic proteinase family that can be sub-categorized into seven groups based on the amino acid sequence identity. This chapter discusses our progress in understanding the biosynthesis, biological functions and enzymatic characteristics of the plasmepsin family. This led to development of various types of plasmepsin-targeted compounds and the assessment of their binding affinity and selectivity, anti-parasitic activity and cytotoxicity. The gained experience and current status in developing plasmepsin-targeted antimalarial drugs are addressed. Finally, a deeper and broader investigation on the functions and characteristics of the plasmepsin family is encouraged.

Keywords: malaria, plasmepsin, drug design, *Plasmodium*, aspartic proteinase

1. Introduction

Malaria, a life-threatening infectious disease, afflicts approximately 3.2 billion people, causes 214 million clinical cases and leads to nearly 440,000 deaths worldwide in 2015 despite the facts that malaria mortality rates decreased by 60% globally and by 66% in Africa between 2000 and 2015, and that malaria incidence rates decreased by 37% globally and by 42% in Africa for the past 15 years [1, 2]. Nearly 90% of the malaria cases and deaths occur in Sub-Saharan Africa in 2015, loading a heavy socio-economic burden to this poorly developed region [1].

Malaria is caused by parasitic protozoa of the genus *Plasmodium*. Hundreds of *Plasmodium* species have been identified to infect reptiles, birds and mammals, including rodents and primates. Four *Plasmodium species pluralis* (spp.), *P. falciparum*, *P. vivax*, *P. malariae* and *P. ovale*, are known to infect man, though other malarial species of non-human primates occasionally infect human as well. Among these species, *P. falciparum* is the most deadly and *P. vivax*, the most prevalent. *P. falciparum* invades both young and mature erythrocytes and provokes malignant disease symptoms. Prevalent mainly in Africa, *P. falciparum* accounts for ~40% of the clinical cases on a global basis [1]. In contrast, *P. vivax* prefers invading young erythrocytes and causes benign symptoms; it has a wider geographical distribution than *P. falciparum* and is responsible for half of the total reported cases [1].

To complete its life cycle, the malaria parasite requires a female mosquito as the transmission vector and a vertebrate host (**Figure 1**). When a blood meal is taken, a parasite-infected mosquito inoculates sporozoites into the human host to start the exo-erythrocytic phase, in which sporozoites infect hepatocytes and mature into schizonts. Of note, in parasites such as *P. vivax* and *P. ovale*, a dormant stage, namely hypnozoites, can maintain in hypatic cells for weeks or even years before invading the bloodstream. Rupture of schizonts releases merozoites, which

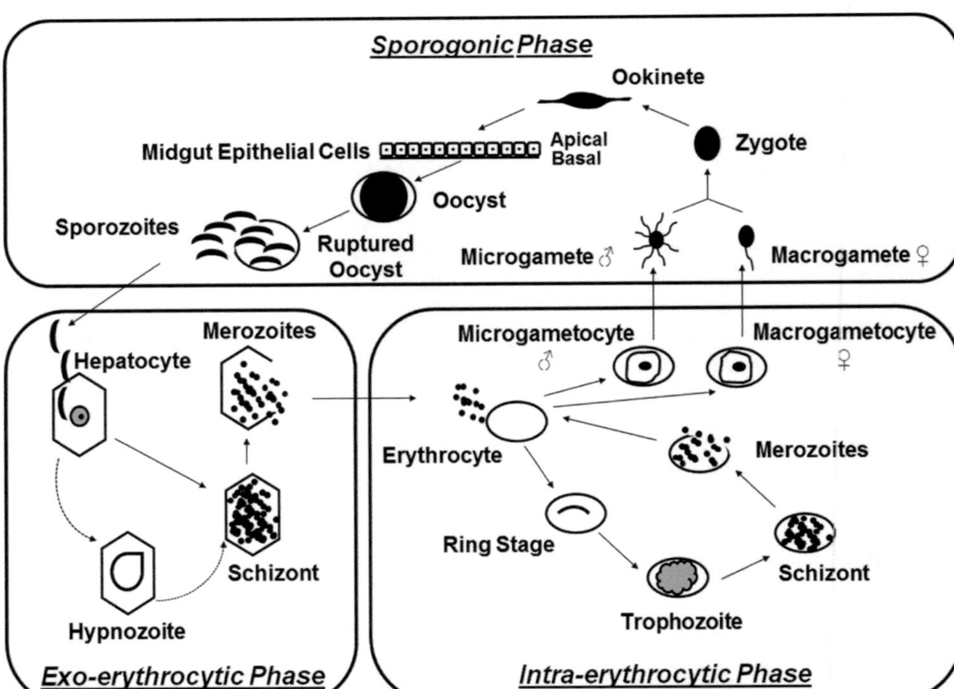

Figure 1. The life cycle of malaria parasites. Malaria parasites require a transmission vector (e.g., mosquito) and a vertebrate host (e.g., human) to complete their life cycle. The exo-erythrocytic and intra-erythrocytic phases occur in the vertebrate host, and the sporogonic phase occurs in the transmission vector.

then infect erythrocytes to initiate the intra-erythrocytic phase. In this phase, the parasite undergoes multiple rounds of asexual replication with each cycle comprising, in sequence, the ring, the trophozoite and the schizont stage. A portion of merozoites infect erythrocyte to differentiate into gametocytes. Microgametocytes and macrogametocytes are ingested by a mosquito to start the sporogonic phase. In the mosquito's stomach, gametocytes further differentiate into gametes. Microgametes fertilize macrogametes to generate zygotes, which subsequently develop into motile and elongated ookinetes. Ookinetes penetrate the midgut of the mosquito and develop into oocysts, from which sporozoites are released and delivered to the mosquito's salivary gland, ready for the next infection.

Malaria control in the modern era arguably starts from the isolation of antimalarial quinine and quinidine from cinchona bark in early nineteenth century [3], while it was not until 1925 that pamaquine (also known as plasmoquine or plasmochin), the first synthetic antimalarial drug, was yielded. Synthesized in 1934, chloroquine (CQ), a 4-aminoquinoline compound, exhibited a strong antimalarial potency and a low toxicity and became the most extensively used drug in malaria prophylaxis and treatment between 1940s and 1960s [4–6]. The massive use of CQ, however, resulted in the emergence of CQ-resistant *P. falciparum* strains, which promoted development of novel antimalarial drugs (e.g., 8-aminoquinolines, antifolates, naphthoquinones and non-antifolate antibiotics). Of particular note among these compounds is artemisinin (AN). Extracted from the herbal plant *Artemisia annua*, AN, has been used for malaria treatment since early 1970s [7]. Though AN and its various derivatives display high antimalarial activities (e.g., [8–12]) and quick attenuation of disease symptoms [13], they have short half lives *in vivo* [14]. The combination of AN and a longer-acting drug (e.g., artemether-lumefantrine and artesunate-mefloquine) is effective for disease treatment and for deferring drug resistance development. Artemisinin-based combination therapies (ACTs) have up till now been used as a standard therapy in many countries and regions despite potentially unmatched pharmacokinetics between drugs and/or widespread resistance against the non-artemisinin components. Malaria control was also carried out by intervention of disease transmission, thanks to the discovery of insecticidal properties of dichloro-diphenyltrichloroethane (DDT) in 1939 [15]. Due to health and environmental risks, DDT was later substituted by other insecticides, such as pyrethroids, chlorfenapyr and pyriproxyfen. While both indoor residual spraying and insecticide-treated bed nets contribute to controlling epidemic outbreaks of malaria, the latter provide more effective protection for people living in temporary shelters. Nonetheless, one cannot ignore the growing emergence of insecticide-resistant vector strains and the lack of interventions targeting outdoor mosquito populations, which constitute major challenges in blocking malaria transmission. Intervention of malaria transmission has also been managed via biological control of mosquitoes at both the larval and the adult stage. Several fish species, such as *Poecilia reticulate* (guppy) and *Gambusia affinis* (mosquitofish), are able to consume mosquito larvae and reduce their population; however, these fish also pose a threat to other native aquatic predators of mosquitoes due to intraguild predation [16, 17]. In contrast, the larval dytiscid beetles *Agabus* do exhibit a selective predation on mosquitoes over alternative prey, although intraguild predation and cannibalism also occur within and between *Agabus* species [18]. In addition, the use of water-dispersible granular formulation of two *Bacillus* species in malaria control results in an efficacious elimination of the larval mosquito population with a negligible environmental impact [19]. Also of note is the use of fungi for malaria control. Ground and aerial application of self-propagating *Lagenidium giganteum* effectively controls the larval mosquito population for at least an entire breeding season [20, 21]. Oil-based formulations of fungal entomopathogens are able to block malaria transmission by reducing adult mosquito survival and altering parasite survival/maturation in the vector [22]. Further, transgenic fungi *Metarhizium anisopliae* targeting sporozoites in mosquitoes inhibit parasite development [23]. These pieces of evidence indicate the potential of fungi as a biocontrol agent of mosquitoes. Natural products are another important source utilized to control malaria transmission. A variety of plant extracts and essential oils (e.g., the neem oil, the fenugreek oil and the extracts from Indian sandalwood) exhibit larvicidal activities and adult mosquito repellency properties (for example, see [24–30]). Moreover, natural product-synthesized silver nanoparticles show a higher potency in mosquitocidal activity than the aqueous extracts but their toxicity against other natural mosquito consumers is negligible (for example, see [31–33]). These, in addition to the time-efficiency, cost-effectiveness and eco-friendliness green-synthesis of nanoparticles, suggest the feasibility and importance of a synergistic mosquito control using botanical nano-insecticides and biological agents. Besides these antimalarial approaches, vaccines against malaria parasites have been under development since 1970s [34, 35]. Malaria vaccines are categorized into three types: exo-erythrocytic vaccines, blood-stage vaccines and transmission-blocking vaccines; sustainable prevention requires a combination of vaccines targeting multiple life stages of the parasite. RTS,S/AS01, the first and thus far the only vaccine that completes a Phase III clinical trial, targets the exo-erythrocytic phase of *P. falciparum*. Though this vaccine demonstrates a decent efficacy for prevention of clinical malaria cases in African children (age 5–17 months, efficacy 50%) and infants (age 6–12 weeks, efficacy 30%) [36], an ideal candidate aiming for global eradication would require a higher efficacy [37].

A major challenge faced by the anti-malaria campaign currently is the emergence and rapid spread of drug-resistant variants of *Plasmodium* spp. [38]. Malaria parasites have developed resistance to virtually every type of antimalarial drugs thus far used, including AN and its derivatives [39]. The lack of effective treatment of symptoms caused by drug-resistant parasites urges us to identify molecular targets, against which novel drugs can be subsequently developed to combat malaria. Plasmepsins (PMs), a family of aspartic proteinases, are considered a promising drug target.

This review focuses on the biosynthesis, biological functions and enzymatic characteristics of the plasmepsin (PM) family from human malaria parasites. The progression of PM-targeted antimalarial drug development is also discussed.

2. Plasmepsin family overview

From comparative genomic analysis of sequence information of seven *Plasmodium* spp. deposited in the *Plasmodium* genome database [40], a cohort of genes that encode PMs were identified and categorized into seven groups based on their amino acid sequence identity [41]. In *P. falciparum*, up to ten PMs have thus far been identified, namely *Pf*PMs 1, 2, 4–10 and *Pf*HAP (Histo-Aspartic Proteinase) [42]. These PMs, encoded by genes located in five different chromosomes, are composed of the pro-segment and the mature enzyme domain. *Pf*PM5 and

*Pf*PM9 also contain extra residues at their C-termini. PMs are distinct in structural and biochemical properties, such as molecular weight and isoelectric point (**Table 1**).

PM	Chr.	Pro	Zymogen				Mature enzyme			
		# a.a.	# a.a.	% i.d.	MW (Da)	pI	# a.a.	% i.d.	MW (Da)	pI
PM1	14	123	452	62	51,461	7.23	329	70	37,050	4.82
PM2	14	124	453	61	51,481	5.29	329	69	36,915	4.62
HAP	14	123	451	52	51,694	8.23	328	59	36,979	4.97
PM4	14	121	449	—	51,047	5.19	328	—	36,955	4.38
PM5	13	83	590	25	68,481	7.66	440	25	50,844	6.50
PM6	3	84	432	29	49,434	7.75	348	29	39,352	6.44
PM7	10	76	450	28	52,329	8.44	374	28	43,317	6.09
PM8	14	45	385	26	44,255	9.38	340	29	38,976	8.85
PM9	14	212	627	27	74,184	9.63	402	25	46,970	9.28
PM10	8	232	573	30	65,115	5.22	341	29	38,604	5.38

The % i.d. data is calculated using the Basic Local Alignment Search Tool [43]. The MW and pI data of zymogens are adopted from the Plasmodium Genomics Resource [44]. The MW and pI data of mature enzymes are calculated using ProtParam [45]. Abbreviations: Pro, pro-segment; # a.a., numbers of amino acids; % i.d., percentage of identity versus PM4.

Table 1. Comparative properties of plasmepsins from the *P. falciparum* 3D7 strain.

Of note, *pfpm4, pfpm1, pfpm2* and *pfhap* cluster in a 20-kb-long region of chromosome 14, and share a high amino acid sequence identity (**Table 1**). Each non-*falciparum* parasite, however, harbors usually one gene (*pm4*) that shares with *pfpm4* the highest sequence identity, which is comparable to those shared among the four *pfpms*. It is believed that the other three PM genes may arise from multiple gene duplication events [41]. Since these four PM paralogs were initially detected in the food vacuole (FV), an acidic organelle unique to the genus *Plasmodium* where degradation of hemoglobin of red blood cells (erythrocytes) occurs [46–48], they are named the FV *Pf*PMs. PM4s of the non-*falciparum* species are also grouped as FV PMs because they are highly homologous to the FV *Pf*PMs. *Pf*PMs 5–10 share a low amino acid sequence identity with the FV *Pf*PMs, and their sequence structures are distinct from each other and from those of the FV *Pf*PMs (**Table 1**), indicating that there exist diverse biological functions and enzymatic features among the PM family members.

3. Biosynthesis

3.1. Food vacuole plasmepsins

FV *Pf*PMs are synthesized as type II integral membrane proteins, with the putative transmembrane motif residing in the N-terminal pro-segment. Using immunoelectron microscopy (immunoEM), *Pf*PM1 and *Pf*PM2 were observed in the lumens of transport vesicles and FVs, in the parasite plasma membrane (PPM), in small vesicular structures near PPM and in the cytostome, a morphologically variable microstructure comprising invaginated parasitophorous vacuolar membrane (PVM) and PPM [46] (**Figure 2**). Further, Klemba and colleagues probed the trafficking of *Pf*PM2 in a transgenic *P. falciparum* culture model [49]. The *Pf*M2-green fluorescence protein (GFP) fusion protein was detected by immunoEM in the membrane and lumen of FVs and in the cytostomes, consistent with the previous finding [46]. Administration of brefeldin A (BFA), an inhibitor blocking anterograde protein traffic from the endoplasmic reticulum (ER), to trophozoites retained *Pf*PM2-GFP in the ER/nuclear envelope (NE); yet this protein was detected in the cytostomes and subsequently the FVs minutes after release of the BFA inhibition. The role of Golgi apparatus in the biosynthesis of FV *Pf*PMs is not yet clear, but is doubtful, since FV *Pf*PMs are known to be unglycosylated. Taken together, these findings suggest that the biosynthesis of FV *Pf*PMs follows an "ER-to-PPM-to-FV" route (**Figure 2**). Interestingly, *Pf*PM2 has also been detected in the cytoplasm of host erythrocytes (see Section 4.2 for more discussion), leading to the hypothesis that there exists an alternative traffic route for the FV PMs.

To gain catalytic activity, FV PMs need to release their pro-segments. The cleavage site is conserved at the motif (Y/H)LG* (S/N)XXD (* represents the scissile bond) [50], which is different from the sites where *in vitro* PM auto-maturation occurs ([48, 51–54], see also discussion

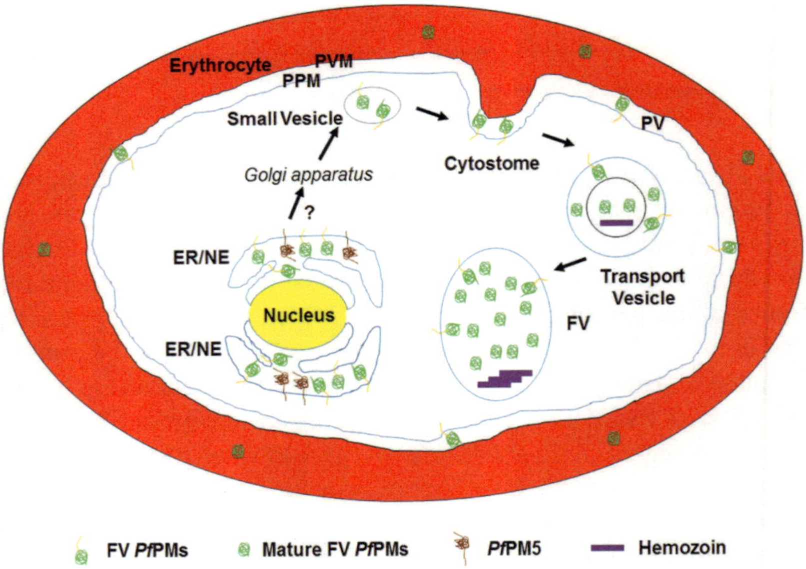

Figure 2. Biosynthesis of plasmepsins in the *P. falciparum* intra-erythrocytic phase. Food vacuole plasmepsins from *P. falciparum* (FV P*f*PMs) are expressed as type II integral membrane proteins with their N-terminal pro-segments (orange threads) spanning the endoplasmic reticulum/nuclear envelope (ER/NE) membrane. FV P*f*PMs are transported via small vesicular structures to the parasite plasma membrane (PPM), where some reside in the cytostomal vacuole. The involvement of Golgi apparatus in this secretory pathway is not clear. Endocytosis of cytostomes retains FV P*f*PMs in transport vesicles, which convey the enzymes eventually to the FV. Maturation of the FV P*f*PMs is carried out in the acidic FVs and transport vesicles. Certain FV P*f*PMs (e.g., PfPM2) are also found functionally active in the host erythrocytes, though how they are secreted outside the parasite is not yet clear. In contrast, P*f*PM5 is an ER-resident, type I integral membrane protein. PV, parasitophorous vacuole; PVM, parasitophorous vacuolar membrane.

in Section 5). This observation suggests that PM maturation in the parasite is a convertase-catalyzed *trans*-processing event. Further studies showed that the pro-segment cleavage of naturally-occurring PMs occurs in an acidic milieu, is largely completed within half an hour in cultured *P. falciparum* at the trophozoite stage, and is inhibited by tripeptide aldehyde *N*-acetyl-Leu-Leu-norleucinal (ALLN) or *N*-acetyl-Leu-Leu-methioninal [50, 55]. The identity of the convertase is believed to be the cysteine proteinases falcipain (FP) -2 and -3 in that (1) both FP-2 and FP-3 catalyze cleavage of peptide substrates at the C-terminus of the conserved glycine; (2) a membrane-permeant derivative of the cysteine proteinase inhibitor E-64 directly binds to FP-2 and FP-3 and, in turn, slows the kinetics of PM maturation in cultured parasites; and (3) both FPs are inhibited by ALLN at low micromolar magnitude *in vitro* [56]. Of note, when FPs are inhibited, the parasite can use PMs (e.g. *Pf*PM2) as alternative convertases [56], though it is not known yet whether and to what degree this alternative processing is employed.

Where does the maturation of FV PMs occur? Evidence from immunoEM shows that antibodies directed against N-terminal epitopes of mature *Pf*PM1 and *Pf*PM2 recognize the enzymes not only in the FV but also in transport vesicles [46, 49]. Of note, hemozoin crystals stemmed from hemoglobin degradation that is initiated and carried out by mature FV PMs are also observed in both the FVs and transport vesicles [57]. These findings indicate that both subcellular compartments contain catalytically active PMs. In addition, the finding that functional vacuolar proton pumps are present in the PPM [58, 59], the outer membrane of transport vesicles, suggests that the vesicular milieu is acidic. Taken together, it is conceivable that the convertase-catalyzed PM maturation also occurs in transport vesicles.

The four FV *Pf*PMs exhibit distinct temporal expression patterns in the intra-erythrocytic phase of the parasite life cycle: *Pf*PM1 and *Pf*PM2 emerge as early as the ring stage, *Pf*PM4 first appears in the early trophozoite stage, and yet *Pf*HAP is not detected until the mid-trophozoite stage; all the four continue to be expressed at the schizont stage [48]. This is expected since the FV *Pf*PMs are key enzymes to hemoglobin processing, and *Pf*PM1 and *Pf*PM2 are believed to initiate that event (for more discussion, see Section 4.1). Importantly, expression of these FV *Pf*PMs is not restricted in trophozoites and schizonts in that mass spectrometry (MS)-based analyses have identified their presence in gametocytes, merozoites, oocysts and sporozoites [60–62].

No studies, to the author's knowledge, have been reported on biosynthesis of the FV PMs from non-*falciparum* species. It is likely that they adopt a similar pattern as the *Pf*PMs due to the high sequence identity shared among these homologs.

3.2. Non-food vacuole plasmepsins

Among the non-FV PMs, PM5 is the most studied. *Pf*PM5 is synthesized as a type I integral membrane protein comprising an N-terminal pro-segment, a catalytic domain, a C-terminal transmembrane domain and a cytoplasmic tail [63]. Notably, the sequence of the pro-segment region of PM5 is highly variable among *Plasmodium* spp. [44]. *Pf*PM5 is almost exclusively detected in the ER/NE (**Figure 2**) [63]. The C-terminal transmembrane domain is essential to the ER/NE residence of *Pf*PM5 [64]. Expression of *Pf*PM5 is detected throughout the life cycle of the parasite [44, 65, 66]; in the intra-erythrocytic phase, *Pf*PM5 expression starts at the early ring stage in a scarce level and continues to increase steadily through the trophozoite and schizont stages, which mirrors the temporal expression patterns of *Pf*PM1 and *Pf*PM2 [48, 63]. Interestingly, in contrast to the rapid maturation of the FV *Pf*PMs, no processing of the N-terminal pro-segment is observed hours after the synthesis of *Pf*PM5; also unlike the FV *Pf*PMs, *Pf*PM5 is catalytically active in the presence of the pro-segment [63].

Few studies have addressed the biosynthesis of PMs 6–10. Genes encoding *Pf*PM9 and *Pf*PM10, but not *Pf*PMs 6–8, are transcribed in parasites infecting erythrocytes [67]. In the intra-erythrocytic phase, *Pf*PM9 and *Pf*PM10 exhibit a diffuse expression pattern throughout the cytoplasm, but are excluded from the FV [48]. Of note, MS-based analysis indicates the presence of *Pf*PM9 in sporozoites and the presence of both *Pf*PM6 and *Pf*PM10 in merozoites and sporozoites [60–62]. In addition, expression of *Pf*PM7 and *Pf*PM10 is detected in zygotes and ookinetes [68, 69].

4. Biological function

4.1. Hemoglobin digestion and degradation

The primary pathological role that FV PMs play is digestion and degradation of the oxygen-carrying hemoglobin that constitutes 95% of cytosolic proteins of human red blood cells (**Figure 3**).

In the intra-erythrocytic phase, hemoglobin digestion and degradation is carried out between the ring and the early schizont stage [70, 71]. A vast majority of hemoglobin, at a millimolar concentration in erythrocytes, however, is processed within the 6–12-hour trophozoite stage [72], indicative of an enzyme-catalyzed event. The processing of hemoglobin occurs mainly

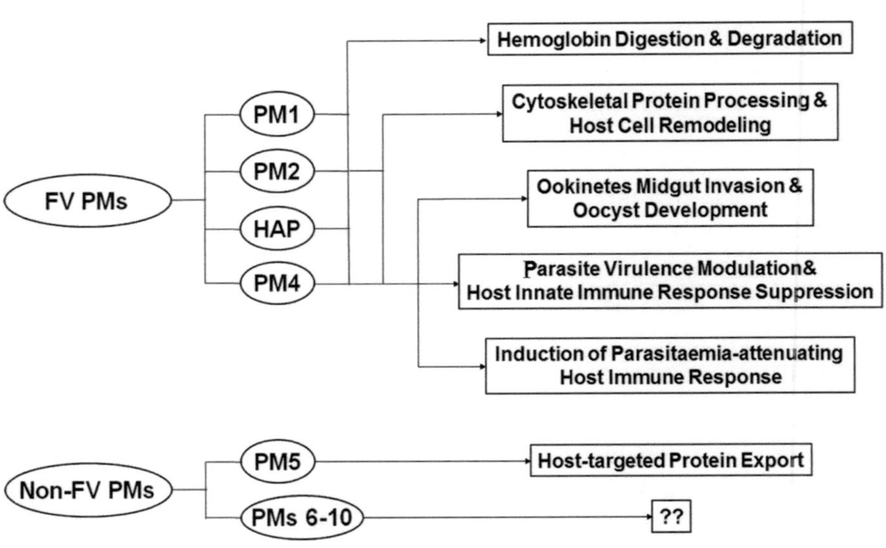

Figure 3. A diagram illustrating the connections of plasmepsins and their known biological functions.

in FVs; however, it is also carried out in vesicles arising either from micropinocytosis of cytoplasm of host cells or from endocytosis of cytostomes [57].

Early investigations establish that aspartic and cysteine proteinase activities are responsible for hemoglobin processing [73–81]. The successful isolation of FV from cultured trophozoites renders possible identification of naturally-occurring hemoglobin-processing enzymes [82]. *Pf*PM1, the first proteinase purified from isolated FVs, exhibits its cleavage specificity at the α-subunit amino acids F33-L34 (α33-34) of native hemoglobin [83]. Located in a highly conserved region among vertebrate species [84], this peptide bond is essential for maintaining the quaternary structure of the hemoglobin tetramer [85]. Breaking the α33-34 bond unravels the molecule and, in turn, leads to additional enzyme cleavages of the α- and β-subunits [47]. Sharing a 73% amino acid sequence identity with *Pf*PM1, *Pf*PM2, the second proteinase purified from FVs, also cleaves native hemoglobin at α33-34, though less efficiently than *Pf*PM1 [47]. SC-50083, a selective inhibitor of *Pf*PM1 over *Pf*PM2 by two orders of magnitude [46], blocks a majority of native hemoglobin degradation by FV protein extracts [47], indicating that *Pf*PM1 initiates the proteolysis. Of note, both *Pf*PM1 and *Pf*PM2 can further digest denatured globin into smaller peptides [47]. A third FV PM, *Pf*HAP, purified from FVs, cleaves native hemoglobin even less efficiently than *Pf*PM2 does and yet shows an efficiency in degrading denatured globin equivalent to *Pf*PM2 [48]. Similar to *Pf*HAP, *Pf*PM4 of the recombinant form prefers degrading denatured globin than native hemoglobin [48]. Other proteolytic enzymes, such as the cysteine proteinase falcipains, the metallo-proteinase falcilysin and aminopeptidases, are actively involved in further degrading hemoglobin fragments to oligopeptides and amino acids [42, 86]. These findings indicate that hemoglobin digestion and degradation in *P. falciparum* is an ordered process, in which *Pf*PM1 and *Pf*PM2 initiate the cleavage and various proteinases are involved in additional processing. Hemoglobin processing in other human malaria parasites may depend on their FV PMs that are homologous to *Pf*PM4.

The purpose of hemoglobin digestion and degradation has been under debate. Some believe that malaria parasites consume hemoglobin as a source of nutrients [87–91], which is supported by their limited capacity to *de novo* synthesis [88, 92] or exogenous amino acid uptake [93]. Nonetheless, hemoglobin degradation alone seems insufficient to maintain parasite metabolism due to its low contents of cysteine, glutamine, glutamic acid and methionine and its lack of isoleucine; in addition, hemoglobin-derived amino acids are found diffused into the host cell [89], indicating an excessive amount of hemoglobin being processed. This leads to a second hypothesis positing that the parasites degrade hemoglobin to empty space for their development and growth [94]. A third hypothesis, supported by an experimental-based modeling study, is that hemoglobin degradation is necessary to maintain the osmotic stability of infected erythrocytes such that the malaria parasite is able to grow and replicate in integrated host cells [95].

4.2. Cytoskeletal protein processing and host cell remodeling

*Pf*PM2 plays a role in remodeling host erythrocytes. In cultured schizonts, *Pf*PM2 was observed in the cytoplasm of the host cell in addition to the parasite [96], suggesting its potential interactions with cytoskeleton proteins. In support of this finding, recombinant

*Pf*PM2 exhibits hydrolysis of spectrin, actin and protein 4.1 at near neutral pH conditions [96]. In addition, schizont-expressed, naturally-occurring *Pf*PM2, but not *Pf*PM1 or falcipains, is enriched in the size exclusion chromatography (SEC) fractions that show proteolytic activity of the SH3 motif of the cytoskeletal protein spectrin [96], thus supporting its host cell remodeling role at the mature stage of the intra-erythrocytic phase. Of note, recombinant *Pf*PM4 hydrolyzes spectrin at pH 6.6 in a similar pattern as recombinant *Pf*PM2 does [97]. Further, a 37-kDa aspartic proteinase purified from the rodent malaria parasite *P. berghei* enables hydrolysis of spectrin and protein 4.1 from human erythrocytes at physiological pH [98]. Based on these pieces of evidence, it is likely that the FV PM-mediated host cell remodeling commonly occurs in the intra-erythrocytic phase of *Plasmodium* spp. (**Figure 3**).

4.3. Ookinetes midgut invasion and oocyst development

PM4 (*Pg*PM4) from the avian malaria parasite *P. gallinaceum* is involved in ookinete invasion of mosquito midguts and oocyst development during the sporogonic phase (**Figure 3**) [99]. In its mosquito host, *P. gallinaceum* expresses *Pg*PM4 in zygotes and ookinetes. In ookinetes, *Pg*PM4 is located at the apical membrane surface as well as in micronemes, an organelle of apicomplexan parasites involving in protein secretion. Monoclonal antibodies directed against *Pg*PM4 block oocyst development, but have no effects on ookinete formation. *Pg*PM4, together with chitinase and other enzymes, is speculated to hydrolyze peritrophic matrix proteins during ookinetes' midgut invasion, a critical step for parasite development. Questions remain elusive, such as how the expression of *Pg*PM4 and its orthologs is spatio-temporally regulated in the life cycle of malaria parasites, whether PM4 orthologs from other *Plasmodium* spp. play a similar role, what the natural substrates of *Pg*PM4 are, and how *Pg*PM4 recognizes and cleaves its substrates.

Of particular note, antibodies directed against the catalytic domain of either *Pf*PM7 or *Pf*PM10 decrease the prevalence of *P. falciparum* invasion of the mosquito and reduce the intensity of developed oocysts [69], indicating the involvement of mature *Pf*PM7 or *Pf*PM10 in parasite development during the sporogonic phase as well.

4.4. Host-targeted protein export

In the intra-erythrocytic phase, malaria parasites express and export hundreds of proteins, collectively named the "exportome," to infected red blood cells in order to acquire nutrients, to remodel the host cell, to avoid host immune detection, and to promote virulence [100–102]. A portion of the exportome shares at the N-terminus a pentameric sequence motif of RxLxE/Q/D (x represents any natural amino acid), known as the *Plasmodium export element* (PEXEL) [101] or the vacuolar transport signal [100]. A cleavage of the PEXEL motif at the C-terminus of leucine triggers the PEXEL-containing proteins to traverse the PPM and PVM, and subsequently reach the host cell [103]. PM5 catalyzes this reaction in the ER following the translation of PEXEL-containing proteins (**Figure 3**) [64, 104].

PM5-mediated PEXEL cleavage is proved to be essential to not only protein export but also parasite survival in that episomal expression of a catalytically inactive PM5 mutant decreases the level of proteins exported to host cells and slows down the parasite growth rate [64]. Interestingly, when the PEXEL motif of the *P. falciparum* erythrocyte membrane protein 3 (*Pf*EMP3) is engineered such that a signal peptidase, but not PM5, is able to conduct the cleavage, the resulting protein is transported to the parasitophorous vacuole rather than the cytoplasm of host cell, even if it has the same acetylated-xQ sequence retaining at the N-terminus as the PM5-cleaved mature *Pf*EMP3 does [104]. Meanwhile, when proteins are engineered to alter the prime side sequence of the PEXEL motif, the processed mature proteins fail to export to host erythrocytes even if PM5 performs the cleavage [105]. These findings highlight the importance of both PM5's involvement in the cleavage and the exposure of appropriate N-terminal sequence of the mature protein in host-targeted protein export. Detailed mechanisms related to how PM5-mediated PEXEL cleavage contributes to host-targeted protein export, and other potential roles of PM5 in the protein export event remain elusive.

Of particular note, the host-targeted malaria protein export is not restricted in the intra-erythrocytic phase but occurs over the course of the parasite life cycle [66, 106, 107], which coincides with the spatio-temporal expression pattern of PM5 [44, 65, 66]. It is thus conceivable that PM5 is also involved in protein export at other stages of the parasite life cycle, though no supporting evidence has been reported yet.

4.5. Other functions

Recent studies from Spaccapelo and colleagues showed the role of PM4 (*Pb*PM4) from the rodent malaria parasite *P. berghei* in maintaining virulence and suppressing innate immune responses of parasite-infected mice (**Figure 3**) [108, 109]. Supporting evidence comes from the observations that (1) the parasite with *pbpm4* genetically ablated (*Δpbpm4*) fails to elicit experimental cerebral malaria (ECM) in the ECM-susceptible mice; (2) the *Δpbpm4* is unable to kill the ECM-resistant mice as the parent strain does, but is cleared from blood after a three-week infection; and (3) after a single infection of naïve hosts by the *Δpbpm4*, these convalescent mice gain immune protection from a later parent strain infection. The mechanism by which *Pb*PM4 contributes to parasite virulence warrants further investigation.

In another study [110], recombinant *Pb*PM4 expressed and purified from *E. coli* was injected intraperitoneally (i.p.) in mice, together with the adjuvant saponin; sera obtained from the immunized mice contain antibodies that can recognize the cultured *P. berghei* strain from which the immunogen-encoding sequence originates. In addition, i.p. injecting erythorcytes infected by this *P. berghei* strain into *Pb*PM4-immunized mice boosts their production of the parasite-recognizing antibodies *in vivo*. Interestingly, three of five *Pb*PM4-immunized mice show resistance to *P. berghei* infection with the parasitaemia percentage reduced by an order of magnitude compared to naïve mice. These findings suggest that PMs are able to serve both as drug targets and as immunogens for malaria control (**Figure 3**). Though whether PM4 homologs residing in the host-infecting parasites are able to elicit a similar immune response as purified recombinant forms is not yet clear, their potential immunogenic role in malaria prevention and treatment merits further investigation.

5. Enzymatic characterization

5.1. Food vacuole plasmepsins

5.1.1. Plasmodium falciparum plasmepsin 1

The naturally-occurring *Pf*PM1 runs as a 37-kDa monomeric protein in SEC, indicative of its mature form [47, 83]. Purified naturally-occurring *Pf*PM1 hydrolyzes native hemoglobin at α33-34 at an optimal pH 5.0 [83], within the pH range of the FV [111, 112]. This reaction is fully inhibited by pepstatin, a typical aspartic proteinase inhibitor, at nanomolar magnitude, but little by serine, cysteine or metallo-proteinase inhibitors in the millimolar range [83].

*Pf*PM1 of the recombinant form was expressed in *E. coli*. To obtain catalytically active mature enzyme, two technical obstacles were overcome: first, to avoid the potential toxicity the putative transmembrane motif exerts to *E. coli*, a truncated construct lacking the N-terminal half of the pro-segment was used [113]; second, to confer the auto-maturation capability on the truncated zymogen, this *Pf*PM1 construct was further engineered by introducing a self-cleavage site in the pro-segment [51, 52], by retaining a longer pro-segment [114], or by co-expressing with thioredoxin in one open reading frame [115]. These engineered *Pf*PM1s conduct auto-maturation at pH 4.0–5.5; however, the resulting mature enzyme retains a 7- or 12-amino-acid pro-segment [51, 52, 115]. Furthermore, the *Pf*PM1 produced by auto-maturation *in vitro* shows unanimously weaker kinetic efficiencies (k_{cat}/K_m) in cleaving hemoglobin-derived substrates than the naturally-occurring, mainly due to lower k_{cat} values [52, 115, 116]. These findings suggest that the presence of a short piece of pro-segment in the *in vitro* auto-matured *Pf*PM1 inhibits the enzyme activity and that the inhibition may occur in a different way than that it directly occupies the active site, like the case of pepsinogen and progastricsin [117–120]. In support of this, a crystal structure of the highly homologous *Pf*PM2 zymogen demonstrates that the pro-segment blocks enzyme activity by harnessing the C-terminal domain away from the N-terminal half to prevent the cooperative action of the catalytic dyad [120, 121].

The subsite specificity of *Pf*PM1 at S3 – S3' was analyzed using combinatorial chemistry-based peptide libraries [52]. In this study, the degree of accommodation of each of the 19 amino acids (i.e., norleucine and the 20 natural amino acids omitting methionine and cysteine) at each of the six subsites was quantitatively assessed. Ultimately, the peptide sequence comprising the best accommodated amino acid at each investigated position, in the order of P3–P3', is FSF*LQF (* represents the scissor bond). By comparing data to those obtained using the same method from analyzing human cathepsin D (hcatD), the most homologous human enzyme to FV PMs, a peptide sequence was deduced comprising at each position an amino acid that is well fit in *Pf*PM1, but better recognized by *Pf*PM1 than by hcatD. A peptidomimetic inhibitor (KPFSLΨLQF, where Ψ = –CH_2–NH–), converted from such peptide sequence by reducing the scissor bond to the non-cleavable methyleneamino (–CH_2–NH–), exhibit an inhibition of *Pf*PM1 with the dissociation constant (K_i) in nanomolar magnitude and a >5-fold selectivity for *Pf*PM1 over hcatD. In another study using a random decamer peptide library, Siripurkpong and colleagues showed that *Pf*PM1 prefers accommodating leucine and serine at S1' and S2', respectively [122]. While the two studies agreed on the S1' subsite specificity, the discrepancy at S2' may arise from difference in enzyme preparation, peptide library composition, or catalytic conditions.

5.1.2. *Plasmodium falciparum plasmepsin 2*

The naturally-occurring *Pf*PM2 is purified as a 36-kDa mature enzyme, separated from *Pf*PM1 by elution at a lower salt concentration [47]. As discussed in Section 3.1, the naturally-occurring *Pf*PM2 cleaves native hemoglobin at α33-34 less efficiently than *Pf*PM1 [47]; however, it digests acid-denatured globin 3-fold more efficiently than *Pf*PM1 [113]. Similar to the naturally-occurring *Pf*PM1, *Pf*PM2 is tightly inhibited by pepstatin with the K_i in sub-nanomolar magnitude [113, 116].

Unlike the case of *Pf*PM1, a recombinantly expressed truncated *Pf*PM2 zymogen lacking the putative transmembrane motif fully converts itself to mature enzyme in acidic conditions [53]. *Pf*PM2 generated from *in vitro* auto-maturation retains a 2- or 12-amino-acid pro-segment; though, the *in vitro* auto-matured enzyme and its naturally-occurring counterpart shares similar kinetic efficiencies in digesting hemoglobin-derived substrates and inhibition by peptidomimetic compounds [113, 116]. Interestingly, *Pf*PM2 can adopt the proper conformation from *in vitro* protein refolding such robustly that deleting part of (e.g. Δ112p–121p) or the entire pro-segment costs no loss of its catalytic activity [123, 124].

Beyer and colleagues studied the subsite specificity of *Pf*PM2 at S3 – S3' using the combinatorial chemistry-based peptide libraries discussed in Section 4.1.1 [125]. *Pf*PM2 prefers accommodating bulky hydrophobic residues (e.g., norleucine, leucine, isoleucine and phenylalanine) in all studied subsites except for the S2', where glutamine is the most favored. The peptide sequence comprising the most favored amino acid at each position, in the order of P3 – P3', is nLInL*LQI (nL = norleucine). A peptidomimetic inhibitor (KPnLSnLΨLQI) designed using the same approach described above exhibits an inhibition of *Pf*PM2 with the K_i at nanomolar magnitude and a >15-fold selectivity for *Pf*PM2 over hcatD. In two earlier studies, the catalytic activity of *Pf*PM2 was assessed in cleaving five sets of chromogenic octapeptides; peptide substrates within a particular set differ in amino acids substituted in one of the P4, P3, P2, P2' and P3' positions [126, 127]. The results showed that peptides with large hydrophobic amino acids (e.g. phenylalanine and leucine) residing in P3, P2 and P3' give rise to the highest k_{cat}/K_m values, consistent with the findings from the combinatorial peptide library study. In addition, Siripurkpong and colleagues reported that *Pf*PM2 digests a library of random decameric peptides most efficiently when leucine is placed in the P1' position and that the enzyme has comparable kinetic efficiencies when residues of different properties (e.g., serine, methionine, alanine and glutamine) are placed in the P2' position [122], again consistent with the previous findings. Of note, an N-terminal extension of peptide substrates to P6 enhances the kinetic efficiency of *Pf*PM2, and yet C-terminally extended peptides manifest no such effect [124]. The possible presence of a similar effect in other PM homologs is unclear yet.

5.1.3. *Plasmodium falciparum histo-aspartic proteinase*

HAP is a PM with the catalytic aspartic acid of the N-terminus replaced by a histidine. Naturally-occurring *Pf*HAP, purified as a monomeric mature enzyme of ~37 kDa, cleaves hemoglobin-derived substrates at an optimal pH 5.7 [48]. *Pf*HAP shows nearly no cleavage of native hemoglobin, but is able to digest acid-denatured globin and to hydrolyze α33-34 in hemoglobin-derived peptide substrates [48]. Nonetheless, *Pf*HAP cleaves α33-34 20-fold less efficiently than *Pf*PM1 and *Pf*PM2 [48, 113]. The naturally-occurring *Pf*HAP can be fully inhibited by isovaleryl-pepstatin (pepstatin A) at 1 μM and by the serine proteinase inhibitor phenylmethylsulfonyl fluoride (PMSF) at 1 mM [48].

Catalytically active *Pf*HAP of the recombinant form was obtained using a similar strategy as the one applied to recombinant *Pf*PM1 [128, 129]. The *in vitro* auto-matured *Pf*HAP retains 4 pro-segment residues [128]. It exhibits an optimal catalytic activity at pH 5.2 and lowers kinetic efficiencies in cleaving hemoglobin-derived peptides than its naturally-occurring counterpart [128]. In addition, though pepstatin A at 1 μM completely inactivate the enzyme, PMSF at 1 mM inhibits enzyme activity by only 25% [128]. The apparent differences in enzymatic features between the naturally-occurring *Pf*HAP and the *in vitro* auto-matured may be attributable to improper folding of the recombinant protein [128] and/or the inhibition effects of the pro-segment [120].

A key question remains elusive is whether *Pf*HAP functions as an aspartic or a serine proteinase. Based on results from computational modeling, some view *Pf*HAP as a serine proteinase with a catalytic triad of H34, S37 and D214 [130], and others consider *Pf*HAP an atypical aspartic proteinase with D214 performing catalysis and H34 stabilizing the intermediate enzyme species [131]. By conducting alanine mutation of these residues related to catalysis, Parr and colleagues showed that D214A renders *Pf*HAP incapable of auto-maturation, whereas H34A and S37A do not affect auto-maturation, but lead to a lower kinetic efficiency in cleaving peptide substrates [132]. These findings support the role of D214 in enzyme catalysis, indicating that *Pf*HAP is an atypical aspartic proteinase.

5.1.4. *Plasmepsin 4 orthologs*

To the author's knowledge, no literatures have thus far reported the characteristics of naturally-occurring *Pf*PM4. The recombinantly expressed *Pf*PM4 zymogen lacking the putative transmembrane motif conducts auto-maturation under acidic conditions, resulting in a mature form retaining 12 pro-segment residues [48]. This mature *Pf*PM4 cleaves hemoglobin-derived peptides at an optimal pH 5.4 [48]. *Pf*PM4 digests native hemoglobin less efficiently than *Pf*PM1 and *Pf*PM2 and prefers cleaving acid-denatured globin [48]. Similar to *Pf*PM1 and *Pf*PM2, but unlike *Pf*HAP, *Pf*PM4 is fully inhibited by pepstatin A at sub-nanomolar magnitude, but not by inhibitors of other types of proteinases [48, 54].

Recombinant PM4s from the other three human malaria parasites and the rodent malarial parasite *P. berghei* were similarly produced and activated [54, 126, 133]. The subsite specificity at S3 – S3' of the five PM4 orthologs (i.e., *Pf*PM4, *Po*PM4, *Pv*PM4, *Pm*PM4 and *Pb*PM4) was investigated using combinatorial peptide libraries [125, 133]. All five PM4s unanimously prefer accommodating phenylalanine or tyrosine at S1 and S1', except that *Pb*PM4 accommodates norleucine best at S1'. At S3, bulky hydrophobic amino acids, such as leucine, norleucine and phenylalanine, are preferred by all five enzymes. At S3', the acceptance of amino acids by the four human PM4s is broad with isoleucine accommodated best, whereas *Pb*PM4 accommodates aromatic phenylalanine and tryptophan best. For S2 and S2', all five PM4s seem to tolerate amino acids of different properties. Glutamic acid, serine and isoleucine are the most favored at S2; while for glutamine, isoleucine, glutamic acid and arginine, when accommodated in S2', each leads to a considerable peptide cleavage. The peptide sequence comprising the most favored residue by each subsite, in the order of P3 – P3', is IQF*YIL for *Pf*PM4, is FEF*YFI for *Po*PM4, is LEF*FII for *Pv*PM4, is FEF*FII for *Pm*PM4, and is FEF*nLSW for *Pb*PM4. Peptidomimetic inhibitors were designed using the same approach described in Section 4.1.1: KPVEFΨRQT for *Pf*PM4, KPLEFΨFRV for *Po*PM4, KPLEFΨYRV for *Pv*PM4, KPFELΨAWT for *Pm*PM4, and KPYEFΨRQF for *Pb*PM4. These compounds unanimously exhibit a selective inhibition of their respective PM4s over hcatD, and inhibit their respective PM4s with the K_i values at sub-nanomolar to nanomolar magnitude, except for the one designed for *Pm*PM4, which inhibits *Pm*PM4 with the K_i at micromolar magnitude. Such a poor inhibition may be due to the incorporation in the P1' position of an alanine that is poorly recognized by *Pm*PM4, indicating the key role of the P1' amino acid in determining the enzyme-ligand interaction. In another two studies, the subsite specificity of the four human PM4s was analyzed at S3, S2, S2' and S3' using chromogenic octapeptides [54, 126]. The results showed that (1) hydrophobic amino acids (e.g., phenylalanine and isoleucine) are more favored at P3 than smaller hydrophobic, polar and charged amino acids, (2) hydrophobic amino acids are favored at P2, and (3) amino acids of different properties at P2' and P3' are well tolerated. These findings are consistent with the data obtained from the combinatorial peptide library study.

5.2. Non-food vacuole plasmepsins

Thus far, enzymatic characterization of non-FV PMs has been focused on the PM5 orthologs. PM5 (*Pf*PM5) immunopurified from cultured *P. falciparum* cleaves PEXEL (RxLxQ/E/D)-containing substrates at the C-terminus of leucine at pH 5–7 [64], resembling the pH of the mammalian ER [134]. The PEXEL-cleaving activity of *Pf*PM5 is partially inhibited by pepstatin A and HIV-1 PIs (i.e., lopinavir, nelfinavir, ritonavir and saquinavir) with the IC_{50} values in the high micromolar range [64, 104]. The presence of P3 R and P1 L is key to *Pf*PM5-catalyzed PEXEL cleavage in that mutations in these two positions (e.g., P3 R-to-A or K and P1 L-to-A or I) unanimously inhibit the cleavage, and abolish the export of PEXEL-containing proteins to host erythrocytes; amino acids in the prime side positions also influence the efficiency of PEXEL cleavage and subsequent protein export [104, 105, 135]. *Pf*PM5 also digests non-canonical PEXEL motifs (e.g., RxLxxE) at the C-terminus of P1 L, which in turn, triggers host-targeted protein export [105]. Likewise, this *Pf*PM5-catalyzed non-canonical PEXEL cleavage and subsequent protein export are blocked by a P3 R-to-A mutation [105]. Of note, though deleting neither the P1' nor the P2' amino acid affects enzyme cleavage, protein export efficiency is reduced by these prime side mutations [105]. Taken together, these findings highlight the essential role of P3 R and P1 L in modulating *Pf*PM5-mediated PEXEL cleavage and the importance of the prime side peptide sequence in directing host-targeted protein export.

Two constructs of *Pf*PM5 encoding a truncated zymogen (amino acids 37–521) and a mature enzyme (amino acids 84–521) have been recombinantly expressed in *E. coli* [136, 137]. Following *in vitro* protein refolding, both the zymogen and the mature enzyme exhibit catalytic activity in cleaving PEXEL-containing peptides at an optimal pH 6.0–6.5 [136, 137]. Indeed, the pro-segment of *Pf*PM5 was shown to be non-essential for guiding the proper folding of protein [137, 138]. Subsite specificity analysis of the recombinant mature *Pf*PM5 on a peptide series of RxLxE at P2 and P1' showed that when the polar serine is placed at P1', the hydrophobic isoleucine is more favored at P2 than the charged glutamic acid and lysine; and vice versa, when isoleucine is placed at P2, serine is better accommodated at S1' than glutamic acid and the hydrophobic valine [136]. Recombinant *Pf*PM5, like the parasite-expressed, can only be partially (<50%) inhibited by pepstatin A, nelfinavir or PMSF at 100 mM; however, its catalytic activity is almost fully blocked by Cu^{2+} or Hg^{2+} at the sub-micromolar level [137]. Furthermore, the zymogen and mature form of PM5 (*Pv*PM5-Thai) from *P. vivax* Thailand

PM	Expression pattern	Subcellular location[a]	Enzymatic characteristics			
			pH[b]	Natural substrates	Subsite specificity[d]	Pepstatin A inhibition
*Pf*PM1	Intra-erythrocytic phase; merizoites; gametocytes	FV, TV	5.0	Hb	FSF*L(Q/S)F	<1 nM (K_i)
*Pf*PM2	Intra-erythrocytic phase; merizoites; gametocytes; oocysts; sporozoites	FV, TV	4.7; ~6.8	Hb; Host cytoskeletal proteins	nLInL*LQI	<1 nM (K_i)
*Pf*HAP	Intra-erythrocytic phase; merizoites; gametocytes; sporozoites	FV, TV	5.7	Hb	n.d.	1 μM (fully inhibition)
*Pf*PM4	Intra-erythrocytic phase; merizoites; gametocytes; oocysts; sporozoites	FV, TV	4.5; ~6.6	Hb[c]; Host cytoskeletal proteins[c]	IQF*YIL	<1 nM (K_i)
*Pv*PM4	Intra-erythrocytic phase	FV, TV	4.5	Hb[c]	LEF*FII	<1 nM (K_i)
*Po*PM4	n.d.	FV, TV	4.5	Hb[c]	FEF*YFI	<1 nM (K_i)
*Pm*PM4	n.d.	FV, TV	4.5	Hb[c]	FEF*FII	<1 nM (K_i)
*Pb*PM4	n.d.	FV, TV	5.0–5.5	Hb[c]; Host cytoskeletal proteins	FEF*nLSW	<1 nM (K_i)
*Pf*PM5	Intra-erythrocytic phase; merizoites; gametocytes; sporozoites	ER/NE	6.0–6.5	PEXEL-containing parasite proteins	RxL*x(Q/E/D); RxL*xxE	~20–30 μM (IC_{50})

[a]This column shows the subcellular locations of catalytically active, mature plasmepsins.
[b]This column shows the optimal catalytic pH; for *Pf*PM2 and *Pf*PM4, digestion of host cytoskeletal proteins is carried out at near neutral pH.
[c]Digestion of these natural substrates were performed *in vitro* using *recombinant* plasmepsins.
[d]This column shows the best amino acids accommodated at subsites in the order of P3 – P3′; * represents scissile bond between P1 and P1′; x represents any natural amino acid; nL = norleucine.

Table 2. Enzymatic properties of plasmepsins.

isolates were recombinantly expressed; the purified *Pv*PM5-Thai exhibits similar enzymatic features as the recombinant *Pf*PM5 does [139].

The enzymatic properties of PMs discussed in this section are summarized in **Table 2**.

6. Plasmepsin-targeted antimalarial drug development

6.1. Evaluation of food vacuole plasmepsins as antimalarial drug targets

The establishment of the role of FV PMs in hemoglobin processing raised the question whether FV PMs can be targets of novel antimalarial drugs. Peptidomimetic compounds developed in the early stage (e.g., pepstatin A, SC-50083, Ro40-4388, and HIV-1 PIs) bind FV PMs tightly and block growth of cultured parasites [46, 51, 140, 141], suggesting that inhibition of FV PMs is a promising antimalarial strategy. Numerous types of FV PM-targeted compounds, synthetic or isolated from natural sources, have been assessed for the past two and a half decades based on criteria involving binding affinity and selectivity, inhibition potency to cultured parasite growth, and cytotoxicity to mammalian cell culture (for reviews, see for example [142, 143]). For example, certain hydroxyethylamine derivatives inhibit *Pf*PM1, *Pf*PM2 and *Pf*PM4 in nanomolar magnitude, exhibit a >30-fold binding selectivity over hcatD, and disrupt growth of cultured *P. falciparum* with IC_{50}s in the low micromolar range [144, 145]. In a series of studies, several allophenylnorstatine-based compounds were found to inhibit all four FV *Pf*PMs in nanomolar magnitude, to block parasite growth with IC_{50}s in the low micromolar range, and to have the TD_{50}s (cytotoxicity) in high micromolar magnitude to rat skeletal myoblasts [146–148]. In addition, clinically used HIV-1 PIs exhibit antimalarial activity on parasites in both the exo-erythrocytic and the intra-erythrocytic phases in the sub-micromolar to low micromolar range [149–151], inhibit *Pf*PM2 and *Pf*PM4 at low micromolar magnitude, and have a >10-fold selectivity over hcatD [141]. Interestingly, using affinity binding probes coupled to a FV PM inhibitor library, a hydroxyethyl-based inhibitor was identified that inhibits all four FV *Pf*PMs and the growth of cultured *P. falciparum* with IC_{50} at ~1 μM [152].

To assess whether FV PMs are appropriate drug targets, *pfpm4*, 1, 2 and *pfhap* were knocked out individually (i.e., Δ*pfpm4*, Δ*pfpm1*, Δ*pfpm2* and Δ*pfhap*), in combination (e.g., Δ*pfpm4/1* and Δ*pfpm1/2/hap*), or together as a whole (i.e., Δ*pfpm4/1/2/hap*). Genetic ablation of any particular gene alters neither the mRNA transcription nor the protein expression of the other three paralogs over the course of the intra-erythrocytic phase [153]. For hemoglobin metabolism, the Δ*pfpm4* strain, but not the Δ*pfpm1*, Δ*pfpm2* or Δ*pfhap*, shows a reduction in hemozoin accumulation in the FV compared to the parent line [154, 155]. Of note, genetic disruption of PM expression does affect the rate of parasite replication in that the Δ*pfpm4*, Δ*pfpm1*, Δ*pfpm2*, Δ*pfpm4/1* and Δ*pfpm4/1/2/hap* strains all exhibit a reduced growth rate in amino-acid-rich media compared to the parent line, and that when cultured in amino-acid-limited media, the Δ*pfhap* strain also demonstrates a slower growth rate [153–157]. As for cell and subcellular organelle morphology, though no morphological abnormalities are apparent in the Δ*pfpm1* and Δ*pfhap* strains, a portion of the Δ*pfpm2* shows enlarged mitochondria, and a portion of the Δ*pfpm4* exhibits a notable accumulation of electron-dense, single-membrane vesicles in the FV

[154, 156]; in addition, ceroid-like multilamellar bodies, and electron-dense, single-membrane vesicles are accumulated in the FV of the *Δpfpm4/1/2/hap* strain [155]. Taken together, genetic ablation of *pfpms* is not lethal to the parasite in cultured conditions despite apparent metabolic and pathological abnormalities, thus it seems that FV PMs may be dispensable for parasite survival; however, one cannot overlook the potential contribution of *Pb*PM4 to the virulence of the parasite in infected mice (see discussion in Section 4.5). Understanding the pathological role of FV PMs in both cell-based and animal models may lead to a better assessment of the feasibility of PM-targeted drug development.

To better understand the relationship between enzyme inhibition and anti-parasitic activity, the effects of known FV PM inhibitors on the growth of PM-knockout parasites were investigated. When pepstatin A was administered to cultured parasite in the intra-erythrocytic phase, growth of the Δ*pfpm1*, Δ*pfpm2*, Δ*pfhap* and Δ*pfpm4/1* strains is even slightly less sensitive to the compound than that of the parent line, and yet growth of the FP-2-knockout strain is at least one order of magnitude more sensitive to pepstatin A [156, 157]. These findings indicate that the parasite may turn to other proteinases to maintain normal function when the activities of FV PMs are blocked. The effects of HIV-1 PIs on *in vitro* PM inhibition and blockage of parasite growth have been well established [141, 158]. However, the Δ*pfpm1/2/hap* and Δ*pfpm4/1/2/hap* strains share a comparable sensitivity to five HIV-1 PIs (i.e., atazanavir, lopinavir, indinavir, ritonavir and saquinavir) with the parent line [155], indicating that FV PMs may not be the target of these inhibitors in the parasite [141]. Such off-target effects are rather common among developed PM inhibitors of distinct classes (e.g., C_2-symmetric 1,2-dihydroxyethylenes [159], hydroxylethylamine transition-state isosteres [145] and amidine-containing diphenylureas [160]). The authentic targets of these inhibitors in the parasite have been under investigation [161].

Despite that FV PMs are not critical to parasite survival at the blood stage and that certain FV PM inhibitors exhibit their anti-parasitic activities with an off-target effect, it is still early to negate FV PM-targeted drug design given our limited understanding of their functions and characteristics. The continuously identified novel functions of FV PMs plus their broad spatio-temporal expression pattern over the course of the parasite life cycle are worthy of further investigation.

6.2. Developing novel antimalarial drugs targeting non-food vacuole plasmepsins

PM5 has been considered an ideal target for novel antimalarial drug design based on a series of findings: first, ablation of the gene encoding PM5 is lethal to cultured *P. berghei* [104], so is mutation of a catalytic aspartic acid of PM5 to cultured *P. falciparum* [64]; second, PM5 is evolutionarily conserved among *Plasmodium* spp. with no identified gene replication or functional redundancy [44]; third, PM5 shares a low amino acid sequence identity with human aspartic proteinases (e.g., 26% with mature hcatD, and 18% with mature human β-secretase 1 (hBACE-1)); and fourth, the expression profile of PM5 spans the entire life cycle of malaria parasites [44, 65, 66].

Two basic components were incorporated in the initial design of PM5 inhibitors: a PEXEL sequence, which provides a moderate fit of compounds to the active site of the enzyme, and a transition-state peptidomimetic moiety, which gives rise to a tight interaction with the catalytic residues of proteinases. WEHI-916, a statine-based compound mimicking the non-prime-side RVL motif of the PEXEL, shows a strong inhibition (IC_{50} = ~20 nM) of *Pf*PM5 and *Pv*PM5, a much weaker inhibition of hcatD (IC_{50} = 25 μM), and a negligible inhibition of hBACE-1 (IC_{50}>100 μM) [162, 163]. Administration of WEHI-916 to cultured *P. falciparum* blocks the PEXEL cleavage in a dose-dependent manner, and impairs protein export to host erythrocytes [162]. Of particular interest, conditioned knockdown of *pfpm5* enhances WEHI-916-mediated inhibition of PEXEL cleavage and the sensitivity of parasite growth to this compound; whereas overexpression of *Pf*PM5 weakens the anti-parasitic potency of WEHI-916 [162]. These findings confirm that PM5 is the target of WEHI-916 in the parasite. Though, WHEI-916 has only a moderate potency (EC_{50} = 2.5 μM to the strain 3D7) in killing cultured *P. falciparum*, which may be attributed to its poor membrane permeability [162, 163]. To enhance the anti-parasitic potency of WEHI-916 while retaining its strong binding to PM5, the highly polar P3 arginine in WEHI-916 was modified to its isostere L-canavanine, and the N-terminal sulfonamide was replaced by a carbamate [164, 165]. The resulting compound WEHI-842 inhibits *Pf*PM5 and *Pv*PM5 more tightly (IC_{50} = 0.2–0.4 nM), and blocks the PEXEL cleavage and protein export more potently than WEHI-916 [165]. Importantly, WEHI-842 kills the chloroquine-sensitive 3D7 strain and multiple chloroquine-resistant *P. falciparum* strains with a potency (EC_{50} = 0.4 μM) one order of magnitude higher than that of WEHI-916, and yet it exhibits a low cytotoxicity against human cells (TD_{50}>50 μM) [165]. Taken together, WEHI-842 represents a promising lead for developing PM5-targeted antimalarial drugs.

Our limited knowledge on PMs 6–10 makes it difficult to assess the necessity and importance of developing drugs targeting these enzymes. However, the detection of these PMs in multiple stages of the parasite life cycle suggests that their role in malaria pathogenesis is non-trivial. For future PM-targeted drug development, the functions and characteristics of PMs 6-10 warrant further study.

7. Concluding remarks

Malaria, one of the deadliest infectious diseases in history, still poses a serious socio-economic problem at present. Malaria control has been effectively undertaken from multiple perspectives, including drug-based disease prevention and treatment, intervention of malaria transmission by the mosquito vector, and usage of vaccine against malaria parasites. Though, the emergence and quick spread of drug-resistant parasite strains urges us to identify new antimalarial drug targets. The subject of this review has focused on the aspartic proteinase PM family, the molecular entities deemed novel and promising targets of next-generation antimalarial drugs.

Discussed here is our understanding of the PM family members on their biosynthesis, biological functions and characteristics for the past two and a half decades. Seven groups of PMs have thus far been identified from genome comparison of a series of *Plasmodium* spp. infecting rodents, birds, humans and non-human primates. These PMs, unique in enzymatic feature and spatio-temporal expression pattern, play multifaceted roles in the pathogenicity of the malaria parasite. Due to the seemingly dispensable role of FV PMs in parasite growth and survival, the focus of PM-targeted drug development is shifting towards non-FV PMs. Selective inhibitors of PM5 have been developed and shown strong inhibition potency to parasite growth.

On the other hand, our knowledge on PMs is still quite limited and much needs to be clarified and explored in the future studies. For example, what is the biological meaning of the presence of four FV PM paralogs in *P. falciparum*? What do the FV PM inhibitors authentically target to exert their anti-parasitic activity? What are other possible roles of PM5 than host-targeted protein export? What are the functions of PMs 6-10, and can these enzymes be antimalarial drug targets? What is the likelihood that PMs are used as immunogens in active immunization and that antibodies directed against PMs are used in passive immunization to protect hosts from malaria parasite infection? Successful PM-targeted drug development replies on a comprehensive understanding of this enzyme family.

List of abbreviations

ACTs	artemisinin-based combination therapies
ALLN	*N*-acetyl-Leu-Leu-norleucinal
AN	artemisinin
BFA	brefeldin A
Chr.	chromosome
CQ	chloroquine
(k)Da	(kilo-)dalton
DDT	dichloro-diphenyltrichloroethane
E. coli	*Escherichia coli*
E-64	L-3-carboxy-2,3-trans-epoxypropionyl-leucylamido(4-guanidino)butane
EC_{50}	half maximal effective concentration
ECM	experimental cerebral malaria
EM	electron microscopy
ER	endoplasmic reticulum
FP	falcipain
FV	food vacuole
GFP	green fluorescence protein
HAP	Histo-Aspartic Proteinase
Hb	hemoglobin
hBACE-1	human β-secretase 1
hcatD	human cathepsin D

HIV-1	human immunodeficiency virus type 1
IC_{50}	half maximal inhibitory concentration
i.p.	intraperitoneally
kb	kilo-base
k_{cat}	turnover number
k_{cat}/K_m	specificity constant
K_i	dissociation/inhibition constant
μM	micromolar
mM	millimolar
MS	mass spectrometry
MW	molecular weight
NE	nuclear envelope
nL	norleucine
nM	nanomolar
P.	*Plasmodium*
Pb	*Plasmodium berghei*
PEXEL	Plasmodium export element
Pf	*Plasmodium falciparum*
*Pf*EMP3	*P. falciparum* erythrocyte membrane protein 3
Pg	*Plasmodium gallinaceum*
pH	negative log of the hydrogen ion concentration
pI	isoelectric point
PIs	proteinase inhibitors
PM	plasmepsin
Pm	*Plasmodium malariae*
PMSF	phenylmethylsulfonyl fluoride
Po	*Plasmodium ovale*
PPM	parasite plasma membrane
PV	parasitophorous vacuole
Pv	*Plasmodium vivax*
PVM	parasitophorous vacuolar membrane
SEC	size exclusion chromatography
spp.	*species pluralis*
TD_{50}	median toxic dose
TV	transport vesicle

Author details

Peng Liu

Address all correspondence to: liuxx726@umn.edu

Department of Neurology, University of Minnesota Medical School, Minneapolis, USA

References

[1] World Health Organization. World malaria report 2015. Brussels: Geneva: World Health Organization; 2015. 280 p.

[2] Benelli G, Mehlhorn H. Declining malaria, rising of dengue and Zika virus: insights for mosquito vector control. Parasitology Research. 2016;**115**(5):1747-1754. doi:10.1007/s00436-016-4971-z

[3] Delepine M. Joseph Pelletier and Joseph Caventou. Journal of Chemical Education. 1951;**28**(9):454. doi:10.1021/ed028p454

[4] Meshnick SR, Dobson MJ. The History of Antimalarial Drugs. In: Rosenthal PJ, editor. Antimalarial Chemotherapy: Mechanisms of Action, Resistance, and New Directions in Drug Discovery. 1st ed. Totowa, New Jersey: Humana Press; 2001. p. 15-25. doi:10.1007/978-1-59259-111-4

[5] Coatney GR. Pitfalls in a discovery: the chronicle of chloroquine. The American Journal of Tropical Medicine and Hygiene. 1963;**12**(2):121-128.

[6] Greenwood D. Conflicts of interest: the genesis of synthetic antimalarial agents in peace and war. Journal of Antimicrobial Chemotherapy. 1995;**36**(5):857-872. doi:10.1093/jac/36.5.857

[7] Haynes RK, Vonwiller SC. From Qinghao, marvelous herb of antiquity, to the antimalarial Trioxane Qinghaosu and some remarkable new chemistry. Accounts of Chemical Research. 1997;**30**(2):73-79. doi:10.1021/ar950058w

[8] Ringwald P, Eboumbou EC, Bickii J, Basco LK. In vitro activities of pyronaridine, alone and in combination with other antimalarial drugs, against *Plasmodium falciparum*. Antimicrobial Agents and Chemotherapy. 1999;**43**(6):1525-1527.

[9] Ramharter M, Noedl H, Thimasarn K, Wiedermann G, Wernsdorfer G, Wernsdorfer WH. In vitro activity of tafenoquine alone and in combination with artemisinin against *Plasmodium falciparum*. The American Journal of Tropical Medicine and Hygiene. 2002;**67**(1):39-43.

[10] Tanariya P, Tippawangkoso P, Karbwang J, Na-Bangchang K, Wernsdorfer WH. In vitro sensitivity of *Plasmodium falciparum* and clinical response to lumefantrine (benflumetol)

and artemether. British Journal of Clinical Pharmacology. 2000;**49**(5):437-444. doi:10.1046/j.1365-2125.2000.00176.x

[11] Pradines B, Tall A, Fusai T, Spiegel A, Hienne R, Rogier C, et al.. In vitro activities of benflumetol against 158 Senegalese isolates of *Plasmodium falciparum* in comparison with those of standard antimalarial drugs. Antimicrobial Agents and Chemotherapy. 1999;**43**(2):418-420.

[12] Brockman A, Price RN, van Vugt M, Heppner DG, Walsh D, Sookto P, et al. *Plasmodium falciparum* antimalarial drug susceptibility on the north-western border of Thailand during five years of extensive use of artesunate-mefloquine. Transactions of The Royal Society of Tropical Medicine and Hygiene. 2000;**94**(5):537-544. doi:10.1016/s0035-9203(00)90080-4

[13] White NJ. Clinical pharmacokinetics and pharmacodynamics of artemisinin and derivatives. Transactions of The Royal Society of Tropical Medicine and Hygiene. 1994;**88**(Supplement 1):41-43. doi:10.1016/0035-9203(94)90471-5

[14] Posner GH, O'Neill PM. Knowledge of the proposed chemical mechanism of action and cytochrome p450 metabolism of antimalarial trioxanes like artemisinin allows rational design of new antimalarial peroxides. Accounts of Chemical Research. 2004;**37**(6):397-404. doi:10.1021/ar020227u

[15] Dr. Paul Müller. Nature. 1965;**208**(5015):1043-1044. doi:10.1038/2081043b0

[16] Bence JR. Indirect effects and biological control of mosquitoes by mosquitofish. Journal of Applied Ecology. 1988;**25**(2):505-521. doi:10.2307/2403840

[17] Chandra G, Bhattacharjee I, Chatterjee SN, Ghosh A. Mosquito control by larvivorous fish. The Indian Journal of Medical Research. 2008;**127**(1):13-27.

[18] Culler LE, Lamp WO. Selective predation by larval Agabus (Coleoptera: Dytiscidae) on mosquitoes: support for conservationbased mosquito suppression in constructed wetlands. Freshwater Biology. 2009;**54**(9):2003-2014. doi:10.1111/j.1365-2427.2009.02230.x

[19] Fillinger U, Knols BGJ, Becker N. Efficacy and efficiency of new Bacillus thuringiensis var. israelensis and Bacillus sphaericus formulations against Afrotropical anophelines in Western Kenya. Tropical Medicine and International Health. 2003;**8**(1):37-47. doi 10.1046/j.1365-3156.2003.00979.x

[20] Jaronski S, Axtell RC. Persistence of the mosquito fungal pathogen Coelomomyces giganteum (Oomycetes; Lagenidiales) after introduction into natural habitats. Mosquito News. 1983;**43**(3):332-337.

[21] Kerwin JL, Washino RK. Ground and aerial application of the asexual stage of Coelomomyces giganteum for control of mosquitoes associated with rice culture in the central valley of California. Journal of the American Mosquito Control Association. 1987;**3**(1):59-64.

[22] Blanford S, Chan BHK, Jenkins N, Sim D, Turner RJ, Read AF, et al.. Fungal pathogen reduces potential for malaria transmission. Science. 2005;**308**(5728):1638-1641. doi:10.1126/science.1108423

[23] Fang W, Vega-Rodríguez J, Ghosh AK, Jacobs-Lorena M, Kang A, St. Leger RJ. Development of transgenic fungi that kill human malaria parasites in mosquitoes. Science. 2011;**331**(6020):1074-1077. doi:10.1126/science.1199115

[24] Schmutterer H. Properties and potential of natural pesticides from the Neem tree, Azadirachta indica. The Annual Review of Entomology. 1990;**35**:271-297. doi:10.1146/annurev.en.35.010190.001415

[25] Mordue (Luntz) AJ, Blackwell A. Azadirachtin: an update. Journal of Insect Physiology. 1993;**39**(11):903-924. doi:10.1016/0022-1910(93)90001-8

[26] Elango G, Rahuman A, Bagavan A, Kamaraj C, Zahir A, Venkatesan C.Laboratory study on larvicidal activity of indigenous plant extracts against Anopheles subpictus and Culex tritaeniorhynchus. Parasitology Research. 2009;**104**(6):1381-1388. doi:10.1007/s00436-009-1339-7

[27] Mathew N, Anitha M, Bala T, Sivakumar S, Narmadha R, Kalyanasundaram M. Larvicidal activity of Saraca indica, Nyctanthes arbor-tristis, and Clitoria ternatea extracts against three mosquito vector species. Parasitology Research. 2009;**104**(5):1017-1025. doi:10.1007/s00436-008-1284-x

[28] Zahir A, Rahuman A, Kamaraj C, Bagavan A, Elango G, Sangaran A, et al. Laboratory determination of efficacy of indigenous plant extracts for parasites control. Parasitology Research. 2009;**105**(2):453-461. doi:10.1007/s00436-009-1405-1

[29] Zhu J, Zeng X, O'Neal M, Schultz G, Tucker B, Coats J, et al. Mosquito larvicidal activity of botanical-based mosquito repellents. Journal of the American Mosquito Control Association. 2008;**24**(1):161-168. doi:10.2987/8756-971x

[30] Khater HF, Shalaby AA. Potential of biologically active plant oils to control mosquito larvae (Culex pipiens, Diptera: Culicidae) from an Egyptian locality. Revista do Instituto de Medicina Tropical de São Paulo. 2008;**50**(2):107-112. doi:10.1590/S0036-46652008000200008

[31] Murugan K, Priyanka V, Dinesh D, Madhiyazhagan P, Panneerselvam C, Subramaniam J, et al. Predation by Asian bullfrog tadpoles, Hoplobatrachus tigerinus, against the dengue vector, Aedes aegypti, in an aquatic environment treated with mosquitocidal nanoparticles. Parasitology Research. 2015;**114**(10):3601-3610. doi:10.1007/s00436-015-4582-0

[32] Govindarajan M, Rajeswary M, Muthukumaran U, Hoti SL, Khater HF, Benelli G. Single-step biosynthesis and characterization of silver nanoparticles using Zornia diphylla leaves: A potent eco-friendly tool against malaria and arbovirus vectors. Journal of Photochemistry and Photobiology B: Biology. 2016;**161**:482-489. doi:10.1016/j.jphotobiol.2016.06.016

[33] Govindarajan M, Khater HF, Panneerselvam C, Benelli G. One-pot fabrication of silver nanocrystals using Nicandra physalodes: A novel route for mosquito vector control with moderate toxicity on non-target water bugs. Research in Veterinary Science. 2016;**107**:95-101. doi:10.1016/j.rvsc.2016.05.017

[34] Rieckmann KH, Carson PE, Beaudoin RL, Cassells JS, Sell KW. Letter: Sporozoite induced immunity in man against an Ethiopian strain of *Plasmodium falciparum*. Transactions of the Royal Society of Tropical Medicine and Hygiene. 1974;**68**(3):258-259. doi:10.1016/0035-9203(74)90129-1

[35] Rieckmann KH, Beaudoin RL, Cassells JS, Sell KW. Use of attenuated sporozoites in the immunization of human volunteers against falciparum malaria. The Bulletin of the World Health Organization. 1979;**57**(Suppl 1):261-265.

[36] Rts, S. Clinical trials partnership. Efficacy and safety of RTS,S/AS01 malaria vaccine with or without a booster dose in infants and children in Africa: final results of a phase 3, individually randomised, controlled trial. Lancet. 2015;**386**(9988):31-45. doi:10.1016/S0140-6736(15)60721-8

[37] Tran TM, Portugal S, Draper SJ, Crompton PD. Malaria vaccines: moving forward after encouraging first steps. Current Tropical Medicine Reports. 2015;**2**(1):1-3. doi:10.1007/s40475-015-0041-3

[38] Bloland PB. Drug Resistance in Malaria. Geneva: World Health Organization; 2001. 32 p.

[39] Noedl H. Combination Therapy in Light of Emerging Artemisinin Resistance. In: Staines HM, Krishna S, editors. Teatment and Prevention of Malaria: Antimalarial Drug Chemistry, Action and Use. 1st ed. Springer, Basel; 2012. pp. 213-225. doi:10.1007/978-3-0346-0480-2

[40] Aurrecoechea C, Brestelli J, Brunk BP, Dommer J, Fischer S, Gajria B, et al. PlasmoDB: a functional genomic database for malaria parasites. Nucleic Acids Research. 2009;**37**(Suppl 1) D539-D543. doi:10.1093/nar/gkn814

[41] Dame JB, Yowell CA, Omara-Opyene L, Carlton JM, Cooper RA, Li T. Plasmepsin 4, the food vacuole aspartic proteinase found in all *Plasmodium* spp. infecting man. Molecular and Biochemical Parasitology. 2003;**130**(1):1-12. doi:10.1016/s0166-6851(03)00137-3

[42] Coombs GH, Goldberg DE, Klemba M, Berry C, Kay J, Mottram JC. Aspartic proteases of *Plasmodium falciparum* and other parasitic protozoa as drug targets. Trends in Parasitology. 2001;**17**(11):532-537. doi:10.1016/s1471-4922(01)02037-2

[43] Altschul SF, Gish W, Miller W, Myers EW, Lipman DJ. Basic local alignment search tool. Journal of Molecular Biology. 1990;**215**(3):403-410. doi:10.1016/S0022-2836(05)80360-2

[44] Silvestrini F, Lasonder E, Olivieri A, Camarda G, van Schaijk B, Sanchez M, et al.. Protein export marks the early phase of gametocytogenesis of the human malaria parasite *Plasmodium falciparum*. Molecular & Cellular Proteomics. 2010;**9**(7):1437-1448. doi:10.1074/mcp.M900479-MCP200

[45] Walker JM, editor. Proteomics Protocols Handbook. Totowa, New Jersey: Humana Press; 2005. 969 p. doi:10.1385/1592598900

[46] Francis SE, Gluzman IY, Oksman A, Knickerbocker A, Mueller R, Bryant ML, et al. Molecular characterization and inhibition of a *Plasmodium falciparum* aspartic hemoglobinase. The EMBO Journal. 1994;**13**(2):306-317.

[47] Gluzman IY, Francis SE, Oksman A, Smith CE, Duffin KL, Goldberg DE. Order and specificity of the *Plasmodium falciparum* hemoglobin degradation pathway. The Journal of Clinical Investigation. 1994;**93**(4):1602-1608. doi:10.1172/JCI117140

[48] Banerjee R, Liu J, Beatty W, Pelosof L, Klemba M, Goldberg DE. Four plasmepsins are active in the *Plasmodium falciparum* food vacuole, including a protease with an active-site histidine. Proceedings of the National Academy of Sciences of the United States of America. 2002;**99**(2):990-995. doi:10.1073/pnas.022630099

[49] Klemba M, Beatty W, Gluzman I, Goldberg DE. Trafficking of plasmepsin II to the food vacuole of the malaria parasite *Plasmodium falciparum*. The Journal of Cell Biology. 2004;**164**(1):47-56. doi:10.1083/jcb200307147

[50] Banerjee R, Francis SE, Goldberg DE. Food vacuole plasmepsins are processed at a conserved site by an acidic convertase activity in *Plasmodium falciparum*. Molecular and Biochemical Parasitology. 2003;**129**(2):157-165. doi:10.1016/s0166-6851(03)00119-1

[51] Moon RP, Tyas L, Certa U, Rupp K, Bur D, Jacquet C, et al. Expression and characterisation of plasmepsin I from *Plasmodium falciparum*. European Journal of Biochemistry/ FEBS. 1997;**244**(2):552-560. doi:10.1111/j.1432-1033.1997.00552.x

[52] Liu P, Marzahn MR, Robbins AH, Gutierrez-de-Teran H, Rodriguez D, McClung SH, et al. Recombinant plasmepsin 1 from the human malaria parasite *plasmodium falciparum*: enzymatic characterization, active site inhibitor design, and structural analysis. Biochemistry. 2009;**48**(19):4086-4099. doi:10.1021/bi802059r

[53] Hill J, Tyas L, Phylip LH, Kay J, Dunn BM, Berry C. High level expression and characterisation of Plasmepsin II, an aspartic proteinase from *Plasmodium falciparum*. FEBS Letters. 1994;**352**(2):155-158. doi:10.1016/0014-5793(94)00940-6

[54] Li T, Yowell CA, Beyer BB, Hung SH, Westling J, Lam MT, et al. Recombinant expression and enzymatic subsite characterization of plasmepsin 4 from the four *Plasmodium* species infecting man. Molecular and Biochemical Parasitology. 2004;**135**(1):101-109. doi:10.1016/s0166-6851(04)00032-5

[55] Francis SE, Banerjee R, Goldberg DE. Biosynthesis and maturation of the malaria aspartic hemoglobinases plasmepsins I and II. The Journal of Biological Chemistry. 1997;**272**(23):14961-14968. doi:10.1074/jbc.272.23.14961

[56] Drew ME, Banerjee R, Uffman EW, Gilbertson S, Rosenthal PJ, Goldberg DE. Plasmodium food vacuole plasmepsins are activated by falcipains. The Journal of Biological Chemistry. 2008;**283**(19):12870-12876. doi:10.1074/jbc.M708949200

[57] Rudzinska MA, Trager W, Bray RS. Pinocytotic uptake and the digestion of hemoglobin in malaria parasites. The Journal of Protozoology. 1965;**12**(4):563-576. doi:10.1111/j.1550-7408.1965.tb03256.x

[58] Saliba KJ, Kirk K. pH regulation in the intracellular malaria parasite, *Plasmodium falciparum*. H(+) extrusion via a V-type H(+)-ATPase. The Journal of Biological Chemistry. 1999;**274**(47):33213-33219. doi:10.1074/jbc.274.47.33213

[59] Hayashi M, Yamada H, Mitamura T, Horii T, Yamamoto A, Moriyama Y. Vacuolar H(+)-ATPase localized in plasma membranes of malaria parasite cells, *Plasmodium falciparum*, is involved in regional acidification of parasitized erythrocytes. The Journal of Biological Chemistry. 2000;**275**(44):34353-34358. doi:10.1074/jbc.m003323200

[60] Florens L, Washburn MP, Raine JD, Anthony RM, Grainger M, Haynes JD, et al. A proteomic view of the *Plasmodium falciparum* life cycle. Nature. 2002;**419**(6906):520-526. doi:10.1038/nature01107

[61] Lindner SE, Swearingen KE, Harupa A, Vaughan AM, Sinnis P, Moritz RL, et al. Total and putative surface proteomics of malaria parasite salivary gland sporozoites. Molecular & Cellular Proteomics. 2013;**12**(5):1127-1143. doi:10.1074/mcp.M112.024505

[62] Lasonder E, Janse CJ, van Gemert GJ, Mair GR, Vermunt AM, Douradinha BG, et al. Proteomic profiling of Plasmodium sporozoite maturation identifies new proteins essential for parasite development and infectivity. PLoS Pathogens. 2008;**4**(10):e1000195. doi:10.1371/journal.ppat.1000195

[63] Klemba M, Goldberg DE. Characterization of plasmepsin V, a membrane-bound aspartic protease homolog in the endoplasmic reticulum of *Plasmodium falciparum*. Molecular and Biochemical Parasitology. 2005;**143**(2):183-191. doi:10.1016/j.molbiopara.2005.05.015

[64] Russo I, Babbitt S, Muralidharan V, Butler T, Oksman A, Goldberg DE. Plasmepsin V licenses Plasmodium proteins for export into the host erythrocyte. Nature. 2010;**463**(7281):632-636. doi:10.1038/nature08726

[65] Lopez-Barragan MJ, Lemieux J, Quinones M, Williamson KC, Molina-Cruz A, Cui K, et al. Directional gene expression and antisense transcripts in sexual and asexual stages of *Plasmodium falciparum*. BMC Genomics. 2011;**12**(1):587. doi:10.1186/1471-2164-12-587

[66] Singh AP, Buscaglia CA, Wang Q, Levay A, Nussenzweig DR, Walker JR, et al. Plasmodium circumsporozoite protein promotes the development of the liver stages of the parasite. Cell. 2007;**131**(3):492-504. doi:10.1016/j.cell.2007.09.013

[67] Le Roch KG, Zhou Y, Blair PL, Grainger M, Moch JK, Haynes JD, et al.. Discovery of gene function by expression profiling of the malaria parasite life cycle. Science. 2003;**301**(5639):1503-1508. doi:10.1126/science.1087025

[68] Zhou Y, Ramachandran V, Kumar KA, Westenberger S, Refour P, Zhou B, et al. Evidence-based annotation of the malaria parasite's genome using comparative expression profiling. PLoS One. 2008;**3**(2):e1570. doi:10.1371/journal.pone.0001570

[69] Li F, Bounkeua V, Pettersen K, Vinetz JM. *Plasmodium falciparum* ookinete expression of plasmepsin VII and plasmepsin X. Malaria Journal. 2016;**15**(1):111. doi:10.1186/s12936-016-1161-5

[70] Asawamahasakda W, Ittarat I, Chang CC, McElroy P, Meshnick SR. Effects of antimalarials and protease inhibitors on plasmodial hemozoin production. Molecular and Biochemical Parasitology. 1994;**67**(2):183-191. doi:10.1016/0166-6851(94)00128-6

[71] Orjih AU, Fitch CD. Hemozoin production by *Plasmodium falciparum*: variation with strain and exposure to chloroquine. Biochimica et Biophysica Acta. 1993;**1157**(3):270-274. doi:10.1016/0304-4165(93)90109-l

[72] Yayon A, Vande Waa JA, Yayon M, Geary TG, Jensen JB. Stage-dependent effects of chloroquine on *Plasmodium falciparum* in vitro. The Journal of Protozoology. 1983;**30**(4):642-647. doi:10.1111/j.1550-7408.1983.tb05336.x

[73] Aissi E, Charet P, Bouquelet S, Biguet J. Endoprotease in *Plasmodium yoelii* nigeriensis. Comparative Biochemistry and Physiology B, Comparative Biochemistry. 1983;**74**(3):559-566. doi:10.1016/0305-0491(83)90229-8

[74] Cook L, Grant PT, Kermack WO. Proteolytic enzymes of the erythrocytic forms of roden and simian species of malarial plasmodia. Experimental Parasitology. 1961;**11**(4):372-379. doi:10.1016/0014-4894(61)90041-8

[75] Gyang FN, Poole B, Trager W. Peptidases from *Plasmodium falciparum* cultured in vitro. Molecular and Biochemical Parasitology. 1982;**5**(4):263-273. doi:10.1016/0166-6851(82)90034-2

[76] Hempelmann E, Wilson RJ. Endopeptidases from *Plasmodium knowlesi*. Parasitology. 1980;**80**(2):323-330. doi:10.1017/s0031182000000780

[77] Levy MR, Chou SC. Activity and some properties of an acid proteinase from normal and Plasmodium berghei-infected red cells. The Journal of Parasitology. 1973;**59**(6):1064-1070. doi:10.2307/3278644

[78] Levy MR, Siddiqui WA, Chou SC. Acid protease activity in *Plasmodium falciparum* and *P. knowlesi* and ghosts of their respective host red cells. Nature. 1974;**247**(5442):546-549. doi:10.1038/247546a0

[79] Rosenthal PJ, McKerrow JH, Aikawa M, Nagasawa H, Leech JH. A malarial cysteine proteinase is necessary for hemoglobin degradation by *Plasmodium falciparum*. The Journal of Clinical Investigation. 1988;**82**(5):1560-1566. doi:10.1172/jci113766

[80] Sherman IW, Tanigoshi L. Purification of Plasmodium lophurae cathepsin D and its effects on erythrocyte membrane proteins. Molecular and Biochemical Parasitology. 1983;**8**(3):207-226. doi:10.1016/0166-6851(83)90044-0

[81] Vander Jagt DL, Hunsaker LA, Campos NM. Characterization of a hemoglobin-degrading, low molecular weight protease from *Plasmodium falciparum*. Molecular and Biochemical Parasitology. 1986;**18**(3):389-400. doi:10.1016/0166-6851(86)90095-2

[82] Goldberg DE, Slater AF, Cerami A, Henderson GB. Hemoglobin degradation in the malaria parasite *Plasmodium falciparum*: an ordered process in a unique organelle. Proceedings of the National Academy of Sciences of the United States of America. 1990;**87**(8):2931-2935. doi:10.1073/pnas.87.8.2931

[83] Goldberg DE, Slater AF, Beavis R, Chait B, Cerami A, Henderson GB. Hemoglobin degradation in the human malaria pathogen *Plasmodium falciparum*: a catabolic pathway initiated by a specific aspartic protease. The Journal of Experimental Medicine. 1991;**173**(4):961-969. doi:10.1084/jem.173.4.961

[84] Dickerson RE, Geis I. Hemoglobin: Structure, Function, Evolution, and Pathology. Menlo Park, CA: The Benjamin/Cummings Publishing Company; 1983. 176 p.

[85] Stamatoyannopoulos G, Nienhuis AW, Leder P, Majerus PW, editors. The Molecular Basis of Blood Diseases. Philadelphia: W.B. Saunders Company; 1987. 747 p.

[86] Chugh M, Sundararaman V, Kumar S, Reddy VS, Siddiqui WA, Stuart KD, et al. Protein complex directs hemoglobin-to-hemozoin formation in *Plasmodium falciparum*. Proceedings of the National Academy of Sciences of the United States of America. 2013;**110**(14):5392-5397. doi:10.1073/pnas.1218412110

[87] Sherman IW, Tanigoshi L. Incorporation of 14C-amino-acids by malaria (*Plasmodium lophurae*) IV. In vivo utilization of host cell haemoglobin. International Journal of Biochemistry. 1970;**1**(5):635-637. doi:10.1016/0020-711x(70)90033-9

[88] Sherman IW. Amino acid metabolism and protein synthesis in malarial parasites. Bulletin of the World Health Organization. 1977;**55**(2-3):265-276.

[89] Zarchin S, Krugliak M, Ginsburg H. Digestion of the host erythrocyte by malaria parasites is the primary target for quinoline-containing antimalarials. Biochemical Pharmacology. 1986;**35**(14):2435-2442. doi:10.1016/0006-2952(86)90473-9

[90] Wernsdorfer WH, McGregor I, editors. Malaria: Principles and Practice of Malatiology, Volume 1. Edinburgh: Churchill Livingstone; 1988. 1818 p.

[91] Naughton JA, Nasizadeh S, Bell A. Downstream effects of haemoglobinase inhibition in *Plasmodium falciparum*-infected erythrocytes. Molecular and Biochemical Parasitology. 2010;**173**(2):81-87. doi:10.1016/j.molbiopara.2010.05.007

[92] Ting IP, Sherman IW. Carbon dioxide fixation in malaria—I. Kinetic studies in *plasmodium lophurae*. Comparative biochemistry and physiology. 1966;**19**(4):855-869. doi 10.1016/0010-406x(66)90441-5

[93] Polet H, Conrad ME. Malaria: extracellular amino acid requirements for in vitro growth of erythrocytic forms of *Plasmodium knowlesi*. Proceedings of the Society for Experimental Biology and Medicine Society for Experimental Biology and Medicine. 1968;**127**(1):251-253 doi:10.3181/00379727-127-32666

[94] Krugliak M, Zhang J, Ginsburg H. Intraerythrocytic *Plasmodium falciparum* utilizes only a fraction of the amino acids derived from the digestion of host cell cytosol for the biosynthesis of its proteins. Molecular and Biochemical Parasitology. 2002;**119**(2):249-256. doi:10.1016/s0166-6851(01)00427-3

[95] Lew VL, Tiffert T, Ginsburg H. Excess hemoglobin digestion and the osmotic stability of *Plasmodium falciparum*-infected red blood cells. Blood. 2003;**101**(10):4189-4194. doi:10.1182/blood-2002-08-2654

[96] Le Bonniec S, Deregnaucourt C, Redeker V, Banerjee R, Grellier P, Goldberg DE, et al. Plasmepsin II, an acidic hemoglobinase from the *Plasmodium falciparum* food vacuole, is active at neutral pH on the host erythrocyte membrane skeleton. The Journal of Biological Chemistry. 1999;**274**(20):14218-14223. doi:10.1074/jbc.274.20.14218

[97] Wyatt DM, Berry C. Activity and inhibition of plasmepsin IV, a new aspartic proteinase from the malaria parasite, *Plasmodium falciparum*. FEBS Letters. 2002;**513**(2-3):159-162. doi:10.1016/s0014-5793(02)02241-x

[98] Deguercy A, Hommel M, Schrevel J. Purification and characterization of 37-kilodalton proteases from *Plasmodium falciparum* and *Plasmodium berghei* which cleave erythrocyte cytoskeletal components. Molecular and Biochemical Parasitology. 1990;**38**(2):233-244. doi:10.1016/0166-6851(90)90026-i

[99] Li F, Patra KP, Yowell CA, Dame JB, Chin K, Vinetz JM. Apical surface expression of aspartic protease Plasmepsin 4, a potential transmission-blocking target of the *plasmodium ookinete*. The Journal of Biological Chemistry. 2010;**285**(11):8076-8083. doi:10.1074/jbc.m109.063388

[100] Hiller NL, Bhattacharjee S, van Ooij C, Liolios K, Harrison T, Lopez-Estrano C, et al. A host-targeting signal in virulence proteins reveals a secretome in malarial infection. Science. 2004;**306**(5703):1934-1937. doi:10.1126/science.1102737

[101] Marti M, Good RT, Rug M, Knuepfer E, Cowman AF. Targeting malaria virulence and remodeling proteins to the host erythrocyte. Science. 2004;**306**(5703):1930-1933. doi:10.1126/science.1102452

[102] Sargeant TJ, Marti M, Caler E, Carlton JM, Simpson K, Speed TP, et al. Lineage-specific expansion of proteins exported to erythrocytes in malaria parasites. Genome Biology. 2006;**7**(2):R12. doi:10.1186/gb-2006-7-2-r12

[103] Boddey JA, Moritz RL, Simpson RJ, Cowman AF. Role of the Plasmodium export element in trafficking parasite proteins to the infected erythrocyte. Traffic. 2009;**10**(3):285-299. doi:10.1111/j.1600-0854.2008.00864.x

[104] Boddey JA, Hodder AN, Gunther S, Gilson PR, Patsiouras H, Kapp EA, et al. An aspartyl protease directs malaria effector proteins to the host cell. Nature. 2010;**463**(7281):627-631. doi:10.1038/nature08728

[105] Boddey JA, Carvalho TG, Hodder AN, Sargeant TJ, Sleebs BE, Marapana D, et al. Role of plasmepsin V in export of diverse protein families from the *Plasmodium falciparum* exportome. Traffic. 2013;**14**(5):532-550. doi:10.1111/tra.12053

[106] Marti M, Baum J, Rug M, Tilley L, Cowman AF. Signal-mediated export of proteins from the malaria parasite to the host erythrocyte. The Journal of Cell Biology. 2005;**171**(4):587-592. doi:10.1083/jcb.200508051

[107] Eksi S, Haile Y, Furuya T, Ma L, Su X, Williamson KC. Identification of a subtelomeric gene family expressed during the asexual-sexual stage transition in *Plasmodium falciparum*. Molecular and Biochemical Parasitology. 2005;**143**(1):90-99. doi:10.1016/j.molbiopara.2005.05.010

[108] Spaccapelo R, Janse CJ, Caterbi S, Franke-Fayard B, Bonilla JA, Syphard LM, et al. Plasmepsin 4-deficient *Plasmodium berghei* are virulence attenuated and induce protective immunity against experimental malaria. The American Journal of Pathology. 2010;**176**(1):205-217. doi:10.2353/ajpath.2010.090504

[109] Spaccapelo R, Aime E, Caterbi S, Arcidiacono P, Capuccini B, Di Cristina M, et al. Disruption of plasmepsin-4 and merozoites surface protein-7 genes in *Plasmodium berghei* induces combined virulence-attenuated phenotype. Scientific Reports. 2011;**1**:39. doi:10.1038/srep00039

[110] Pirta C, Sharma NN, Banyal HS. A 43 kDa recombinant plasmepsin elicits immune response in mice against *Plasmodium berghei* malaria. Acta Parasitologica. 2016;**61**(1):102-107. doi:10.1515/ap-2016-0013

[111] Yayon A, Cabantchik ZI, Ginsburg H. Identification of the acidic compartment of *Plasmodium falciparum*-infected human erythrocytes as the target of the antimalarial drug chloroquine. The EMBO Journal. 1984;**3**(11):2695-2700.

[112] Krogstad DJ, Schlesinger PH, Gluzman IY. Antimalarials increase vesicle pH in *Plasmodium falciparum*. The Journal of Cell Biology. 1985;**101**(6):2302-2309. doi:10.1083/jcb.101.6.2302

[113] Luker KE, Francis SE, Gluzman IY, Goldberg DE. Kinetic analysis of plasmepsins I and II aspartic proteases of the *Plasmodium falciparum* digestive vacuole. Molecular and Biochemical Parasitology. 1996;**79**(1):71-78. doi:10.1016/0166-6851(96)02651-5

[114] Lolupiman S, Siripurkpong P, Yuvaniyama J. Disulfide linkages in *Plasmodium falciparum* plasmepsin-i are essential elements for its processing activity and multi-milligram recombinant production yield. PLoS One. 2014;**9**(2):e89424. doi:10.1371/journal.pone.0089424

[115] Xiao H, Tanaka T, Ogawa M, Yada RY. Expression and enzymatic characterization of the soluble recombinant plasmepsin I from *Plasmodium falciparum*. Protein Engineering, Design & Selection. 2007;**20**(12):625-633. doi:10.1093/protein/gzm066

[116] Tyas L, Gluzman I, Moon RP, Rupp K, Westling J, Ridley RG, et al. Naturally-occurring and recombinant forms of the aspartic proteinases plasmepsins I and II from the human malaria parasite *Plasmodium falciparum*. FEBS Letters. 1999;**454**(3):210-214. doi:10.1016/s0014-5793(99)00805-4

[117] James MN, Sielecki AR. Molecular structure of an aspartic proteinase zymogen, porcine pepsinogen, at 1.8Å resolution. Nature. 1986;**319**(6048):33-38. doi:10.1038/319033a0

[118] Moore SA, Sielecki AR, Chernaia MM, Tarasova NI, James MN. Crystal and molecular structures of human progastricsin at 1.62Å resolution. Journal of Molecular Biology. 1995;**247**(3):466-485. doi:10.1006/jmbi.1994.0154

[119] Khan AR, Cherney MM, Tarasova NI, James MN. Structural characterization of activation 'intermediate 2' on the pathway to human gastricsin. Nature Structural Biology. 1997;**4**(12):1010-1015. doi:10.1038/nsb1297-1010

[120] Khan AR, Khazanovich-Bernstein N, Bergmann EM, James MN. Structural aspects of activation pathways of aspartic protease zymogens and viral 3C protease precursors. Proceedings of the National Academy of Sciences of the United States of America. 1999;**96**(20):10968-10975. doi:10.1073/pnas.96.20.10968

[121] Bernstein NK, Cherney MM, Yowell CA, Dame JB, James MN. Structural insights into the activation of *P. vivax* plasmepsin. Journal of Molecular Biology. 2003;**329**(3):505-524. doi:10.1016/s0022-2836(03)00444-3

[122] Siripurkpong P, Yuvaniyama J, Wilairat P, Goldberg DE. Active site contribution to specificity of the aspartic proteases plasmepsins I and II. The Journal of Biological Chemistry. 2002;**277**(43):41009-41013. doi:10.1074/jbc.M204852200

[123] Gulnik SV, Afonina EI, Gustchina E, Yu B, Silva AM, Kim Y, et al. Utility of (His)6 tag for purification and refolding of proplasmepsin-2 and mutants with altered activation properties. Protein Expression and Purification. 2002;**24**(3):412-419. doi:10.1006/prep.2001.1590

[124] Istvan ES, Goldberg DE. Distal substrate interactions enhance plasmepsin activity. The Journal of Biological Chemistry. 2005;**280**(8):6890-6896. doi:10.1074/jbc.M412086200

[125] Beyer BB, Johnson JV, Chung AY, Li T, Madabushi A, Agbandje-McKenna M, et al. Active-site specificity of digestive aspartic peptidases from the four species of Plasmodium that infect humans using chromogenic combinatorial peptide libraries. Biochemistry. 2005;**44**(6):1768-1779. doi:10.1021/bi047886u

[126] Westling J, Yowell CA, Majer P, Erickson JW, Dame JB, Dunn BM. *Plasmodium falciparum, P. vivax,* and *P. malariae*: a comparison of the active site properties of plasmepsins cloned and expressed from three different species of the malaria parasite. Experimental Parasitology. 1997;**87**(3):185-193. doi:10.1006/expr.1997.4225

[127] Westling J, Cipullo P, Hung SH, Saft H, Dame JB, Dunn BM. Active site specificity of plasmepsin II. Protein Science: a Publication of the Protein Society. 1999;**8**(10):2001-2009. doi:10.1110/ps.8.10.2001

[128] Xiao H, Sinkovits AF, Bryksa BC, Ogawa M, Yada RY. Recombinant expression and partial characterization of an active soluble histo-aspartic protease from *Plasmodium falciparum*. Protein Expression and Purification. 2006;**49**(1):88-94. doi:10.1016/j.pep.2006.02.022

[129] Xiao H, Briere LA, Dunn SD, Yada RY. Characterization of the monomer-dimer equilibrium of recombinant histo-aspartic protease from *Plasmodium falciparum*. Molecular and Biochemical Parasitology. 2010;**173**(1):17-24. doi:10.1016/j.molbiopara.2010.04.008

[130] Andreeva N, Bogdanovich P, Kashparov I, Popov M, Stengach M. Is histoaspartic protease a serine protease with a pepsin-like fold?. Proteins. 2004;**55**(3):705-710. doi:10.1002/prot.20078

[131] Bjelic S, Aqvist J. Computational prediction of structure, substrate binding mode, mechanism, and rate for a malaria protease with a novel type of active site. Biochemistry. 2004;**43**(46):14521-14528. doi:10.1021/bi048252q

[132] Parr CL, Tanaka T, Xiao H, Yada RY. The catalytic significance of the proposed active site residues in *Plasmodium falciparum* histoaspartic protease. The FEBS Journal. 2008;**275**(8):1698-1707. doi:10.1111/j.1742-4658.2008.06325.x

[133] Liu P, Robbins AH, Marzahn MR, McClung SH, Yowell CA, Stevens SM, Jr., et al. Enzymatic Characterization of recombinant food Vacuole Plasmepsin 4 from the Rodent Malaria Parasite *Plasmodium berghei*. PLoS One. 2015;**10**(10):e0141758. doi:10.1371/journal.pone.0141758

[134] Kim JH, Johannes L, Goud B, Antony C, Lingwood CA, Daneman R, et al. Noninvasive measurement of the pH of the endoplasmic reticulum at rest and during calcium release. Proceedings of the National Academy of Sciences of the United States of America. 1998;**95**(6):2997-3002. doi:10.1073/pnas.95.6.2997

[135] Tarr SJ, Cryar A, Thalassinos K, Haldar K, Osborne AR. The C-terminal portion of the cleaved HT motif is necessary and sufficient to mediate export of proteins from the malaria parasite into its host cell. Molecular Microbiology. 2013;**87**(4):835-850. doi:10.1111/mmi.12133

[136] Boonyalai N, Sittikul P, Yuvaniyama J. *Plasmodium falciparum* Plasmepsin V (PfPMV): insights into recombinant expression, substrate specificity and active site structure. Molecular and Biochemical Parasitology. 2015;**201**(1):5-15. doi:10.1016/j.molbiopara.2015.05.004

[137] Xiao H, Bryksa BC, Bhaumik P, Gustchina A, Kiso Y, Yao SQ, et al. The zymogen of plasmepsin V from *Plasmodium falciparum* is enzymatically active. Molecular and Biochemical Parasitology. 2014;**197**(1-2):56-63. doi:10.1016/j.molbiopara.2014.10.004

[138] Bedi RK, Patel C, Mishra V, Xiao H, Yada RY, Bhaumik P. Understanding the structural basis of substrate recognition by *Plasmodium falciparum* plasmepsin V to aid in the design of potent inhibitors. Scientific Reports. 2016;**6**:31420. doi:10.1038/srep31420

[139] Sappakhaw K, Takasila R, Sittikul P, Wattana-Amorn P, Assavalapsakul W, Boonyalai N. Biochemical characterization of plasmepsin V from *Plasmodium vivax* Thailand isolates: substrate specificity and enzyme inhibition. Molecular and Biochemical Parasitology. 2015;**204**(2):51-63. doi:10.1016/j.molbiopara.2016.01.003

[140] Bailly E, Jambou R, Savel J, Jaureguiberry G. *Plasmodium falciparum*: differential sensitivity in vitro to E-64 (cysteine protease inhibitor) and Pepstatin A (aspartyl protease inhibitor). The Journal of Protozoology. 1992;**39**(5):593-599. doi:10.1111/j.1550-7408.1992.tb04856.x

[141] Andrews KT, Fairlie DP, Madala PK, Ray J, Wyatt DM, Hilton PM, et al. Potencies of human immunodeficiency virus protease inhibitors in vitro against *Plasmodium falciparum* and in vivo against murine malaria. Antimicrobial Agents and Chemotherapy. 2006;**50**(2):639-648. doi:10.1128/AAC.50.2.639-648.2006

[142] Meyers MJ, Goldberg DE. Recent advances in plasmepsin medicinal chemistry and implications for future antimalarial drug discovery efforts. Current Topics in Medicinal Chemistry. 2012;**12**(5):445-455. doi:10.2174/156802612799362959

[143] Ersmark K, Samuelsson B, Hallberg A. Plasmepsins as potential targets for new antimalarial therapy. Medicinal Research Reviews. 2006;**26**(5):626-666. doi:10.1002/med.20082

[144] Noteberg D, Schaal W, Hamelink E, Vrang L, Larhed M. High-speed optimization of inhibitors of the malarial proteases plasmepsin I and II. Journal of Combinatorial Chemistry. 2003;**5**(4):456-464. doi:10.1021/cc0301014

[145] Noteberg D, Hamelink E, Hulten J, Wahlgren M, Vrang L, Samuelsson B, et al. Design and synthesis of plasmepsin I and plasmepsin II inhibitors with activity in *Plasmodium falciparum*-infected cultured human erythrocytes. Journal of Medicinal Chemistry. 2003;**46**(5):734-746. doi:10.1021/jm020951i

[146] Nezami A, Luque I, Kimura T, Kiso Y, Freire E. Identification and characterization of allophenylnorstatine-based inhibitors of plasmepsin II, an antimalarial target. Biochemistry. 2002;**41**(7):2273-2280. doi:10.1021/bi0117549

[147] Nezami A, Kimura T, Hidaka K, Kiso A, Liu J, Kiso Y, et al. High-affinity inhibition of a family of *Plasmodium falciparum* proteases by a designed adaptive inhibitor. Biochemistry. 2003;**42**(28):8459-8464. doi:10.1021/bi034131z

[148] Hidaka K, Kimura T, Ruben AJ, Uemura T, Kamiya M, Kiso A, et al. Antimalarial activity enhancement in hydroxymethylcarbonyl (HMC) isostere-based dipeptidomimetics targeting malarial aspartic protease plasmepsin. Bioorganic & Medicinal Chemistry. 2008;**16**(23):10049-10060. doi:10.1016/j.bmc.2008.10.011

[149] Skinner-Adams TS, McCarthy JS, Gardiner DL, Hilton PM, Andrews KT. Antiretrovirals as antimalarial agents. Journal of Infectious Diseases. 2004;**190**(11):1998-2000. doi:10.1086/425584

[150] Skinner-Adams TS, Andrews KT, Melville L, McCarthy J, Gardiner DL. Synergistic interactions of the antiretroviral protease inhibitors saquinavir and ritonavir with chloroquine and mefloquine against *Plasmodium falciparum* in vitro. Antimicrobial Agents and Chemotherapy. 2007;**51**(2):759-762. doi:10.1128/AAC.00840-06

[151] Hobbs CV, Voza T, Coppi A, Kirmse B, Marsh K, Borkowsky W, et al.. HIV protease inhibitors inhibit the development of preerythrocytic-stage plasmodium parasites. Journal of Infectious Diseases. 2009;**199**(1):134-141. doi:10.1086/594369

[152] Liu K, Shi H, Xiao H, Chong AG, Bi X, Chang YT, et al. Functional profiling, identification, and inhibition of plasmepsins in intraerythrocytic malaria parasites. Angewandte Chemie International Edition in English. 2009;**48**(44):8293-8297. doi:10.1002/anie.200903747

[153] Bonilla JA, Moura PA, Bonilla TD, Yowell CA, Fidock DA, Dame JB. Effects on growth, hemoglobin metabolism and paralogous gene expression resulting from disruption of genes encoding the digestive vacuole plasmepsins of *Plasmodium falciparum*. International Journal for Parasitology. 2007;**37**(3-4):317-327. doi:10.1016/j.ijpara.2006.11.008

[154] Omara-Opyene AL, Moura PA, Sulsona CR, Bonilla JA, Yowell CA, Fujioka H, et al.. Genetic disruption of the *Plasmodium falciparum* digestive vacuole plasmepsins demonstrates their functional redundancy. The Journal of Biological Chemistry. 2004;**279**(52):54088-54096. doi:10.1074/jbc.M409605200

[155] Bonilla JA, Bonilla TD, Yowell CA, Fujioka H, Dame JB. Critical roles for the digestive vacuole plasmepsins of *Plasmodium falciparum* in vacuolar function. Molecular Microbiology. 2007;**65**(1):64-75. doi:10.1111/j.1365-2958.2007.05768.x

[156] Liu J, Gluzman IY, Drew ME, Goldberg DE. The role of *Plasmodium falciparum* food vacuole plasmepsins. The Journal of Biological Chemistry. 2005;**280**(2):1432-1437. doi:10.1074/jbc.M409740200

[157] Liu J, Istvan ES, Gluzman IY, Gross J, Goldberg DE. *Plasmodium falciparum* ensures its amino acid supply with multiple acquisition pathways and redundant proteolytic enzyme systems. Proceedings of the National Academy of Sciences of the United States of America. 2006;**103**(23):8840-8845. doi:10.1073/pnas.0601876103

[158] Parikh S, Gut J, Istvan E, Goldberg DE, Havlir DV, Rosenthal PJ. Antimalarial activity of human immunodeficiency virus type 1 protease inhibitors. Antimicrobial Agents and Chemotherapy. 2005;**49**(7):2983-2985. doi:10.1128/AAC.49.7.2983-2985.2005

[159] Ersmark K, Feierberg I, Bjelic S, Hamelink E, Hackett F, Blackman MJ, et al. Potent inhibitors of the *Plasmodium falciparum* enzymes plasmepsin I and II devoid of cathepsin D inhibitory activity. Journal of Medicinal Chemistry. 2004;**47**(1):110-122. doi:10.1021/jm030933g

[160] Guatam B, Lucia G, Suping J, Karl AW. Activity of Amidine-containing Diphenylureas Against *P. falciparum*. Letters in Drug Design & Discovery. 2005;**2**(2):162-164. doi:10.2174/1570180053175061

[161] Moura PA, Dame JB, Fidock DA. Role of *Plasmodium falciparum* digestive vacuole plasmepsins in the specificity and antimalarial mode of action of cysteine and aspartic protease inhibitors. Antimicrobial Agents and Chemotherapy. 2009;**53**(12):4968-4978. doi:10.1128/AAC.00882-09

[162] Sleebs BE, Lopaticki S, Marapana DS, O'Neill MT, Rajasekaran P, Gazdik M, et al. Inhibition of Plasmepsin V activity demonstrates its essential role in protein export, PfEMP1 display, and survival of malaria parasites. PLoS Biology. 2014;**12**(7):e1001897. doi:10.1371/journal.pbio.1001897

[163] Sleebs BE, Gazdik M, O'Neill MT, Rajasekaran P, Lopaticki S, Lackovic K, et al. Transition state mimetics of the Plasmodium export element are potent inhibitors of Plasmepsin V from *P. falciparum* and *P. vivax*. Journal of Medicinal Chemistry. 2014;**57**(18):7644-7662. doi:10.1021/jm500797g

[164] Gazdik M, Jarman KE, O'Neill MT, Hodder AN, Lowes KN, Jousset Sabroux H, et al. Exploration of the P3 region of PEXEL peptidomimetics leads to a potent inhibitor of the Plasmodium protease, plasmepsin V. Bioorganic & Medicinal Chemistry. 2016;**24**(9):1993-2010. doi:10.1016/j.bmc.2016.03.027

[165] Hodder AN, Sleebs BE, Czabotar PE, Gazdik M, Xu Y, O'Neill MT, et al. Structural basis for plasmepsin V inhibition that blocks export of malaria proteins to human erythrocytes. Nature Structural & Molecular Biology. 2015;**22**(8):590-596. doi:10.1038/nsmb.3061

Chapter 9

Vaccination against *Trichinella spiralis*: Potential, Limitations and Future Directions

Jonathan I. Andrade-Becerra,
Ericka N. Pompa-Mera,
Rosa María Ribas-Aparicio and Lilián Yépez-Mulia

Additional information is available at the end of the chapter

http://dx.doi.org/10.5772/66499

Abstract

Trichinellosis is a food-borne parasitic disease caused by round worms of the genus *Trichinella*. The majority of human outbreaks are attributed to consumption of raw or undercooked pork meat contaminated with *T. spiralis* muscle larvae. A blocking-transmission vaccine against trichinellosis will allow preventing swine infection and will contribute to disease control. In this chapter, different vaccine candidates so far developed against *T. spiralis*, including first-, second-, and third-generation vaccines, are discussed. Most vaccine candidates are based on a unique antigen mainly from the muscle larva stage, inducing with some exceptions, partial protection although a mix Th1/Th2 immune response is elicited. Therefore, the need for identification of new antigens from different parasite stages focusing on infective intestinal larvae, adult, and newborn larvae stages as well as the evaluation of their protective capacity in pigs is presented. The design of multi-epitope vaccines and the use of adjuvants or immunomodulatory molecules capable to polarize the immune response to a Th2-type-protective response are discussed as imperative elements of modern vaccines. Plant-based vaccines and probiotics as excellent tools for vaccine development against *T. spiralis* are also presented as an attractive platform for veterinary vaccines.

Keywords: *Trichinella spiralis*, DNA vaccine, live carriers, edible vaccines, probiotics

1. Introduction

Trichinellosis is a significant global zoonotic disease produced by the nematode species of the genus *Trichinella*. Trichinellosis is an emerging and reemerging disease in many countries [1]. In the international ranking of food-borne parasites, *T. spiralis* was ranked among the top 10 [2]. *T. spiralis* is the best characterized member of *Trichinella* genus since it is highly infective for sylvatic and domestic animals as well as for humans. Besides, its life cycle can be maintained in experimental animals, providing information about host-parasite relationships and immunity. Infection with *T. spiralis* initiates when the host ingests raw or undercooked meat contaminated with encysted muscle larvae (ML) (**Figure 1**). The larvae are released from muscle tissue by host digestive enzymes in the stomach. Then, ML migrates to the small intestine where they penetrate the intestinal mucosa and undergo four successive molts, becoming mature adult worms. This intestinal phase is the first stage in the host-parasite interplay. At days 1 and 2 post infection, newborn larvae (NBL) are released by female adult worm and spread via the blood and lymphatic systems to striated muscle, where they invade the myofibers, develop into ML, and induce the transformation of infected cells to the nurse-cell complex.

T. spiralis continues to be the causative agent in most outbreaks in humans. The majority of outbreaks are attributed to domestic pork maintained in small farms or non-controlled outdoor backyard pigs, where poor husbandry conditions place pigs at high risk. From 1986 to 2009, there were 65,818 cases and 42 deaths reported from 41 countries, 50% of those occurred in Romania, mainly during 1990–1999 [3]. In China, from 2005 to 2009, 15 outbreaks of human trichinellosis with 1387 cases and four deaths were recorded in three provinces of southwestern China. Twelve of these 15 outbreaks were caused by the eating of raw or undercooked pork meat [4]. The animal health situation varies between different countries being Argentina and some Eastern European countries where most of the cases were reported in pigs in 2015 [5].

T. spiralis infection induces a complex host immune response against a diversity of stage-specific antigens. Up to now, it is well known that during the intestinal phase of infection, the immune response involves a Th1/Th2 response with predominance of the Th2 phenotype characterized by the production of high levels of cytokines IL-4, IL-5, IL-9, and IL-10 as well as IgE, IgG1, and the mobilization of eosinophils and mast cells. Furthermore, the long-lasting

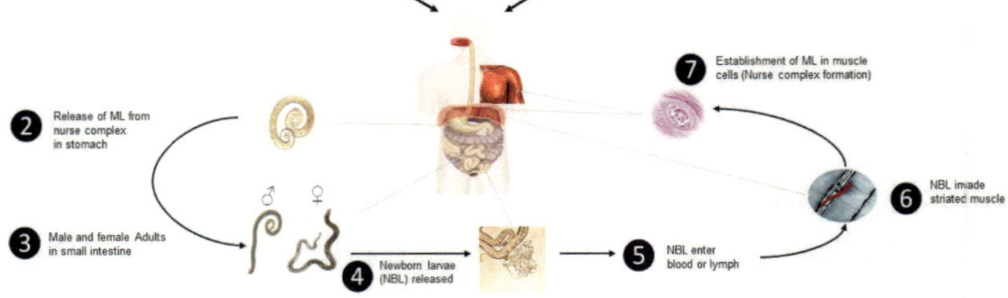

Figure 1. *Trichinella spiralis* life cycle.

http://dx.doi.org/10.5772/66499

infection of muscles with *Trichinella* reflects successful immunomodulation of the immune response, mainly characterized by a Th2 phenotype [6].

Despite the availability of effective and relatively safe drugs such as albendazole and mebendazole for trichinellosis treatment, chemotherapy has several disadvantages such as treatment failure, parasite drug resistance, poor drug absorption in the intestinal lumen, and low bioavailability. Besides, traditional anthelminthic drugs are active against enteric stages of *T. spiralis*, but currently no anthelminthic drug has proven to be effective against the parasite systemic stages [7, 8]. Furthermore, serious side effects including bone marrow suppression and teratogenic effects are observed [7, 8].

An alternative for trichinellosis control is vaccination of livestock. Indeed, veterinary vaccines have already made enormous impacts not only on animal health, welfare, and production but also on human health [9]. Vaccines have been demonstrated to be efficient, reliable, and sustainable method to control parasitic infections, and have been referred as a green solution [10].

The aim of this chapter is to update the advances so far achieved in the development of a transmission-blocking vaccine against trichinellosis to prevent swine infection. Trichinellosis vaccine would make a practical contribution to disease control, reducing the production of residues in meat and food chain, eliminating the risk for the consumer and in some cases to improve the productivity of the individual animal.

The first part of the review presents an overview of *T. spiralis* antigenic molecules proposed as first- and second-generation vaccines, discussing the need for identifying and characterizing antigenic molecules from NBL and adult worm, mainly recognized by *T. spiralis*-infected swine, administered with adjuvants or delivered by carrier systems. The second part provides a description of third-generation vaccines (DNA vaccines) delivered as naked DNA or by carrier systems. Some experimental data recently obtained by our research group using second- and third-generation vaccines will be presented. Finally, the alternative use of adjuvants, multi-epitope vaccines, plants as a system to express antigenic molecules, and probiotics to protect against parasite infection will be discussed too.

2. First- and second-generation vaccines against trichinellosis

The biggest challenge for vaccine development is the identification of the best *T. spiralis* antigens that elicit host-protective immunity in terms of safety and protection at the both enteral and systemic levels. Different antigenic preparations from different parasite stages using different adjuvants have been tested as vaccine candidates. Most information related to immunity elicited by vaccine candidates have been mainly obtained from rodent models and only few studies have been performed in pigs.

2.1. First-generation vaccines

First-generation vaccines developed against trichinellosis include the use of autoclaved *T. spiralis* larvae and inactivated ML administered with complete Freund's adjuvant (CFA). These types of vaccines induced in immunized mice significant ML burden reduction, as well as degeneration and hyalinization of the nurse-cell structure, accompanied by early pericystic fibrosis [11, 12]. In addition, antigenic preparations from the different stages of *T. spiralis* have been used in protection assays in mice. In this way, adult total extracts and ML total extracts provided protection against adult (89–74%) and ML (80%) stages. Importantly, ML total extracts induced the reduction of female fecundity (74%). The combination of adult and ML total extracts reduced the adult and ML load by 96% and 86%, respectively, and 73% reduction in female fecundity [13]. Protection assays performed in pigs have explored the use of excretory/secretory (E/S) antigens from *T. spiralis* ML and NBL total extracts [14, 15]. E/S products administered with CFA or aluminum hydroxide induced moderate protection mainly directed against the fecundity of female worms [14]. On the other hand, NBL killed by freezing and thawing combined with CFA were highly protective in swine (78%) against *T. spiralis* challenge, compared to 40% protection elicited with E/S products of ML [15]. These assays established that in pigs the immune response is mainly directed against fecundity of female worms and to the NBL.

It is worth mentioning that most of the studies have focused on ML antigens. Indeed, ML antigens are released and presented to the host immune system twice: by ingested ML in the intestine, and again when the new generation of ML becomes resident in muscle cells. Besides, ML antigens play an important role in the invasion of intestinal epithelium and therefore in the establishment of the infection in muscle cells. Even more, *T. spiralis* ML surface and E/S antigens are recognized by a wide range of hosts [16]. The carbohydrate epitope tyvelose confers the immunodominance to surface and E/S ML antigens [17]. Anti-tyvelose antibodies inhibit parasite invasion of an *in vitro* model of epithelial cells [18, 19]; however, tyvelose failed to elicit in mice a protective immune response against the enteral phase of infection [20].

Because of their antigenicity, the protection induced by ML surface and E/S products was extensively evaluated in mice [21–23]. In all these assays, partial protection against *T. spiralis* challenge was obtained as assessed by the reduction of adult and ML burden as well as female worm fecundity (35–58%).

A further step was achieved with surface and E/S stage-specific antigens purified by specific monoclonal antibodies [21, 24]. These antigens administered with CFA protected mice against parasite challenge, as determined by ML load reduction (29.6 and 50%, respectively). Protection induced by purified E/S products (49 and 55 kDa) was similar to that achieved when total E/S products were used [21].

Other E/S products, mainly glycoprotein of Mr 53 kDa (gp53) and 43 kDa (gp43), were widely investigated as first-generation vaccines. The role of these glycoproteins as mediators of intestinal epithelial cell invasion and niche establishment of *T. spiralis* has been suggested [18]. Even more, it was shown that antibodies against these glycoproteins inhibit *in the vitro* invasion of intestinal epithelial by *T. spiralis* [19]. Therefore, gp43 and gp53 are considered good vaccine candidates.

2.2. Second-generation vaccines

The 40- and 30-mer peptides derived from gp43 were synthesized and tested in protection assays [25, 26], giving rise to the development of second-generation vaccines against trichinellosis. The 40- and 30-mer synthetic peptides were administered to mice by intranasal (i.n.) or subcutaneous route with adjuvants such as the subunit B of cholera toxin (CTB) or incomplete Freund's adjuvant (IFA). The 40- and 30-mer synthetic peptides induced a significant reduction of adult worm burden against *T. spiralis* infection in comparison to control (36 and 64%, respectively). The immune response was characterized by the production of IgG1. Although the use of the synthetic peptides represents an innovative strategy for vaccine development, protection induced was not higher than that elicited with crude total extracts.

The induction of mucosal immunity plays an important aspect to be considered in the design of a blocking-transmission vaccine in which the use of liposomes, viral particles, and bacterial carriers has been used to deliver the selected antigen [27–31].

In this regard, *Salmonella*-based vaccine systems are considered among the most advanced and promising technologies developed to induce immunological protection against enteric pathogens because of their ability to both colonize the small intestine and invade non-phagocytic epithelial cells, thus allowing access to the underlying lymphoid tissue [32]. Taking advance of the use of *Salmonella* as live bacterial carrier, our group developed a *Salmonella* vaccine candidate expressing the 30-mer peptide derived from gp43 (amino acid residues 210–239, designated as Ag30) from *T. spiralis* ML. The autotransporter ShdA was employed to translocate Ag30 peptide to the surface of *S. enterica* serovar Typhimurium SL3261 [27]. Mice immuzed by i.n. route with the recombinant *Salmonella* pAg30 elicited a protective immune response against *T. spiralis* challenge, with 61.83% reduction of the adult burden and production of antigen-specific IgG1 and IL-5 (**Figure 2**). The use of the autotransporter MisL has also been used to translocate Ag30 to the surface of *S. enterica* serovar Typhimurium SL3261. The immunization of mice with the recombinant vaccine (i.n. route) in combination with an intraperitoneal (i.p.) boost with the recombinant protein induced a higher level of protection (76%) against the enteral phase of *T. spiralis* infection [28]. In addition, our group explore the use of the 40-mer peptide of *T. spiralis* gp43 protein (named Ag40) expressed on the surface of *S. enterica* serovar Typhimurium SL3261 using the autotransporter ShdA (*Salmonella* pAg40). Partial protection against *T. spiralis* infection at the enteral level was induced (47%). The use of *Salmonella* pAg30 together with *Salmonella* pAg40 did not elicit higher protection against *T. spiralis* infection (58%) [33].

To enhance the humoral and cellular antigen-specific immune response against *T. spiralis* infection, multiple copies of the minimum binding domain of complement C3 component (P28) were used as molecular adjuvant. For this, *Salmonella* pAg30 vaccine was engineered to express the Ag30 peptide from *T. spiralis* fused to three copies of P28 adjuvant (Ag30-P28$_3$) and was either expressed on the bacterial surface or secreted to the milieu [31]. *Salmonella* vaccines were administered to mice by i.n. route. Data showed that *Salmonella* strains secreting Ag30-P28$_3$ or Ag30 reduced the adult worm burden by 92.8 and 72%, respectively, following the challenge with *T. spiralis* ML compared to 42% achieved by recombinant *Salmonella* displaying Ag30-P28$_3$ on the surface (**Figure 2**). The protection induced by secreted Ag30-P28$_3$ was associated with a mixed Th1/Th2 with predominance of Th2 phenotype, characterized by the production of IgG1, intestinal IgA antibodies, and IL-5 secretion.

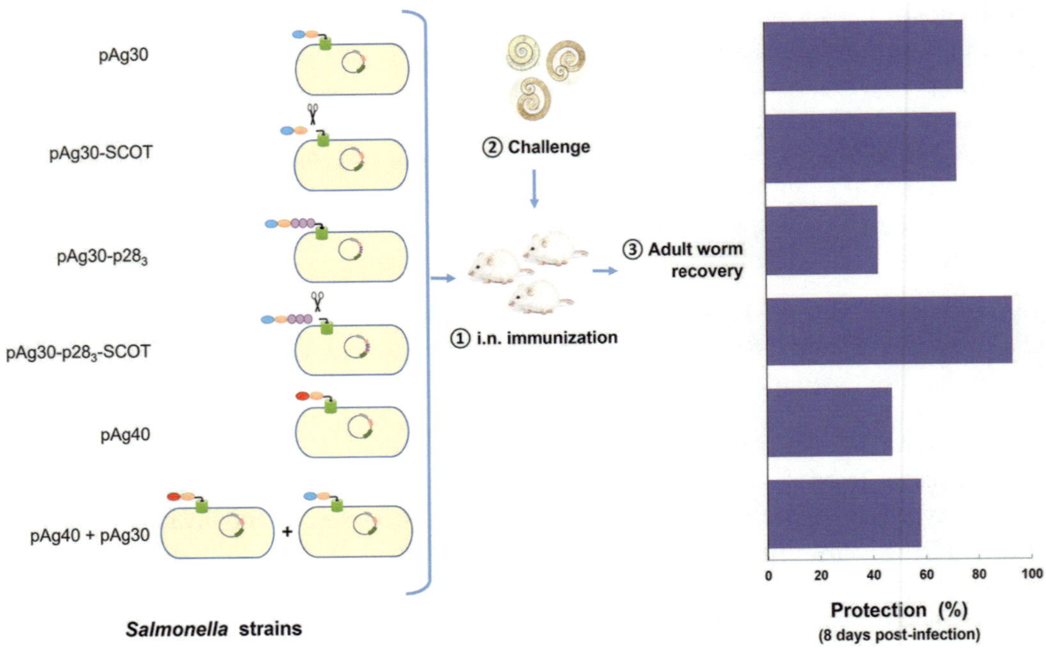

Figure 2. Protection in mice induced by recombinant *Salmonella enterica* serovar Typhimurium strains against the challenge with *Trichinella spiralis* muscle larvae. Attenuated *Salmonella* expresses Ag30 or Ag40 derived from the gp43 of *T. spiralis* muscle larvae displayed on the surface of recombinant *Salmonella* strains. In addition, Ag30 was fused to three copies of the molecular adjuvant P28 (Ag30-P28$_3$) and it was expressed on the bacterial surface or secreted to the medium through OmpT protease site (SCOT).

Some new surface and E/S proteins from ML (some of them expressed in other stages of the parasite) have been identified and their recombinant proteins evaluated as vaccine candidates. The surface protein 28.9 kDa (Ts14-3-3) [34], the E/S protein of 35.5 kDa (TspSP1.2) [35], 54.7 kDa amino peptidase (TsAP) also expressed by adult worms and NBL, located primarily at the cuticle and internal organs of the parasite [36], the protein of 20 kDa (Ts-ES-1) existing in the E/S products of *T. spiralis* adult and ML [37], and paramyosin (Ts-Pmy) [38] among others have been tested in mice. In all cases, partial protection assessed against the enteral and muscle phase of the infection was elicited (35–55%). Interestingly, a multiple epitope vaccine was developed including a highly antigenic epitope of Ts-Pmy (8F7) and an epitope (M7) from Ts-87 antigen (present in adult worm). Epitopes were conjugated to KLH and mixed to formulate a multi-epitope vaccine. This vaccine induced partial protection (35%) against *T. spiralis* infection in mice [30]. Protection elicited was not higher than that obtained with 8F7 or M7 alone.

Importantly, it was shown that ML cannot invade the intestinal epithelial cells *in vitro* cultured unless they are exposed to the intestinal milieu or bile and activated into the intestinal infective larvae (IIL) [39–41]. The identification of IIL molecules provides attractive information not only to elucidate the mechanism of parasite invasion and immune evasion but also to

http://dx.doi.org/10.5772/66499

identify possible molecular targets for vaccine. Following this purpose, several IIL molecules have been identified and their protective capacity evaluated. The Tsp10 polypeptide of *T. spiralis* IIL displayed on the surface of T7 phage was injected i.p. and intradermally at different sites of the abdomen, and elicited in immunized mice a Th2-protective response against parasite challenge, reducing the adult and ML load by 62.8 and 78.6%, respectively [29].

Other proteins with significant higher expression in IIL than in ML such as a putative copper/zinc superoxide dismutase (SODC), adult-specific DNase II, putative low-density lipoprotein receptor domain class A (LDLRA), and secreting receptor (SR) have been identified [41]. More recently, some important proteins were identified in E/S from IIL, such as the gp53 kDa with serine protease activity, multi-cystatin-like domain and cystatin-like protein, deoxyribonuclease II family protein, among others [42]. The protective evaluation of recombinant cystatin-like protein from *T. spiralis* IIL administered in mice with CFA and boosted with recombinant protein with IFA showed 62 and 64% reduction in the number of ML and adult worm, respectively. Interestingly, it was recognized by pig antiserum as early as 15 days post infection [43].

T. spiralis protein Nudix hydrolase (TsNd) is an up-regulated gene in IIL compared to ML. Recombinant TsNd emulsified with CFA displayed in mice a 57.7 and 56.9% reduction in adult worms and in ML burden, respectively, after a challenge infection with *T. spiralis* with high IgG1 levels [44].

Although rodent models have provided important knowledge about the immune response elicited against *T. spiralis* and immunogenic molecules recognized by sera from infected animals, it is important to mention two important aspects of trichinellosis that should be taken into account for the development of a vaccine. First, domestic pork consumption still accounts for many trichinellosis outbreaks, mostly in Eastern Europe and Argentina, where backyard pigs are raised under high-risk-rearing practices, especially the feeding of food waste. Second, a small number of studies have characterized adult antigens that stimulate immunity during an early infection and could be effective in host protection. In this way, recent studies have identified proteins from adult and ML that are recognized by sera of pigs experimentally infected with *T. spiralis* [45, 46]. Some proteins common from adult and ML stage have been identified, among them heat-shock proteins (HSPs), enolase, and 5'-nucleotidase. It was shown that HSP70 and a 38 kDa protein (Ts87) that is present in E/S products and on the adult cuticle induced protective immunity in mice assessed by ML burden reduction (38.4 and 29%, respectively) [46, 47].

It is worth noting that another important aspect that has to be considered is the anti-fecundity effects and immunity to the NBL described in *T. spiralis*-infected pigs [48]. Therefore, the identification of immunogenic proteins characteristic of NBL is important for the induction of protection and vaccine development that could be applied in swine. In this regard, an immunodominant serine protease, named NBL1, has been identified in NBL, embryos, and larvae before birth within the gravid females [49]. Importantly, sera from pigs experimentally infected with *Trichinella* and pigs immunized with the recombinant C terminal part of NBL1 allowed the recognition and identification of six immunodominant linear epitopes on the protein [50]. These epitopes could be used for the development of subunit and multiple epitope vaccines.

2.3. Third-generation vaccines

DNA vaccines allow the *in vivo* expression of antigens in their native conformation, persistent expression of the desired antigen, and the induction of both humoral and cellular immunity [51]. Up to date, three DNA vaccines for veterinary use have been licensured (against West Nile equine virus, melanoma in dogs, and hematopoietic necrosis virus in salmon) [52], encouraging the improvement of experimental DNA vaccines against trichinellosis.

Several DNA vaccines using the eukaryotic expression vector pcDNA3.1 have been designed against *T. spiralis* infection and the induced immune response in mice evaluated. The 31 kDa E/S antigen of ML (TspE1) and TsNd, an up-regulated gene in IIL compared to ML, have been cloned in pcDNA3.1 vector [53, 54]. Recombinant pcDNA3.1-TsNd vaccine conferred higher levels of protection against *T. spiralis* infection in comparison to pcDNA3.1-TsE1. Vaccination of mice with pcDNA3.1-TsNd showed 40.44% reduction in worm adults and 53.9% reduction in ML burden with the production of a mixed Th1/Th2 systemic immune response and IgA production at the mucosal level [54]. In this case, the use of pcDNA3.1/TsNd did not increase the protection previously conferred by recombinant TsNd (57.7 and 56.9% reduction in adult and ML burden, respectively) [44].

The eukaryotic expression vector pVAX1 has also been used to express different *T. spiralis* antigens such as macrophage migration inhibitory factor (MIF) of *T. spiralis* (TsMIF), the protein domain of multi-cystatin-type 1 (MCD-1) (TsMCD-1), and the co-expression of TsMIF and TsMCD-1. Vaccination of mice with the recombinant vaccines induced low levels of protection (23.17% reduction of ML load) [55]. Slightly higher protection was achieved when pVAX1-ubiquitin vaccine was used (37.95%) [56]. In addition, the recombinant vaccines pVAX1-Ts87 and pVAX1-TsPmy conferred 9.7 and 46.6% protection against parasite challenge [57, 58]. Higher levels of protection (43.8%) were obtained when animals were co-immunized with pVAX1-Ts87 and recombinant Ts87. In both cases, a Th1/Th2 immune response was induced [57].

To avoid degradation of DNA vaccines by nucleases, the use of live carriers has been investigated. In this way, pVAX1-Ts87 and pcDNA3.1/TsNd were delivered by *S.* typhimurium strains SL7207 and SL1344, respectively [59, 60]. Mice immunized with *Salmonella* pcDNA3.1/TsNd showed higher levels of protection assessed by adult (73.32%) and ML (49.5%) load reduction [60]. In this case, higher protection at the enteral level was achieved than with the use of the DNA vaccine alone (73.32 vs. 40.44%).

2.3.1. DNA vaccine encoding Ag30

Since DNA vaccines have several advantages over protein vaccines, our research group developed a DNA vaccine encoding Ag30 using the pVAX1 vector (pVAX1-Ag30). The intramuscular administration of 50-μg pVAX1-Ag30 induced 54% reduction of adult burden in mice.

The use of *Salmonella* to deliver pVAX1-Ag30 failed to elicit higher protection levels at the intestinal level (22%) (data not published).

The use of liposomes as carriers of plasmid DNA has been used for vaccination purposes in various studies, because they act as adjuvants and protect plasmids from the attack of host enzymes [61]. It was our interest to assess the protection elicited by lipoplexes formed with 3-μg pVAXAg30 and cationic liposomes (LLO-LLE plus cholesterol, L-lysyl-octadecanol, and L-lysyl eicosanol). The intranasal administration of the lipoplexes induced in mice very low levels of protection against *T. spiralis* infection (7 and 9% reduction of adult and ML burden) (data not published).

Second generation	**Protection %**	**Reference**
Recombinant TsPmy	ML 36.2	[38]
Recombinant TsNd	A 57.7 ML 56.9	[44]
Recombinant Ts87	ML 39.7	[57]
30-mer synthetic peptide (Ag30)	A 36	[26]
Salmonella pAg30	A 61.8	[27]
Salmonella pAg30 (secreted)	A 72	[31]
Salmonella pAg30-p28$_3$ (secreted)	A 92.8	[31]
Salmonella pAg30-p28$_3$ (surface)	A 42	[31]
Phage T7-Tsp10	A 62.8 ML 78.6	[29]
Multi-epitope (Tspmy, TS87)	ML 35	[30]
Third generation		
pcDNA3.1-TsNd	A 40.44 ML 53.9	[54]
pVAX1-Ts87	ML 9.7	[57]
pVAX1-Ag30	A 54	Personal communication
Third generation + carrier		
Salmonella pVAX1-TsPmy	A 44.8 ML 46.6	[58]
Salmonella pcDNA3.1-TsNd	A 73.32 ML 49.5	[60]
Salmonella pVAX1-Ts87	A 29.8 ML 34.2	[59]
Salmonella pVAX1-Ag30	A 22	Personal communication

A, adult; ML, muscle larvae.

Table 1. Protection in mice induced by some second- and third-generation vaccines administered alone or delivered by carriers.

2.3.2. Protection induced by some candidate antigens as second- and third-generation vaccines delivered alone or by live carriers

A summary of protection elicited in mice by some candidate antigens proposed as second- and third-generation vaccines is presented in **Table 1**. Antigen and delivery systems are critical elements that influence the protection level induced by the candidate vaccines. Some antigens such as Ts87 used as second-generation vaccine or as third-generation vaccine delivered by *Salmonella* elicit similar protection against *T. spiralis* infection. In the case of Ag30, it improves the protection induced against the enteral stage of *T. spiralis* when it is administered as second-generation vaccine delivered by attenuated *Salmonella*, particularly when it is fused to the molecular adjuvant P28 and secreted to the medium. For TsNd, no differences in protection are observed with second- and third-generation vaccines; however, it elicits higher protection against *T. spiralis* adult as third-generation vaccine delivered by *Salmonella*. On the other hand, Tsp10, an IIL antigen displayed on the surface of T7 phage, induced the highest protection against the systemic stage of *T. spiralis*; however, at the enteral level the protection was lower. An important aspect to mention is the administration route of these candidate vaccines that is correlated with the protection elicited against the parasite challenge. The second-generation vaccine, *Salmonella* pAg30-p28$_3$ (secreted) administered by i.n. route, afforded at the intestinal level the highest protection against *T. spiralis* challenge (92.8%), followed by *Salmonella* pAg30 displayed by MisL (second-generation vaccine) (76%), also administered by i.n. route and *Salmonella* pcDNA3.1-TsNd (third-generation vaccine) (73.2%) administered by oral route. On the other hand, Tsp10, an IIL antigen displayed by T7 phage, provided the highest protection against *T. spiralis* ML (78.6%); it was administered by i.p. and intradermal via at multiple sites of mice abdomen. Therefore, the administration route also plays an important aspect to be considered in the vaccine development.

3. Adjuvants

The induction of mucosal immunity plays an important aspect to be considered in the design of a vaccine against *T. spiralis* infection. Therefore, it is desirable that vaccine formulations contain adjuvants or immunomodulatory molecules capable to polarize the immune response to a Th2-type response. Indeed, adjuvants can influence the balance of the induced antibody and cell-mediated immunity so constitute an imperative element of modern vaccines [62].

An adjuvant with documented *in vitro* and *in vivo* Th2-skewing properties is the cholera toxin subunit B (CTB) [63]. CTB has been used as potent immunological adjuvant in the induction of protective Th2-type response by first- and second-generation vaccines against *T. spiralis*. More recently, the second-generation vaccine, gp53 of *T. spiralis* ML, contained into virus-like particles with the influenza matrix protein 1 (M1) as a core protein was administered to mice together with CTB, inducing protective immunity against the parasite challenge [64].

Aluminum hydroxide adjuvant (alum) has also been administered with first- and second-generation vaccines. When administered with E/S products from *T. spiralis* ML, although it has been documented in mice to induce Th2 responses, no production of IL-5 was detected [65].

The use of the adjuvant water in oil emulsions Montanide® ISA70 (Seppic, France) has been recommended for administration with first-generation vaccines, since its administration together with ML total extracts induced high level of protection (84.5%) against *T. spiralis* infection [66].

In order to enhance immunity, cytokines genes such as IL-4 have been included into third-generation vaccines (DNA vaccines) and have demonstrated to evoke a Th2-type response [67]. Interestingly, porcine IL-4 has been successfully evaluated as an immunological adjuvant in a vaccine candidate against porcine reproductive and respiratory syndrome virus (PRRSV) [68]. The cytokine IL-33 plays an important role at the mucosal level, inducing expansion of a multipotent progenitor cell population with differentiation into macrophages, basophils, and mast cell populations that promote the development of Th2 cytokine responses [69]. Further studies are necessary to determine the potential of IL-4 and IL-33 as molecular adjuvants in the induction of mucosal-protective immunity against *T. spiralis*.

4. Perspectives and future directions

4.1. Multi-epitope or polyvalent vaccines against trichinellosis

T. spiralis has a complex life cycle; the immune response elicited by a vaccine based on a unique antigen may not be strong enough to combat the challenging infection, and therefore multi-epitope vaccines against *T. spiralis* have been proposed. In this regard, the combination of three selected epitopes from Ts-Pmy and Ts87 from *T. spiralis* adult elicited in immunized mice IgG and IgG1 production and higher protection (35%) against the parasite challenge in comparison to that induced by individual epitope peptides [47]. To accomplish higher protective immune responses against *T. spiralis*, it will be necessary to design a vaccine with multi-epitopes from different parasite stages focusing on NBL and adult stages.

4.2. Probiotics in protection against *T. spiralis* infection

It has been demonstrated that probiotics modulate the intestinal environment preventing enteric infections. The lactic acid bacteria *Lactobacillus* is considered as probiotic; they are part of the commensal bacteria and contribute to the maintenance of immune homeostasis in the gut [70]. The protective role of *L. casei* against high infection dose of *T. spiralis* has been demonstrated in mice inoculated intraperitoneally with the bacteria as assessed by adult (76.7%) and ML (80.9%) load reduction, production of high IgA and IgG anti-*T. spiralis* antibody levels as well as IL-4 [71]. More recently, the protection conferred by different *Lactobacillus* strains, *L. casei, L. plantarum*, and *L. acidophilus*, against *T. spiralis* infection was analyzed. The highest protection was elicited by *L. plantarum*, against adult (69.02%) and ML (87.92%). Interestingly, the authors demonstrated an amelioration of inflammation and damage in the intestine of *T. spiralis*-infected mice inoculated with *L. plantarum* with respect to non-treated-infected animals [72]. So far, the use of probiotics is considered as a new tool for trichinellosis control.

4.3. Plant-based veterinary vaccine

Plant-based vaccines might be used as edible vaccines for sustainable prophylaxis against various important parasitic diseases, including trichinellosis. Recombinant proteins based in plants can be produced in nuclear-transformed plants, synthesized in the cytoplasm, and can be accumulated in different subcellular organelles, or secreted, once an appropriate transit or signal peptides are used [73, 74]. Plants are considered an attractive platform for veterinary vaccines, due to low-cost production, sterile delivery, and cold storage/transportation at ambient temperature, compared to traditional attenuated vaccines, which present some inconvenience in terms of insufficient mass production, residual toxicity, means of transportation, and safety [75]. Antigens administered by oral route are subject to proteolysis in gastrointestinal tract, reducing their bioavailability, and therefore affecting the quality of immune response. Then, vaccine antigens can be protected by plant cell walls from further degradation in the digestive tract, enabling them to reach the gut-associated lymphoid tissue [73].

Many species of plants, including tobaccos, alfalfa, spinach, potatoes, rice, beans, maize, tomatoes, strawberries, and carrots, can be used in plant biotechnology for the expression and production of foreign proteins, remaining stable without the loss of activity for years at room temperature. Hence, plants could be suitable for direct consumption and useful for the development of animal vaccines [74]. In fact, edible vaccines produced in papaya and corn seed induced protection against porcine-cysticercosis (70–90%) and porcine-transmissible gastroenteritis virus (50%) [76, 77]. Even more, edible vaccines can include adjuvants as it was the case for As16-an antigen protective against the roundworm *Ascaris suum* fused with CTB in transgenic rice seeds, resulting in an antibody response [78].

Plant-based vaccines represent an excellent tool for mass prevention especially at the veterinary field; their use in vaccine development against *T. spiralis* remains to be explored.

5. Conclusions

Different vaccine candidates based on antigens from different stages of *T. spiralis*, used as recombinant proteins or as DNA vaccines, delivered alone or by live carriers have been proposed. Most of them with some exceptions have induced partial protection against the enteral and muscle phase of the infection. In these studies, a mixed Th1/Th2 immune response with predominance of a Th2 response has been elicited. Up to now, the second-generation vaccines, *Salmonella* pAg30-p28$_3$ (secreted) and T7-Tsp10, have afforded at the intestinal and systemic level, respectively, the highest protection against *T. spiralis* challenge. Protection elicited by the candidate vaccines is influenced by the candidate antigen, delivery system, and administration route. Importantly, search for more useful vaccine candidates that could elicit high protection against *T. spiralis* infection in pigs is required. These vaccines may include antigens from IIL, NBL, and from pre-adult and adult stages of infection, administered alone or as multi-epitope vaccine. The use of adjuvants or immunomodulatory molecules capable to polarize the immune response to a Th2 type should be taken into account in a way to improve the protection induced by candidate vaccines. On the other hand, plant-based vaccines represent an excellent tool that needs to be explored in vaccine development against *T. spiralis* with application at the veterinary field.

Acknowledgment

This work was supported by grant FIS/IMSS/PROT/G11/961.

http://dx.doi.org/10.5772/66499

Abbreviations

Ag30	30-mer peptide derived from gp43 from *T. spiralis* ML
Ag30-P28$_3$	Ag30 fused to three copies of P28 adjuvant
Ag40	40-mer peptide derived from gp43 from *T. spiralis* ML
CTB	Cholera toxin subunit B
CFA	Complete Freund's adjuvant
E/S	Excretion/secretion products
gp43	Glycoprotein with molecular weight of 53 kDa from *T. spiralis* ML
gp53	Glycoprotein with molecular weight of 43 kDa from *T. spiralis* ML
HSP70	Heat-shock protein 70
IFA	Incomplete Freund's adjuvant
IIL	Intestinal infective larvae
i.n.	Intranasal
i.p.	Intraperitoneal
KLH	Keyhole limpet hemocyanin
ML	Muscle larvae
NBL	Newborn larvae
P28	Minimum binding domain of complement C3 component
TsAP	54.7 kDa amino peptidase
Ts-ES-1	Protein of 20 kDa existing in the E/S products of *T. spiralis* adult and ML
Ts14-3-3	Surface protein 28.9 kDa
TsMCD-1	Protein domain of multi-cystatin-type 1 of *T. spiralis*
Ts-Pmy	Paramyosin
Ts87	38 kDa protein that is present in E/S products and on the adult cuticle
TsMIF	Macrophage migration inhibitory factor of *T. spiralis*
TsNd	*Trichinella spiralis* Nudix hydrolase
TspE1	31 kDa E/S antigen of ML
TspSP1.2	E/S protein of 35.5 kDa

Author details

Jonathan I. Andrade-Becerra[1,2], Ericka N. Pompa-Mera[2], Rosa María Ribas-Aparicio[1] and Lilián Yépez-Mulia[2*]

*Address all correspondence to: lilianyepez@yahoo.com

1 Laboratory of Production and Biological Control, Department of Microbiology, National School of Biological Sciences, National Polytechnic Institute, Mexico City, Mexico

2 Investigation Unit in Infectious and Parasitic Diseases, Pediatric Hospital, Mexican Institute of Social Security, Mexico City, Mexico

References

[1] Pozio E. 2007. Taxonomy, biology and epidemiology of *Trichinella* parasites. In: Dupouy-Camet J, Murrel KD, editor. Fao/who/oie Guidelines for the Surveillance, Management, Prevention and Control of Trichinellosis. World Organisation for Animal Health Press, Paris, pp. 1-35.

[2] FAO/WHO [Food and Agriculture Organization of the United Nations/World Health Organization]. 2014. Multicriteria-based ranking for risk management of food-borne parasites. Microbiological Risk Assessment Series No. 23. WHO Press, Rome. 302 pp.

[3] Murrell KD, Pozio E. Worldwide occurrence and impact of human trichinellosis, 1986-2009. Emerg Infect Dis. 2011; 17:2194-2202. doi: 10.3201/eid1712.110896

[4] Cui J, Wang ZQ, Xu BL. The epidemiology of human trichinellosis in China during 2004-2009. Acta Trop. 2011; 118(1):1-5. doi: 10.1016/j.actatropica.2011.02.005

[5] OIE World Animal Health Information System [Internet]. 2015. Available from: http://www.oie.int/wahis_2/public/wahid.php/Diseaseinformation/statusdetail [Accessed: 2016-09-09].

[6] Bruschi F, Chiumiento L. *Trichinella* inflammatory myopathy: host or parasite strategy? Parasit Vectors. 2011; 4:42. doi: 10.1186/1756-3305-4-42

[7] Sharma N, Singh V, Shyma KP. Role of parasitic vaccines in integrated control of parasitic diseases in livestock. Vet World. 2015; 8(5):590-8. doi: 10.14202/vetworld.2015.590-598

[8] Shimoni Z, Froom P. Uncertainties in diagnosis, treatment and prevention of trichinellosis. Expert Rev Anti Infect Ther. 2015; 13(10):1279-1288.

[9] Meeusen EN, Walker J, Peters A, Pastoret PP, Jungersen G. Current status of veterinary vaccines. Clin Microbiol Rev. 2007; 20(3):489-510.

[10] Ramaswamy K. Role of parasite vaccines in sustained animal health and production. Proceedings of the XXIVth National Congress of Veterinary Parasitology held at Trichur (5-7 Feb. 2014), p. 22-30.

[11] Eissa MM, el-Azzouni MZ, Baddour NM, Boulos LM. Vaccination trial against experimental trichrinellosis using autoclaved *Trichinella spiralis* larvae vaccine (ATSLV). J Egypt Soc Parasitol. 2003; 33(1):219-228.

[12] Ali SM, El-Zawawy LA, El-Said D, Gaafar MR. Immunization against trichinellosis using microwaved larvae of *Trichinela spiralis*. J Egypt Soc Parasitol. 2007; 37(1):121-133.

[13] Darwish RA, Sanad MM, Youssef SM. Immunization against *Trichinella spiralis* using antigens from different life-cycle stages experimental study in mice. J Egypt Soc Parasitol. 1996; 26(1):19-26.

[14] Gamble HR, Murrell KD, Marti HP. Inoculation of pigs against *Trichinella spiralis*, using larval excretory-secretory antigens. Am J Vet Res. 1986; 47(11):2396-2399.

[15] Marti HP, Murrell KD, Gamble HR. *Trichinella spiralis*: immunization of pigs with newborn larval antigens. Exp Parasitol. 1987; 63(1):68-73.

[16] Yépez-Mulia L, Arriaga C, Peña MA, Gual F, Ortega-Pierres MG. Serologic survey of trichinellosis in wild mammals kept in a Mexico City Zoo. Vet Parasitol. 1996; 67:237-246.

[17] Wisnewski N, McNeil M, Grieve RB, Wassom DL. Characterization of novel fucosyl containing glycoconjugates from *Trichinella spiralis* muscle stage larvae. Mol Biochem Parasitol. 1993; 61:25-35.

[18] McVay CS, Bracken P, Gagliardo LF, Appleton J. Antibodies to tyvelose exhibit multiple modes of interference with the epithelial niche of *Trichinella spiralis*. Infect Immun. 2000; 68(4):1912-1918.

[19] ManWarren T, Gagliardo L, Geyer J, McVay C, Pearce-Kelling S, Appleton J.Invasion of intestinal epithelia in vitro by the parasitic nematode *Trichinella spiralis*. Infect Immun. 1997; 65(11):4806-4812.

[20] Goyal PK, Wheatcroft J, Wakelin D. Tyvelose and protective responses to the intestinal stages of *Trichinella spiralis*. Parasitol Int. 2002; 51: 91-98.

[21] Gamble HR. *Trichinella spiralis*: immunization of mice using monoclonal antibody affinity-isolated antigens. Exp Parasitol. 1985; 59:398-404.

[22] Grencis RK, Crawford C, Pritchard DI, Behnke JM, Wakelin D. Immunization of mice with surface antigens from the muscle larvae of *Trichinella spiralis*. Parasite Immunol. 1986; 8(6):587-596.

[23] Dea-Ayuela MA, Rama-Iñiguez S, Bolás-Fernández F. Vaccination of mice against intestinal *Trichinella spiralis* infections by oral administration of antigens microencapsulated in methacrilic acid copolymers. Vaccine. 2006; 24:2772-2780.

[24] Ortega-Pierres G, Muñiz E, Coral-Vázquez R, Parkhouse RM. Protection against *Trichinella spiralis* induced by purified stage-specific surface antigens of infective larvae. Parasitol Res. 1989; 75(7):563-567.

[25] Robinson K, Bellaby T, Chan WC, Wakelin D. High levels of protection induced by a 40-mer synthetic peptide vaccine against the intestinal nematode parasite *Trichinella spiralis*. Immunology. 1995; 86(4):495-498.

[26] McGuire C, Chan WC, Wakelin D. Nasal immunization with homogenate and peptide antigens induces protective immunity against *Trichinella spiralis*. Infect Immun. 2002; 70(12):7149-7152.

[27] Pompa-Mera EN, Yepez-Mulia L, Ocana-Mondragon A, Garcia-Zepeda EA, Ortega-Pierres G, Gonzalez-Bonilla CR. *Trichinella spiralis*: intranasal immunization with attenuated *Salmonella enterica* carrying a gp43 antigen derived 30mer epitope elicits protection in BALB/c mice. Exp Parasitol. 2011; 129, 393-401. doi: 10.1016/j.exppara.2011.08.013

[28] Castillo-Alvarez AM, Vaquero-Vera A, Fonseca-Liñan R, Ruiz-Perez F, Villegas-Sepulveda N, Ortega-Pierres G. A prime-boost vaccination of mice with attenuated

Salmonella expressing a 30-mer peptide from the *Trichinella spiralis* gp43 antigen. Vet Parasitol. 2013; 194:202-206. doi: 10.1016/j.vetpar.2013.01.056

[29] Cui J, Ren HJ, Liu RD, Wang L, Zhang ZF, Wang ZQ. Phage-displayed specific polypeptide antigens induce significant protective immunity against *Trichinella spiralis* infection in BALB/c mice. Vaccine. 2013; 31(8):1171-1177. doi: 10.1016/j.vaccine.2012.12.070

[30] Gu Y, Wei J, Yang J, Huang J, Yang X, Zhu X. Protective immunity against *Trichinella spiralis* infection induced by a multi-epitope vaccine in a murine model. PLoS One. 2013; 8(10):e77238. doi: 10.1371/journal.pone.0077238. eCollection 2013

[31] Pompa-Mera EN, Arroyo-Matus P, Ocaña-Mondragón A, González-Bonilla CR, Yépez-Mulia L. Protective immunity against enteral stages of *Trichinella spiralis* elicited in mice by live attenuated Salmonella vaccine that secretes a 30-mer parasite epitope fused to the molecular adjuvant C3d-P28. Res Vet Sci. 2014; 97(3):533-545. doi: 10.1016/j.rvsc.2014.09.010

[32] Jazayeri SD, Ideris A, Zakaria Z, Omar AR. Attenuated *Salmonella typhimurium* SV4089 as a potential carrier of oral DNA vaccine in chickens. J Biomed Biotechnol. 2012; 264986. doi: 10.1155/2012/264986

[33] Alvarado-Yaah J. Evaluación de la cepa vacunal pAg40 de *Salmonella entérica* serovar Typhimurium que expresa en su superficie un antígeno de *Trichinella spiralis*. [Thesis]. Centro de Investigación y de Estudios Avanzados del Instituto Politécnico Nacional, Mexico, D.F.; 2008.

[34] Yang J, Zhu W, Huang J, Wang X, Sun X, Zhan B, Zhu X. Partially protective immunity induced by the 14-3-3 protein from *Trichinella spiralis*. Vet Parasitol. 2016; S0304-4017(16)30236-9. doi: 10.1016/j.vetpar.2016.06.028

[35] Wang B, Wang ZQ, Jin J, Ren HJ, Liu LN, Cui J. Cloning, expression and characterization of a *Trichinella spiralis* serine protease gene encoding a 35.5 kDa protein. Exp Parasitol. 2013; 134(2):148-154. doi: 10.1016/j.exppara.2013.03.004

[36] Zhang Y, Wang Z, Li L, Cui J. Molecular characterization of *Trichinella spiralis* aminopeptidase and its potential as a novel vaccine candidate antigen against trichinellosis in BALB/c mice. Parasit Vectors. 2013; 6:246. doi: 10.1186/1756-3305-6-246

[37] Bi K, Yang J, Wang L, Gu Y, Zhan B, Zhu X. Partially protective immunity induced by a 20 kDa protein secreted by *Trichinella spiralis* stichocytes. PLoS One. 2015; 10(8):e0136189. doi: 10.1371/journal.pone.0136189. eCollection 2015

[38] Yang J, Yang Y, Gu Y, Li Q, Wei J, Wang S, Boireau P, Zhu X. Identification and characterization of a full-length cDNA encoding paramyosin of *Trichinella spiralis*. Biochem Biophys Res Commun. 2008; 365(3):528-533.

[39] Ren HJ, Liu RD, Wang ZQ, Cui J. Construction and use of a *Trichinella spiralis* phage display library to identify the interactions between parasite and host enterocytes. Parasitol Res. 2013; 112:1857-1863.

[40] Wang ZQ, Wang L, Cui J. Proteomic analysis of *Trichinella spiralis* proteins in intestinal epithelial cells after culture with their larvae by shotgun LC-MS/MS approach. J Proteomics. 2012;75(8):2375-2383. doi: 10.1016/j.jprot.2012.02.005

[41] Liu RD, Cui J, Liu XL, Jiang P, Sun GG, Zhang X, Long SR, Wang L, Wang ZQ. Comparative proteomic analysis of surface proteins of *Trichinella spiralis* muscle larvae and intestinal infective larvae. Acta Trop. 2015; 150:79-86. doi: 10.1016/j.actatropica.2015.07.002

[42] Liu RD, Jiang P, Wen H, Duan JY, Wang LA, Li JF, Liu CY, Sun GG, Wang ZQ, Cui J. Screening and characterization of early diagnostic antigens in excretory-secretory proteins from *Trichinella spiralis* intestinal infective larvae by immunoproteomics. Parasitol Res. 2016; 115:615-622.

[43] Tang B, Liu M, Wang L, Yu S, Shi H, Boireau P, Cozma V, Wu X, Liu X. Characterisation of a high-frequency gene encoding a strongly antigenic cystatin-like protein from *Trichinella spiralis* at its early invasion stage. Parasit Vectors. 2015;8:78. doi: 10.1186/s13071-015-0689-5

[44] Long SR, Wang ZQ, Liu RD, Liu LN, Li LG, Jiang P, Zhang X, Zhang ZF, Shi HN, Cui J. Molecular identification of *Trichinella spiralis* nudix hydrolase and its induced protective immunity against trichinellosis in BALB/c mice. Parasit Vectors. 2014; 7: 600. doi: 10.1186/s13071-014-0600-9

[45] Bien J, Cabaj W, Moskwa B. Proteomic analysis of potential immunoreactive proteins from muscle larvae and adult worms of *Trichinella spiralis* in experimentally infected pigs. Folia Parasitol (Praha). 2015; 62. pii: 2015.022. doi: 10.14411/fp.2015.022

[46] Fang L, Sun L, Yang J, Gu Y, Zhan B, Huang J, Zhu X. Heat shock protein 70 from *Trichinella spiralis* induces protective immunity in BALB/c mice by activating dendritic cells. Vaccine. 2014; 32(35):4412-4419. doi: 10.1016/j.vaccine.2014.06.055

[47] Gu Y, Li J, Zhu X, Yang J, Li Q, Liu Z, Yu S, Li Y. *Trichinella spiralis*: characterization of phage-displayed specific epitopes and their protective immunity in BALB/c mice. Exp Parasitol. 2008; 118(1):66-74.

[48] Marti HP, Murrell KD. *Trichinella spiralis*: antifecundity and antinewborn larvae immunity in swine. Exp Parasitol. 1986; 62(3):370-375.

[49] Liu M, Wang X, Fu B, Li C, Wu X, Le Rhun D, Chen Q, Boireau P. Identification of stage specifically expressed genes of *Trichinella spiralis* by suppression subtractive hybridization. Parasitology. 2007; 134:1443-1455.

[50] Yang Y, Vallée I, Lacour SA, Boireau P, Cheng SP, Liu MY. Identification and characterization of immunodominant linear epitopes on the antigenic region of a serine protease in newborn *Trichinella* larvae. J Helminthol. 2016;90(2):232-237. doi: 10.1017/S0022149X15000267

[51] Prichard R, Tait A. The role of molecular biology in veterinary parasitology. Vet Parasitol. 2001; 98(1-3):169-194.

[52] Kutzler MA, Weiner DB. DNA vaccines: ready for prime time? Nat Rev Genet. 2008; 9(10):776-788. doi: 10.1038/nrg2432

[53] Wang ZQ, Cui J, Wei HY, Han HM, Zhang HW, Li YL. Vaccination of mice with DNA vaccine induces the immune response and partial protection against *T. spiralis* infection. Vaccine. 2006; 24(8):1205-1212.

[54] Liu P, Cui J, Liu RD, Wang M, Jiang P, Liu LN, Long SR, Li LG, Zhang SB, Zhang XZ, Wang ZQ. Protective immunity against *Trichinella spiralis* infection induced by TsNd vaccine in mice. Parasit Vectors. 2015;8:185. doi: 10.1186/s13071-015-0791-8

[55] Tang F, Xu L, Yan R, Song X, Li X. Evaluation of the immune response induced by DNA vaccines expressing MIF and MCD-1 genes of *Trichinella spiralis* in BALB/c mice. J Helminthol. 2012; 86(4):430-439. doi: 10.1017/S0022149X11000654

[56] Tang F, Xu L, Yan R, Song X, Li X. A DNA vaccine co-expressing *Trichinella spiralis* MIF and MCD-1 with murine ubiquitin induces partial protective immunity in mice. J Helminthol. 2013; 87(1):24-33. doi: 10.1017/S0022149X1100068X

[57] Yang Y, Yang X, Gu Y, Wang Y, Zhao X, Zhu X. Protective immune response induced by co-immunization with the *Trichinella spiralis* recombinant Ts87 protein and a Ts87 DNA vaccine. Vet Parasitol. 2013; 194(2-4):207-210. doi: 10.1016/j.vetpar.2013.01.057

[58] Wang L, Wang X, Bi K, Sun X, Yang J, Gu Y, Huang J, Zhan B, Zhu X. Oral vaccination with attenuated *Salmonella* typhimurium-delivered TsPmy DNA vaccine elicits protective immunity against *Trichinella spiralis* in BALB/c mice. PLoS Negl Trop Dis. 2016; 10(9):e0004952. doi: 10.1371/journal.pntd.0004952

[59] Yang Y, Zhang Z, Yang J, Chen X, Cui S, Zhu X. Oral vaccination with Ts87 DNA vaccine delivered by attenuated *Salmonella typhimurium* elicits a protective immune response against *Trichinella spiralis* larval challenge. Vaccine. 2010; 28(15):2735-2742. doi: 10.1016/j.vaccine.2010.01.026

[60] Liu P, Wang ZQ, Liu RD, Jiang P, Long SR, Liu LN, Zhang XZ, Cheng XC, Yu C, Ren HJ, Cui J. Oral vaccination of mice with *Trichinella spiralis* nudix hydrolase DNA vaccine delivered by attenuated *Salmonella* elicited protective immunity. Exp Parasitol. 2015; 153:29-38. doi: 10.1016/j.exppara.2015.02.008

[61] Hebishima T, Yuba E, Kono K, Takeshima SN, Ito Y, Aida Y. The pH-sensitive fusogenic 3-methyl-glutarylated hyperbranched poly(glycidol)-conjugated liposome induces antigen-specific cellular and humoral immunity. Clin Vaccine Immunol. 2012; 19(9):1492-1498. doi: 10.1128/CVI.00273-12

[62] Tandrup Schmidt S, Foged C, Korsholm KS, Rades T, Christensen D. Liposome-based adjuvants for subunit vaccines: formulation strategies for subunit antigens and immunostimulators. Pharmaceutics. 2016; 8(1). pii: E7. doi:10.3390/pharmaceutics8010007

[63] Stratmann T. Cholera toxin subunit B as adjuvant—an accelerator in protective immunity and a break in autoimmunity. Vaccines (Basel). 2015; 3(3):579-596. doi: 10.3390/vaccines3030579

[64] Lee SH, Kim SS, Lee DH, Kim AR, Quan FS. Evaluation of protective efficacy induced by virus-like particles containing a *Trichinella spiralis* excretory-secretory (ES) protein in mice. Parasit Vectors. 2016; 9(1):384. doi: 10.1186/s13071-016-1662-7

[65] Robinson K, Bellaby T, Wakelin D. Vaccination against the nematode *Trichinella spiralis* in high- and low-responder mice. Effects of different adjuvants upon protective immunity and immune responsiveness. Immunology. 1994; 82(2):261-267.

[66] Deville S, Pooter Ad, Aucouturier J, Lainé-Prade V, Cote M, Boireau P, Vallée I. Influence of adjuvant formulation on the induced protection of mice immunized with total soluble antigen of *Trichinella spiralis*. Vet Parasitol. 2005; 132(1-2):75-80.

[67] Ma Y, An HJ, Wei XQ, Xu Q, Yu YZ, Sun ZW. Enhanced potency of replicon vaccine using one vector to simultaneously co-express antigen and interleukin-4 molecular adjuvant. Hum Vaccin Immunother. 2013; 9(2):242-249.

[68] Li Z, Wang G, Wang Y, Zhang C, Wang X, Huang B, Li Q, Li L, Xue B, Ding P, Syed SF, Wang C, Cai X, Zhou EM. Rescue and evaluation of a recombinant PRRSV expressing porcine Interleukin-4. Virol J. 2015; 12:185. doi: 10.1186/s12985-015-0380-7

[69] Saenz SA, Noti M, Artis D. Innate immune cell populations function as initiators and effectors in Th2 cytokine responses. Trends Immunol. 2010; 31(11):407-413. doi: 10.1016/j.it.2010.09.001

[70] Artis D. Epithelial-cell recognition of commensal bacteria and maintenance of immune homeostasis in the gut. Nat Rev Immunol. 2008; 8: 411-420.

[71] Martínez-Gómez F, Fuentes-Castro BE, Bautista-Garfias CR. The intraperitoneal inoculation of *Lactobacillus casei* in mice induces total protection against *Trichinella spir*alis infection at low challenge doses. Parasitol Res. 2011; 109(6):1609-1617. doi: 10.1007/s00436-011-2432-2

[72] El Temsahy MM, Ibrahim IR, Mossallama SF, Mahrousb H, Baryc AA, Abdel Salama SA. Evaluation of newly isolated probiotics in the protection against experimental intestinal trichinellosis. Vet Parasitol. 2015; 214:303-314. doi.org/10.1016/j.vetpar.2015.08.029

[73] Pniewski T. The twenty-year story of a plant-based vaccine against hepatitis B: stagnation or promising prospects? Int J Mol Sci. 2013; 14(1):1978-1998. doi: 10.3390/ijms14011978

[74] Liew PS, Hair-Bejo M. Farming of plant-based veterinary vaccines and their applications for disease prevention in animals. Adv Virol. 2015; 2015:936940. doi: 10.1155/2015/936940

[75] Shahid N, Daniell H. Plant-based oral vaccines against zoonotic and non-zoonotic diseases. Plant Biotechnol J. 2016; 14(11):2079-2099. doi:10.1111/pbi.12604

[76] Hernández M, Cabrera-Ponce JL, Fragoso G, López-Casillas F, Guevara-García A, Rosas G, León-Ramírez C, Juárez P, Sánchez-García G, Cervantes J, Acero G, Toledo A, Cruz C, Bojalil R, Herrera-Estrella L, Sciutto E. A new highly effective anticysticercosis vaccine expressed in transgenic papaya. Vaccine. 2007; 25(21):4252-4260.

[77] Streatfield SJ, Jilka JM, Hood EE, Turner DD, Bailey MR, Mayor JM, Woodard SL,Beifuss KK, Horn ME, Delaney DE, Tizard IR, Howard JA. Plant-based vaccines: unique advantages. Vaccine. 2001; 19(17-19):2742-2748.

[78] Matsumoto Y, Suzuki S, Nozoye T, Yamakawa T, Takashima Y, Arakawa T, Tsuji N, Takaiwa F, Hayashi Y. Oral immunogenicity and protective efficacy in mice of transgenic rice plants producing a vaccine candidate antigen (As16) of *Ascaris suum* fused with cholera toxin B subunit. Transgenic Res. 2009; 18(2):185-192. doi: 10.1007/s11248-008-9205-4